Thyroid Cancer

David S. Cooper • Cosimo Durante
Editors

Thyroid Cancer

A Case-Based Approach

Springer

Editors
David S. Cooper, MD
Division of Endocrinology
Diabetes, and Metabolism
The Johns Hopkins University
School of Medicine
Baltimore, MD, USA

Cosimo Durante, MD
Department of Internal Medicine
and Medical Specialties
University of Rome "Sapienza"
Rome, Italy

ISBN 978-3-319-22400-8 ISBN 978-3-319-22401-5 (eBook)
DOI 10.1007/978-3-319-22401-5

Library of Congress Control Number: 2015953101

Springer Cham Heidelberg New York Dordrecht London

Printed on acid-free paper

Springer International Publishing AG Switzerland is part of Springer Science+Business Media (www.springer.com)

Preface

There have been few instances in the field of thyroidology as startling and dramatic as the epidemic of differentiated thyroid cancer in virtually all developed and developing countries around the world. Whether this is due, as many suspect, to increases in radiologic procedures and screening, or to environmental factors, such as radiation, or both continues to be a matter of intense debate. However, for the clinicians caring for the large number of new and prevalent thyroid cancer patients, there is no debate about the need for current, practical, and evidence-based information on management. This is especially the case for those with low-risk papillary thyroid cancer, who represent the vast majority of thyroid cancer patients in the twenty-first century. In this group, we are learning that "less is more" in terms of the traditional treatments of surgery and radioiodine and thyroxine-suppressive therapy. On the other end of the spectrum, patients with more advanced disease are benefitting from new targeted therapies with a host of new pharmaceutical agents, as well as local treatments directed at individual metastatic lesions. In addition, new approaches to less common forms of thyroid malignancy, including medullary thyroid cancer, anaplastic cancer, and lymphoma, are also being developed.

There are textbooks of thyroid disease in general and of thyroid cancer specifically; they provide the reader with a vast amount of important information related to etiology, epidemiology, diagnosis, and management. We also know that there is a vast amount of information now available electronically that provides helpful information with the click of a mouse. The object of this text, however, is to provide the practitioner with clinically relevant information in the context of the classical medical learning tool, the case history. These illustrative thyroid cancer cases have been selected to cover the various clinical issues encountered in the care of thyroid cancer patients. The text begins with cases highlighting the diagnostic difficulties in patients with indeterminate thyroid nodules and then provides case histories of patients with the whole range of differentiated thyroid cancer, including special circumstances, such as thyroid cancer in children and in pregnancy. Case histories of patients with advanced thyroid cancer, including those with metastatic disease receiving high-dose radioiodine and those with radioiodine-refractory disease being treated with new "targeted therapies," are also included. All the case histories are written by an international group of authorities in the field of thyroid cancer, and all recommendations are based on evidence-based clinical practice guidelines and data from the recent published literature.

We wish to thank all the contributors to the book. They have done what we asked: to ensure that their case reports were brief, succinct, and current and to provide guidance in areas of controversy. We also wish to thank Ms. Susan Westendorf of Springer for her superb assistance and support in the production of the book. We hope this novel text will provide guidance to those who seek to increase their understanding of thyroid cancer management.

Baltimore, MD, USA
Rome, Italy
10-May-2015

David S. Cooper, MD
Cosimo Durante, MD

Contents

Contributors

Teresa Alonso-Gordoa Medical Oncology Department, Hospital Ramón y Cajal, Madrid, Spain

Monica L. Arango, MD, FAAP Division of Pediatric Endocrinology, The University of Texas, Health Science Center at Houston, Houston, TX, USA

Victor J. Bernet, MD Division of Endocrinology, Mayo Clinic Florida, Mayo Clinic College of Medicine, Rochester, MN, USA

Keith C. Bible, MD, PhD Mayo Clinic, Rochester, MN, USA

Justin A. Bishop, MD The Johns Hopkins University School of Medicine, Baltimore, MD, USA

Valeria Bottici Endocrine Unit, Department of Clinical and Experimental Medicine, University of Pisa, Pisa, Italy

Sarah J. Bottomley, MSN, RN, CPNP The Children's Cancer Hospital, MD Anderson Cancer Center, University of Texas, Houston, TX, USA

James Brierley, MB Department of Radiation Oncology, University of Toronto, Toronto, ON, Canada

Department of Radiation Oncology, Princess Margaret Cancer Centre, Toronto, ON, Canada

Lucia Brilli, MD Department of Medical, Surgical and Neurological Sciences, University of Siena, Siena, Italy

Policlinico Santa Maria alle Scotte, Siena, Italy

Virginia Cappagli Endocrine Unit, Department of Clinical and Experimental Medicine, University of Pisa, Pisa, Italy

Maria Grazia Castagna, MD Department of Medical, Surgical and Neurological Sciences, University of Siena, Siena, Italy

Policlinico Santa Maria alle Scotte, Siena, Italy

Ana-Maria Chindris, MD Division of Endocrinology, Mayo Clinic Florida, Mayo Clinic College of Medicine, Rochester, Minnesota, USA

David S. Cooper, MD Division of Endocrinology, Diabetes, and Metabolism, The Johns Hopkins University School of Medicine, Baltimore, MD, USA

Patricia Cortez Medical Oncology Department, Hospital Ramón y Cajal, Madrid, Spain

Giuseppe Costante, MD Endocrinology Clinic, Medicine Department, Institut Jules Bordet, Comprehensive Cancer Center, Brussels, Belgium

Ramona Dadu, MD Department of Endocrine Neoplasia and Hormonal Disorders, The University of Texas MD Anderson Cancer Center, Houston, TX, USA

Désirée Deandreis, MD Nuclear Medicine and Endocrine Oncology, Gustave Roussy, Villejuif, France

Gerard M. Doherty, MD Department of Surgery, Boston University, Boston, MA, USA

Henning Dralle, MD, FRCS, FACS, FEBS Department of General, Visceral, and Vascular Surgery, University Hospital, Halle (Saale), Germany

Medical Faculty, University of Halle-Wittenberg, Halle (Saale), Germany

Farouk Drissi Clinique de Chirurgie Digestive et Endocrinienne (CCDE), Institut des Maladies de l'Appareil Digestif (IMAD), Hôtel Dieu, , CHU Nantes, Nantes cedex 1, France

Cosimo Durante, MD Department of Internal Medicine and Medical Specialties, University of Rome "Sapienza", Rome, Italy

Rossella Elisei, MD Endocrine Unit, Department of Clinical and Experimental Medicine, University Hospital of Pisa, Pisa, Italy

Sebastiano Filetti, MD Department of Internal Medicine and Medical Specialties, University of Rome "Sapienza", Rome, Italy

Robert F. Gagel, MD Department of Endocrine Neoplasia and Hormonal Disorders, The University of Texas MD Anderson Cancer Center, Houston, TX, USA

Carlotta Giani Endocrine Unit, Department of Clinical and Experimental Medicine, University Hospital of Pisa, Pisa, Italy

Meredith Giuliani, MB Department of Radiation Oncology, University of Toronto, Toronto, ON, Canada

Department of Radiation Oncology, Princess Margaret Cancer Centre, Toronto, ON, Canada

Paolo Goffredo, MD Endocrine Neoplasia, Duke Clinical Research Institute, Duke University, Durham, NC, USA

Alyse S. Goldberg, MD Toronto General Hospital, Toronto, ON, Canada

Adam D. Goodale, MD University of Cincinnati College of Medicine, Department of Otolaryngology - Head & Neck Surgery, Cincinnati, OH, USA

Roberta Granata Head and Neck Cancer Medical Oncology Unit, Fondazione IRCCS Istituto Nazionale dei Tumori, Milan, Italy

Enrique Grande Medical Oncology Department, Hospital Ramón y Cajal, Madrid, Spain

Dana M. Hartl, MD, PhD Thyroid Surgery Unit, Department of Head and Neck Oncology, Institut de Cancérologie Gustave Roussy, Paris-Sud University, Villejuif Cedex, France

Ian D. Hay, MD, PhD, FACE, FACP, FRCP Division of Endocrinology and Internal Medicine, Mayo Clinic and College of Medicine, Rochester, MN, USA

Mimi I. Hu, MD Department of Endocrine Neoplasia and Hormonal Disorders, The University of Texas MD Anderson Cancer Center, Houston, TX, USA

Yasuhiro Ito, MD, PhD Clinical Trial Management Center, Kuma Hospital, Center for Excellence in Thyroid Care, Kobe, Japan

Department of Surgery, Kuma Hospital, Center for Excellence in Thyroid Care, Kobe, Japan

Emad Kandil, MD, FACS, FACE Division of Endocrine Surgery, Department of Surgery, Tulane University School of Medicine, New Orleans, LA, USA

Michele Klain Gustave Roussy and University Paris Sud, Villejuif, France

Livia Lamartina, MD Department of Internal Medicine and Medical Specialties, University of Rome “Sapienza”, Rome, Italy

Stephanie Lee, MD, PhD Division of Endocrinology, Boston Medical Center, Boston, MA, USA

Lisa Licitra Head and Neck Cancer Medical Oncology Unit, Fondazione IRCCS Istituto Nazionale dei Tumori, Milan, Italy

Laura Locati Head and Neck Cancer Medical Oncology Unit, Fondazione IRCCS Istituto Nazionale dei Tumori, Milan, Italy

Cristina Luongo Gustave Roussy and University Paris Sud, Villejuif, France

Andreas Machens, MD Department of General, Visceral, and Vascular Surgery, University Hospital, Halle (Saale), Germany

Medical Faculty, University of Halle-Wittenberg, Halle (Saale), Germany

Susan J. Mandel, MD, MPH Division of Endocrinology, Diabetes and Metabolism, Perelman School of Medicine, University of Pennsylvania, Philadelphia, PA, USA

Antonio Matrone Endocrine Unit, Department of Clinical and Experimental Medicine, University Hospital of Pisa, Pisa, Italy

Donald S.A. McLeod, MBBS (Hon I), FRACP, MPH, PhD Department of Endocrinology and Diabetes, Royal Brisbane and Women's Hospital, Herston, QLD, Australia

Department of Population Health, QIMR Berghofer Medical Research Institute, Herston, QLD, Australia

Salvatore Minisola, MD Department of Internal Medicine and Medical Disciplines, "Sapienza", University of Rome, Rome, Italy

Eric Mirallié Clinique de Chirurgie Digestive et Endocrinienne (CCDE), Institut des Maladies de l'Appareil Digestif (IMAD), Hôtel Dieu, CHU Nantes, Nantes cedex 1, France

Akira Miyauchi, MD, PhD Department of Surgery, Kuma Hospital, Center for Excellence in Thyroid Care, Kobe, Japan

Salem I. Noureldine, MD Division of Head and Neck Endocrine Surgery, Department of Otolaryngology – Head and Neck Surgery, The Johns Hopkins University School of Medicine, Baltimore, MD, USA

Furio Pacini, MD Department of Medical, Surgical and Neurological Sciences, University of Siena, Siena, Italy

Policlinico Santa Maria alle Scotte, Siena, Italy

Jessica Pepe, MD, PhD Department of Internal Medicine and Medical Disciplines, "Sapienza", University of Rome, Rome, Italy

Douglas S. Ross, MD Thyroid Unit WAC 730 S, Massachusetts General Hospital, Boston, MA, USA

Lorne E. Rotstein, MD Toronto General Hospital, Toronto, ON, Canada

Anna M. Sawka, MD, PhD Toronto General Hospital, Toronto, ON, Canada

Martin Schlumberger Gustave Roussy and University Paris Sud, Villejuif, France

Steven I. Sherman, MD University of Texas MD Anderson Cancer Center, Houston, TX, USA

Robert C. Smallridge, MD Mayo Clinic, Jacksonville, FL, USA

Julie Ann Sosa, MD, MA Section of Endocrine Surgery, Department of Surgery, Endocrine Neoplasia Diseases Group, Duke Cancer Institute and Duke Clinical Research Institute, Duke University, Durham, NC, USA

David L. Steward, MD University of Cincinnati College of Medicine, Department of Otolaryngology - Head & Neck Surgery, Cincinnati, OH, USA

Fabiana Trulli, MD Gustave Roussy and University Paris Sud, Villejuif, France

Ralph P. Tufano, MD, MBA, FACS Division of Head and Neck Endocrine Surgery, Department of Otolaryngology–Head and Neck Surgery, The Johns Hopkins University School of Medicine, Baltimore, MD, USA

Fernanda Vaisman, MD, PhD Instituto Nacional do Cancer do Rio de Janeiro (INCA)- Endocrinology, Rio de Janeiro, Brazil

Steven G. Waguespack, MD, FAAP, FACE Department of Endocrine Neoplasia and Hormonal Disorders, MD Anderson Cancer Center, University of Texas, Houston, TX, USA

Tracy S. Wang, MD, MPH Section of Endocrine Surgery, Division of Surgical Oncology, Department of Surgery Medical College of Wisconsin, Milwaukee, WI, USA

Leonard Wartofsky, MD MedStar Washington Hospital Center, Washington, DC, USA

Georgetown University School of Medicine, Washington, DC, USA

Swaytha Yalamanchi, MD Division of Endocrinology, Diabetes, and Metabolism, Johns Hopkins Hospital, Baltimore, MD, USA

Part I
Low Risk Differentiated Thyroid Cancer: *Preoperative Diagnosis*

Chapter 1
A Patient with a Single Thyroid Nodule Suspicious for Follicular Neoplasm According to the Bethesda System for Reporting Thyroid Cytopathology: Molecular Evaluation

Katie B. Guttenberg and Susan J. Mandel

Case Presentation

A 76-year-old woman presents for the evaluation of a thyroid nodule that was found incidentally on carotid ultrasound. She denies a family history of thyroid cancer or exposure to external beam radiation as a child. Her serum TSH level is 2.3 mIU/L. On physical exam, there is a 1 cm palpable left thyroid nodule. A bedside ultrasound reveals a $9 \times 13 \times 18$ mm solid, isoechoic nodule without either microcalcifications or increased intranodular vascularity (Fig. 1.1). No abnormal lymph nodes are visualized in the central or lateral neck. A fine-needle aspiration (FNA) with ultrasound guidance is "suspicious for follicular neoplasm" (Bethesda Class IV).

Assessment and Literature Review

The risk of malignancy for a nodule with a cytologic diagnosis of "suspicious for follicular neoplasm" is approximately 25 % [1, 2]. The standard of care has been diagnostic lobectomy followed by completion thyroidectomy if the nodule is malignant on histopathology. However, most (~75 %) patients who undergo surgery have a benign nodule.

Once a clinician is confronted with a patient with a follicular cytologic diagnosis, the relevant clinical question is that patient's risk of cancer. The application of molecular diagnostic tools to nodules with follicular neoplasm cytology is predicated upon the assumption that results can further refine malignancy risk in these

K.B. Guttenberg, MD • S.J. Mandel, MD, MPH (✉)
Division of Endocrinology, Diabetes and Metabolism, Perelman School of Medicine, University of Pennsylvania, TRC Building 12th Floor, 3400 Civic Center Blvd., Philadelphia, PA 19104, USA
e-mail: Susan.Mandel@uphs.upenn.edu

D.S. Cooper, C. Durante (eds.), *Thyroid Cancer*,
DOI 10.1007/978-3-319-22401-5_1

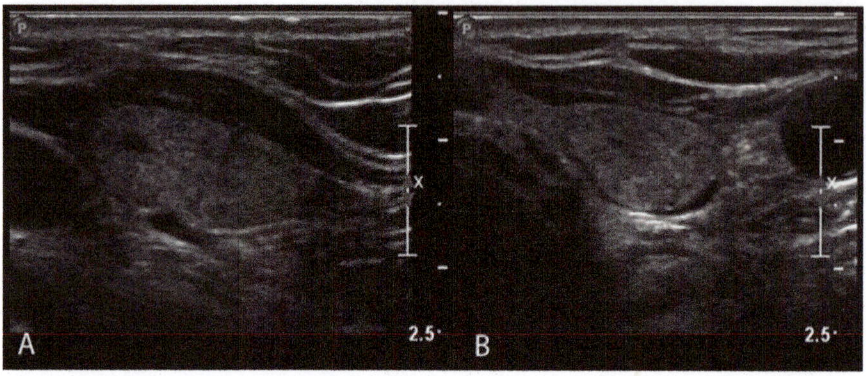

Fig. 1.1 Longitudinal (**a**) and transverse (**b**) grayscale sonographic appearance of a 9×13×18 mm solid, isoechoic, noncalcified nodule with regular margins

patients where cytology is not definitive. If molecular testing techniques were 100 % sensitive and specific for the diagnosis of all thyroid cancer histologies, this technology could replace cytologic analysis. Perhaps future testing strategies will achieve this goal, but current commercially available molecular diagnostics do not. Therefore, to interpret results of these molecular tests for an individual patient, the clinician must understand the reported negative and positive predictive values and their derivation from recently published studies.

A high negative predictive value (NPV) signifies that the cancer risk is very low when the test result is negative, e.g., NPV of 97 % is associated with a cancer risk of only 3 %. On the other hand, a high positive predictive value (PPV) indicates that the likelihood of malignancy is high when the test is positive, e.g., PPV of 90 % means that cancer is present in 90 % of patients with this result. The point estimates for NPV and PPV for a given test vary based upon the prevalence of disease (thyroid cancer) in the tested population. For example, when the cancer risk is low, e.g., 10 %, even a test with a sensitivity of 60 % will be associated with an NPV of over 95 %. Here, because there are so few cancers in the population, the absolute number of cases where the test fails to accurately diagnose cancer is very low, and this does not significantly decrease the NPV. But, as the cancer rate rises, this same test with 60 % sensitivity will miss more diagnoses leading to a higher false-negative rate and lowering the NPV. On the other hand, the PPV rises as the population disease risk increases because false-positive results decrease when there are fewer patients without thyroid cancer.

Therefore, for a given patient, the application and interpretation of results from currently available molecular diagnostics for prediction of malignancy or benignity are predicated upon that patient's baseline malignancy risk after cytologic diagnosis, i.e., the "pretest probability." Although overall the risk of malignancy associated with a "follicular neoplasm" cytologic result is approximately 25 % [1, 2], certain factors may modify this estimate and could potentially alter the interpretation of subsequent molecular diagnostic results. Prior to the discussion of the recent publications about the application of molecular testing, we will review the literature on patient demographics and nodule sonographic features that may alter malignancy risk associated with a nodule with a "suspicious for follicular neoplasm" diagnosis, henceforth referred to as an FN nodule.

Part I: Risk of Malignancy

Limitations of Cytologic and Histologic Interpretation

The diagnosis of "suspicious for follicular neoplasm" (FN) is rendered in approximately 10–15 % of FNAs performed. A 2012 meta-analysis including eight studies showed center-specific rates ranging from 1.2 to 25.3 % [1]. Of the three indeterminate cytology classifications defined by the Bethesda System for Reporting Thyroid Cytopathology [3], follicular neoplasm is the most reliably reproducible. Interobserver diagnostic agreement is considered fair (kappa 0.5), based on Fleiss' criteria for interpreting kappa values [4].

The standard of care for patients with such indeterminate cytology has been diagnostic lobectomy followed by completion thyroidectomy if histology is malignant. In this meta-analysis, 70 % of patients with FN nodules underwent surgery, similar to the rate of resection for cytology suspicious or indicative of malignancy [1]. Approximately 25 % of FN nodules are malignant on histology [1, 2], with center-specific rates ranging from 14 to 49 % [2]. Of these cancers, 16–36 % are follicular carcinomas, but most (55–84 %) are papillary thyroid cancers, with follicular variant as the most common subtype [5–8]. Although clinicians consider pathology the diagnostic "gold standard," even expert pathologists may disagree about the distinction between benign and malignant nodules on histology in up to 10 % of cases [2, 9].

Demographic and Sonographic Features Predictive of Malignancy

Once a nodule has a cytologic diagnosis of "suspicious for follicular neoplasm," some studies have reported that certain clinical features, including male gender, age, and the presence of a solitary nodule, are predictive of malignancy, but these findings have not been consistent [10–18] (Table 1.1). Large nodule size, in contrast, may be a reliable predictor of follicular thyroid carcinoma [11, 12]. Nodule size greater than or equal to 2.8 cm has been associated with an 11-fold increased risk of follicular thyroid carcinoma, but not with an increased risk of papillary thyroid carcinoma, which is typically smaller [11]. For example, in one study [12], nodule size only achieved statistical significance as a predictor of malignancy in FN nodules after papillary carcinoma was excluded from analysis. Consistent with these findings,

Table 1.1 Clinical features predictive of malignancy in a nodule with a cytologic diagnosis of suspicious for follicular neoplasm

Clinical feature	Predictive	Not predictive
Male gender	Tuttle [10]	Lubitz [12]
	Lee [11]—FTC only	Glucelik [13]
		Choi [14]
		Rago [16]
		Raber [17]
		McHenry [18]
Younger age	Schlinkert [15]	Tuttle [10]
		Lee [11]
		Lubitz [12]
		Glucelik [13]
		Choi [14]
		Rago [16]
		Raber [17]
		McHenry [18]
Nodule size	Lee [11] ≥2.8 cm—FTC only	Glucelik [13]
	Lubitz [12] ≥4.0 cm—when PTC excluded from analysis	Choi [14]
		Rago [16]
		Raber [17]
Solitary nodule	Raber [17]	Lubitz [12]
		Glucelik [13]
		Rago [16]

FTC follicular thyroid cancer, *PTC* papillary thyroid cancer

nodule size was not predictive in three studies when the malignant histologic diagnoses were predominately papillary [13, 16, 17]. Only a single study with predominately follicular cancers failed to show nodule size as a significant predictor [14].

For the initial evaluation of a thyroid nodule, certain sonographic features are consistently predictive of malignancy and can be used to determine the size threshold for FNA. These include hypoechoic echogenicity, solid composition, the presence of microcalcifications, irregular borders, and "taller than wide" shape [19]. However, once a "suspicious for follicular neoplasm" cytology is diagnosed, the reliability of ultrasound features to predict malignancy is less robust [11, 13, 14, 16, 17, 20] (Table 1.2).

The presence of microcalcifications in an FN nodule has been associated with an increased but variable (32–84 %) malignancy risk [13, 16]. This variability may be explained by higher proportions of classic versus follicular variant papillary carcinomas. Microcalcifications are thought to correspond to psammoma bodies on histology, and these are commonly found in classic variant papillary thyroid carcinomas, but not in follicular variant papillary carcinomas or follicular carcinomas [21, 22].

Hypoechogenicity in FN nodules correlated with a 33–43 % risk of malignancy in two studies [13, 17], but it was not predictive of malignancy in three other studies [11, 14, 16]. When the histologic diagnoses included a higher proportion of classic variant papillary thyroid carcinomas, which are typically hypoechoic [23], this

Table 1.2 Grayscale and Doppler sonographic features predictive of malignancy in a nodule with a cytologic diagnosis of suspicious for follicular neoplasm

Sonographic feature	Predictive	Not predictive
Hypoechoic echogenicity	Glucelik [13]	Lee [11][a]
	Raber [17]	Choi [14]
		Rago [16]
Solid composition	Glucelik [13]	Lee [11]
		Choi [14]
Microcalcifications	Glucelik [13]	
	Rago [16]	
Internal blood flow	Choi [14]	
	De Nicola [20]	

[a]Isoechoic echogenicity was predictive of follicular thyroid cancer

association was observed. Conversely, the characteristic grayscale sonographic appearance of both follicular carcinoma and follicular variant papillary carcinoma is an iso- or hyperechoic nodule [23, 24]. In one study with a higher percentage of follicular cancer in FN nodules, isoechogenicity was predictive of follicular carcinoma but not papillary carcinoma [11].

Nodule composition (solid versus cystic) may also relate to histopathology because papillary cancers are more likely to be solid than follicular cancers [24]. Solid nodule composition was associated with a 38 % risk of malignancy in the study with the highest proportion of papillary cancers in FN nodules [13].

In addition to the grayscale sonographic features typically considered hallmarks of malignancy, the presence of internal blood flow, as assessed by Doppler examination, may be a predictor in nodules with a cytologic diagnosis of "suspicious for follicular neoplasm." Internal blood flow was associated with a 28–50 % risk of malignancy in two studies [14, 20]. This finding is likely due to the high proportion of follicular cancers diagnosed in these studies. Follicular carcinomas have been shown to exhibit penetrating, intranodular blood flow, while follicular adenomas frequently exhibit peripheral blood flow [25, 26], although no difference was found in a recent study from the Mayo Clinic [27].

In summary, grayscale and Doppler sonographic features may further refine the malignancy risk of an FN nodule. However, the application of these findings to one's clinical practice depends upon the institution-specific proportion of follicular versus papillary carcinomas diagnosed histologically in nodules with a cytologic diagnosis of "suspicious for follicular neoplasm."

Part II: Molecular Evaluation

Molecular Genetics in Thyroid Cancer

Gene point mutations and rearrangements are identified in 61–75 % of thyroid cancers [5, 28, 29]. Mutations are generally mutually exclusive. The MAPK and PI3K-AKT signaling pathways, which regulate cell proliferation, differentiation, and survival, are the main pathways involved in tumor genesis. Activating mutations in the MAPK pathway are common in papillary carcinomas, whereas activating mutations in the PI3K-AKT pathway are more common in follicular carcinomas [30]. *RAS* point mutations and *PAX8/PPARγ* rearrangements are the most common mutations identified in follicular carcinomas and follicular variant papillary carcinomas, the cancers most frequently diagnosed in nodules which are cytologically "follicular neoplasm" [5, 29].

NRAS, *HRAS*, and *KRAS* genes encode intracellular G proteins involved in both pathways. The most common *RAS* mutations occur in *NRAS* codon 61 and *HRAS* codon 61. *RAS* mutations occur in 40–50 % of follicular thyroid cancers and 10–20 % of papillary cancers, most of which are follicular variant. *RAS* mutations are also identified in 20–40 % of follicular adenomas [5, 30]. The *PAX8/PPARγ* rearrangement leads to the fusion of the *PAX8* gene coding for a thyroid-specific transcription factor and the peroxisome proliferation-activated receptor. The mechanism by which this rearrangement promotes carcinogenesis is not entirely clear. It occurs in 30–35 % of follicular cancers as well as up to 13 % of benign follicular adenomas. In addition, it is found in 1–5 % of papillary cancers but only in the follicular variant [30]. The occurrence of *RAS* and *PAX8/PPARγ* mutations in both benign and malignant nodules has led some to suggest that adenomas harboring these mutations are premalignant, but this is unproved [5, 30, 31].

In contrast, *BRAF* point mutations, which are the most common mutations identified in papillary carcinomas, are only found in malignant nodules [5, 29]. BRAF is an intracellular serine-threonine kinase involved in the MAPK pathway. The most common mutation is V600E, accounting for 98–99 % of all *BRAF* mutations. It is found in 40–45 % of classic and tall cell variant papillary thyroid carcinomas. It is rarely found in follicular variant papillary carcinomas. K601E is the most common *BRAF* mutation in follicular variant papillary carcinomas [30].

The *RET* gene codes for a cell-membrane receptor tyrosine kinase involved in the MAPK pathway. *RET* activation occurs via *RET/PTC* chromosomal rearrangement, in which a portion of the *RET* gene fuses to the promoter portion of one of several unrelated genes. *RET/PTC1* and *RET/PTC3* are the most common rearrangements, in which *RET* fuses to *CCDC6* and *NCOA4*, respectively. *RET/PTC* rearrangements can occur clonally in the majority of cells or in a small fraction of cells alone. Clonal rearrangements occur in 10–20 % of papillary thyroid carcinomas, while nonclonal rearrangements have been found in other cancers and benign adenomas [30, 32].

Clinical Performance and Proposed Utility of Molecular Testing

Commercially available diagnostic tests include several mutation panels and the Veracyte Afirma Gene Expression Classifier. The diagnostic use of a mutational analysis panel in nodules with indeterminate cytology, including "suspicious for follicular neoplasm," has been reported by Nikiforov [5] in 2011 prior to commercial availability and more recently by Beaudenon-Huibregtse [28] in a postmarketing study. In both studies, panels included *BRAF* V600E, *NRAS* codon 61, *HRAS* codon 61, and *KRAS* codon 12 and 13 point mutations as well as *RET/PTC1*, *RET/PTC3*, and *PAX8/PPARγ* rearrangements. Specificity was 92 % or greater in surgically resected FN nodules. Due to this high reported specificity, the proposed utility of this molecular analysis panel is to guide surgical management. For example, patients with mutation-positive nodules may be referred for total thyroidectomy instead of diagnostic lobectomy. However, the sensitivity of only 57–66 % is not sufficient to recommend conservative management with close follow-up and avoid surgery for a mutation-negative nodule (i.e., the false-negative rate is too high).

In addition, the following limitations should be considered when evaluating these reports. First, surgical resection was not performed for all nodules that underwent molecular testing. Because of selection bias, NPV and PPV cannot be ascertained. Second, mutations were detected in only a small proportion (16–18 %) of FN nodules, and of these, *RAS* point mutations accounted for 80–100 % of positive results. Third, *RAS* mutations are least specific for cancer detection, and the false-positive rate in this cytologic category was up to 20 % [5, 28].

ThyroSeq v.2® is a custom mutational panel created at the University of Pittsburgh in 2013 to identify new mutations in thyroid cancer using next-generation sequencing, which may in turn increase the sensitivity of mutational analysis [29, 33]. With the increased detection ability of ThyroSeq v.2® compared to the more basic mutation analysis panel used by the University of Pittsburgh earlier in 2011 [5], the rate of mutation-positive FN nodules increased from 18 to 29 %. Again, the most common finding was a point mutation in one of the *RAS* genes, but additional unique gene fusions and mutations were detected. Overall, molecular alterations were found in 90 % of cancers and only 7 % of benign nodules, which leads to promising test performance characteristics for nodules with a "follicular neoplasm" diagnosis. A 2014 study from the University of Pittsburgh using ThyroSeq v.2® reported a calculated NPV of 96 % (95 % CI 92–95 %) and PPV of 83 % (95 % CI 72–95 %), potentially allowing for nonoperative surveillance for mutation-negative nodules with "follicular neoplasm" cytology [33]. The prospective validation study that involves multiple centers is currently enrolling patients. Overall clinical utility of the test cannot be assessed until this study is completed.

Afirma Gene Expression Classifier

The Afirma gene expression classifier is a proprietary test based upon gene array expression that was developed by private industry and then validated in a prospective multicenter study involving both academic centers and community practices [34]. The aim of test development was to define a gene expression profile diagnostic test with high sensitivity for cancer detection when applied to nodules with indeterminate cytologic diagnoses. The final gene expression classifier (GEC) involves an initial screen with 25 genes to filter out rare neoplasms (e.g., metastatic disease, medullary cancer), with subsequent analysis of 142 genes in the main classifier that is reported as either benign or suspicious if nucleic acid quantity is adequate. Sample collection requires two FNA passes rinsed in an RNA-preserving solution because of the higher nondiagnostic rate with only one pass.

In the validation study [34], the NPV was 94 % [95 % CI 79–99 %] for a benign GEC result for FN nodules. However, the influence of the nodule's baseline cancer risk on the NPV is clearly evident from this study because the NPV declined to 85 % [95 % CI 55–98 %] for nodules classified as "suspicious for malignancy," which was associated with a cancer prevalence of 62 %, compared with a prevalence of 25 % among nodules classified as "suspicious for follicular neoplasm." And because PPV and NPV are directly related to the disease prevalence, just as NPV decreases with higher cancer prevalence, PPV will increase. Therefore, the PPV for a suspicious GEC result rose from 37 % [95 % CI 23–52 %] to 76 % [95 % CI 61–88 %] for nodules classified as "follicular neoplasm" and "suspicious for malignancy," respectively. The proposed utility of the GEC is that a benign result decreases the malignancy risk in an FN nodule so that observation rather than surgery can be recommended. However, the clinician must remember that the 6 % false-negative rate of a benign GEC result has a 95 % confidence interval of 1–20 %, and both the NPV and PPV can be altered by the baseline cancer risk for FN cytologic nodules in that clinician's population.

Since the Afirma GEC became commercially available in 2011, one multicenter study and three single-center studies have evaluated its application in clinical practice [35–38]. The use of GEC for nodules with indeterminate cytology, including "follicular neoplasm," has clearly impacted clinical management. While the standard of care for cytologically indeterminate nodules has been diagnostic lobectomy, only 2–25 % of Afirma-benign nodules were resected versus 73–86 % of Afirma-suspicious nodules. Because surgery was not routinely performed in all patients with nodules classified as "suspicious for follicular neoplasm," the NPV and PPV estimates cannot be calculated and compared to the initial validating study. However, the reported cancer risks in resected GEC-suspicious nodules can be compared to the PPV reported in the validation study to get some insight into GEC performance. Six centers demonstrated overall concordance in surgical malignancy rates with the validation study [35, 36, 38], but the results were discrepant from two centers: one was significantly higher (67 %) [35] and the other lower (15 %) [37] (Table 1.3). Additional validation studies should be considered, especially given demonstrated variability in diagnostic performance.

A recent single-center publication from one of these sites reported the extended experience with GEC since the multicenter publication and confirmed that center's overall 37 % cancer rate in GEC-suspicious FN nodules. Interestingly, this was the first study to systematically analyze GEC-suspicious cancer rates separately in nodules with "suspicious for follicular neoplasm" cytology (53 %) versus those interpreted as "follicular neoplasm with oncocytic features" (15 %). The hypothesis for the lower malignancy rate in GEC-suspicious nodules with oncocytic follicular cytology is that the presence of abundant mitochondrial DNA in these oncocytic neoplasms, both benign and malignant, may alter GEC performance [38]. If this

Table 1.3 Cancer rate in GEC-suspicious nodules with a cytologic diagnosis of suspicious for follicular neoplasm

	Cancer rate (%)
Alexander 2012 [34] Afirma GEC validation study	37
Alexander 2014 [35]	37
Site 1	38
Site 2	33
Site 3	35
Site 4	33
Site 5	67
Harrell [36]	38
McIver [37]	15
Lastra [38]	37

finding is confirmed in future studies, this would alter how a clinician might counsel a patient about GEC performance when the nodule demonstrates oncocytic follicular cytology.

Before utilizing molecular diagnostics, one must consider the applicability of published findings to the patient being tested. The primary consideration is the baseline risk of malignancy of an FN nodule because this impacts the positive and negative predictive values. Therefore, a clinician must be cognizant of both the practice-specific cancer risk associated with a cytologic diagnosis of follicular neoplasm and the histologic distribution of malignant diagnoses (follicular cancer versus papillary cancer subtypes). Although the average risk of malignancy is approximately 25 % [1, 2], center-specific rates range from 14 to 49 % [2]. This variability is likely contributed to by poor inter- and intraobserver agreement for cytologic and histologic interpretation [2, 4, 9]. In addition, FN nodule size and the presence of certain sonographic features increase the baseline risk of malignancy to 28–84 %, depending on the feature and the malignant histology [11–14, 16, 17, 20].

Potential applications of molecular testing include the following scenarios for FN nodules:

1. If based upon sonographic features and size, the likelihood of malignancy is 25 % or less, a benign Afirma GEC result will have a relatively high NPV, and observation can be recommended.
2. If the majority of cancers diagnosed in resected FN nodules are papillary histology in a clinician's practice, then the cancer risk of a hypoechoic, solid nodule with microcalcifications will be significantly higher than 25 %. Therefore, the NPV of a benign GEC result will be significantly lower than 94 %, and this test is not optimally used here. Rather, surgical resection, potentially guided by mutational analysis results, is generally indicated.
3. Similarly, if the majority of cancers diagnosed in resected FN nodules are follicular carcinomas in a clinician's practice, then the cancer risk of a large, isoechoic nodule with increased intranodular vascularity exceeds 25 %.

Again, a benign GEC result will not be associated with a sufficiently high NPV to avoid surgery, and mutational analysis may inform the extent of surgical resection.

4. When considering published findings, one should also note that there has only been a single validation study for the Afirma GEC (34) and none for the commercially available mutational analysis panel or the new ThyroSeq v.2® test. In all other studies [5, 28, 33, 35–38], the positive and negative predictive values are unknown because surgery was not universally performed. Additional validation studies may be necessary to optimally interpret results from molecular testing and apply these to practice.

Management of the Case

This patient has a follicular neoplasm cytologic diagnosis without known risk factors for thyroid cancer or sonographic features that increase concern for malignancy. The risk of malignancy (~25 %) associated with this diagnosis was reviewed with the patient. In our institution, follicular variant papillary cancer accounts for 80 % of the cancer diagnoses, and this nodule was not hypoechoic on sonographic imaging. The patient elected to proceed with molecular testing with the Afirma GEC for risk stratification. Her result was "benign." A repeat ultrasound 9 months later documented stability in size.

Clinical Pearls

- The risk of malignancy for a nodule with a cytologic diagnosis of "suspicious for follicular neoplasm" is approximately 25 %, although there is significant variability between institutions.
- A high negative predictive value signifies that the risk of malignancy is low when the test is negative, while a high positive predictive value signifies that the risk of malignancy is high when the test is positive.
- As the baseline risk of cancer (i.e., the "pretest probability") increases, the negative predictive value decreases and the positive predictive value increases.
- Grayscale and Doppler sonographic features may be used to refine the baseline risk of malignancy. However, application to one's clinical practice depends upon the institution-specific proportion of follicular versus papillary carcinomas diagnosed in FN nodules.
- The proposed utility of the GEC is that a benign result decreases the malignancy risk in an FN nodule so that observation rather than surgery can be recommended.
- The proposed utility of mutational analysis is to guide surgical management. A patient with a mutation-positive nodule may be referred for total thyroidectomy

instead of diagnostic lobectomy given the increased risk of malignancy associated with this result.
- If the risk of malignancy is greater than 25 %, the NPV associated with a benign GEC result decreases, and this test cannot be used to avoid surgery. Rather, surgical resection, potentially guided by mutational analysis, may be considered.
- Newer molecular diagnostics using next-generation sequencing may have higher sensitivity, but validation studies are lacking.

References

1. Bongiovanni M, Spitale A, Faquin WC, Mazzucchelli L, Baloch ZW. The Bethesda system for reporting thyroid cytopathology: a meta-analysis. Acta Cytol. 2012;56(4):333–9.
2. Wang CC, Friedman L, Kennedy GC, Wang H, Kebebew E, Steward DL, et al. A large multicenter correlation study of thyroid nodule cytopathology and histopathology. Thyroid. 2011;21(3):243–51.
3. Baloch ZW, LiVolsi VA, Asa SL, Rosai J, Merino MJ, Randolph G, et al. Diagnostic terminology and morphologic criteria for cytologic diagnosis of thyroid lesions: a synopsis of the National Cancer institute thyroid fine-needle aspiration state of the science conference. Diagn Cytopathol. 2008;36(6):425–37.
4. Walts AE, Bose S, Fan X, Frishberg D, Scharre K, de Peralta-Venturina M, et al. A simplified Bethesda system for reporting thyroid cytopathology using only four categories improves intra- and inter-observer diagnostic agreement and provides non-overlapping estimates of malignancy risks. Diagn Cytopathol. 2012;40 Suppl 1:E62–8.
5. Nikiforov YE, Ohori NP, Hodak SP, Carty SE, LeBeau SO, Ferris RL, et al. Impact of mutational testing on the diagnosis and management of patients with cytologically indeterminate thyroid nodules: a prospective analysis of 1056 FNA samples. J Clin Endocrinol Metab. 2011;96(11):3390–7.
6. Yassa L, Cibas ES, Benson CB, Frates MC, Doubilet PM, Gawande AA, et al. Long-term assessment of a multidisciplinary approach to thyroid nodule diagnostic evaluation. Cancer. 2007;111(6):508–16.
7. Yang J, Schnadig V, Logrono R, Wasserman PG. Fine-needle aspiration of thyroid nodules: a study of 4703 patients with histologic and clinical correlations. Cancer. 2007;111(5):306–15.
8. Theoharis CG, Schofield KM, Hammers L, Udelsman R, Chhieng DC. The Bethesda thyroid fine-needle aspiration classification system: year 1 at an academic institution. Thyroid. 2009;19(11):1215–23.
9. Cibas ES, Baloch ZW, Fellegara G, LiVolsi VA, Raab SS, Rosai J, et al. A prospective assessment defining the limitations of thyroid nodule pathologic evaluation. Ann Intern Med. 2013;159(5):325–32.
10. Tuttle RM, Lemar H, Burch HB. Clinical features associated with an increased risk of thyroid malignancy in patients with follicular neoplasia by fine-needle aspiration. Thyroid. 1998;8(5):377–83.
11. Lee SH, Baek JS, Lee JY, Lim JA, Cho SY, Lee TH, et al. Predictive factors of malignancy in thyroid nodules with a cytological diagnosis of follicular neoplasm. Endocr Pathol. 2013;24(4):177–83.
12. Lubitz CC, Faquin WC, Yang J, Mekel M, Gaz RD, Parangi S, et al. Clinical and cytological features predictive of malignancy in thyroid follicular neoplasms. Thyroid. 2010;20(1):25–31.
13. Gulcelik NE, Gulcelik MA, Kuru B. Risk of malignancy in patients with follicular neoplasm: predictive value of clinical and ultrasonographic features. Arch Otolaryngol Head Neck Surg. 2008;134(12):1312–5.

14. Choi YJ, Yun JS, Kim DH. Clinical and ultrasound features of cytology diagnosed follicular neoplasm. Endocr J. 2009;56(3):383–9.
15. Schlinkert RT, van Heerden JA, Goellner JR, Gharib H, Smith SL, Rosales RF, et al. Factors that predict malignant thyroid lesions when fine-needle aspiration is "suspicious for follicular neoplasm". Mayo Clin Proc. 1997;72(10):913–6.
16. Rago T, Di Coscio G, Basolo F, Scutari M, Elisei R, Berti P, et al. Combined clinical, thyroid ultrasound and cytological features help to predict thyroid malignancy in follicular and Hupsilonrthle cell thyroid lesions: results from a series of 505 consecutive patients. Clin Endocrinol (Oxf). 2007;66(1):13–20.
17. Raber W, Kaserer K, Niederle B, Vierhapper H. Risk factors for malignancy of thyroid nodules initially identified as follicular neoplasia by fine-needle aspiration: results of a prospective study of one hundred twenty patients. Thyroid. 2000;10(8):709–12.
18. McHenry CR, Thomas SR, Slusarczyk SJ, Khiyami A. Follicular or Hurthle cell neoplasm of the thyroid: can clinical factors be used to predict carcinoma and determine extent of thyroidectomy? Surgery. 1999;126(4):798–802; discussion 802–4.
19. Brito JP, Gionfriddo MR, Al Nofal A, Boehmer KR, Leppin AL, Reading C, et al. The accuracy of thyroid nodule ultrasound to predict thyroid cancer: systematic review and meta-analysis. J Clin Endocrinol Metab. 2014;99(4):1253–63.
20. De Nicola H, Szejnfeld J, Logullo AF, Wolosker AM, Souza LR, Chiferi Jr V. Flow pattern and vascular resistive index as predictors of malignancy risk in thyroid follicular neoplasms. J Ultrasound Med. 2005;24(7):897–904.
21. Triggiani V, Guastamacchia E, Licchelli B, Tafaro E. Microcalcifications and psammoma bodies in thyroid tumors. Thyroid. 2008;18(9):1017–8.
22. Leung CS, Hartwick RW, Bedard YC. Correlation of cytologic and histologic features in variants of papillary carcinoma of the thyroid. Acta Cytol. 1993;37(5):645–50.
23. Kim DS, Kim JH, Na DG, Park SH, Kim E, Chang KH, et al. Sonographic features of follicular variant papillary thyroid carcinomas in comparison with conventional papillary thyroid carcinomas. J Ultrasound Med. 2009;28(12):1685–92.
24. Jeh SK, Jung SL, Kim BS, Lee YS. Evaluating the degree of conformity of papillary carcinoma and follicular carcinoma to the reported ultrasonographic findings of malignant thyroid tumor. Korean J Radiol. 2007;8(3):192–7.
25. Fukunari N, Nagahama M, Sugino K, Mimura T, Ito K, Ito K. Clinical evaluation of color Doppler imaging for the differential diagnosis of thyroid follicular lesions. World J Surg. 2004;28(12):1261–5.
26. Miyakawa M, Onoda N, Etoh M, Fukuda I, Takano K, Okamoto T, et al. Diagnosis of thyroid follicular carcinoma by the vascular pattern and velocimetric parameters using high resolution pulsed and power Doppler ultrasonography. Endocr J. 2005;52(2):207–12.
27. Sillery JC, Reading CC, Charboneau JW, Henrichsen TL, Hay ID, Mandrekar JN. Thyroid follicular carcinoma: sonographic features of 50 cases. AJR Am J Roentgenol. 2010; 194(1):44–54.
28. Beaudenon-Huibregtse S, Alexander EK, Guttler RB, Hershman JM, Babu V, Blevins TC, et al. Centralized molecular testing for oncogenic gene mutations complements the local cytopathologic diagnosis of thyroid nodules. Thyroid. 2014;24(10):1479–87.
29. Nikiforova MN, Wald AI, Roy S, Durso MB, Nikiforov YE. Targeted next-generation sequencing panel (ThyroSeq) for detection of mutations in thyroid cancer. J Clin Endocrinol Metab. 2013;98(11):E1852–60.
30. Nikiforov YE, Nikiforova MN. Molecular genetics and diagnosis of thyroid cancer. Nat Rev Endocrinol. 2011;7(10):569–80.
31. Eszlinger M, Hegedus L, Paschke R. Ruling in or ruling out thyroid malignancy by molecular diagnostics of thyroid nodules. Best Pract Res Clin Endocrinol Metab. 2014;28(4):545–57.
32. Ciampi R, Nikiforov YE. RET/PTC rearrangements and BRAF mutations in thyroid tumorigenesis. Endocrinology. 2007;148(3):936–41.
33. Nikiforov YE, Carty SE, Chiosea SI, Coyne C, Duvvuri U, Ferris RL, et al. Highly accurate diagnosis of cancer in thyroid nodules with follicular neoplasm/suspicious for a follicular

neoplasm cytology by ThyroSeq v2 next-generation sequencing assay. Cancer. 2014;120: 3627–34.

34. Alexander EK, Kennedy GC, Baloch ZW, Cibas ES, Chudova D, Diggans J, et al. Preoperative diagnosis of benign thyroid nodules with indeterminate cytology. N Engl J Med. 2012; 367(8):705–15.
35. Alexander EK, Schorr M, Klopper J, Kim C, Sipos J, Nabhan F, et al. Multicenter clinical experience with the Afirma gene expression classifier. J Clin Endocrinol Metab. 2014; 99(1):119–25.
36. Harrell RM, Bimston DN. Surgical utility of Afirma: effects of high cancer prevalence and oncocytic cell types in patients with indeterminate thyroid cytology. Endocr Pract. 2014; 20(4):364–9.
37. McIver B, Castro MR, Morris JC, Bernet V, Smallridge R, Henry M, et al. An Independent study of a gene expression classifier (Afirma) in the evaluation of cytologically indeterminate thyroid nodules. J Clin Endocrinol Metab. 2014;99(11):4069–77.
38. Lastra RR, Pramick MR, Crammer CJ, LiVolsi VA, Baloch ZW. Implications of a suspicious afirma test result in thyroid fine-needle aspiration cytology: an institutional experience. Cancer Cytopathol. 2014;122(10):737–44.

Part II
Low Risk Differentiated Thyroid Cancer:
Initial Management: Extent of Surgery and Use of Radioactive Iodine Therapy

Chapter 2
A Case of a Small (1–2 cm) Papillary Thyroid Cancer in a Young Patient: Lobectomy Versus Total Thyroidectomy

Gerard M. Doherty

Case Presentation

A 35-year-old woman was referred to a thyroid clinic due to a newly identified palpable nodule in the left thyroid lobe. She had no history of neck surgery, voice changes, prior thyroid nodules, significant radiation exposure, or family history of thyroid disease. Physical examination included a palpable firm left thyroid nodule, a normal voice, and no cervical adenopathy. Thyroid ultrasound confirmed that the palpable nodule was a solitary hypoechoic 18 mm left thyroid nodule with irregular borders and scattered microcalcifications. A formal ultrasound nodal survey showed no abnormal lymph nodes, and fine needle aspiration cytology of the dominant nodule revealed papillary thyroid cancer. Molecular testing of the FNA sample showed no BRAF mutation. After discussion, the patient elected a strategy of left thyroid lobectomy with intraoperative node assessment, including a planned intraoperative switch to total thyroidectomy and level 6 node dissection only if there were higher-risk features detected during the procedure, such as gross lymph node metastases. The operation was an uncomplicated left thyroid lobectomy under local anesthesia with sedation done as an ambulatory procedure. At 8-week follow-up, her TSH without exogenous thyroid hormone was 1.1 mU/L, and thyroglobulin was 1.8 ng/mL without antithyroglobulin antibodies.

G.M. Doherty, MD (✉)
Department of Surgery, Boston University,
88 East Newton St, Collamore Suite 500, Boston, MA 02116, USA
e-mail: dohertyg@bu.edu

D.S. Cooper, C. Durante (eds.), *Thyroid Cancer*,
DOI 10.1007/978-3-319-22401-5_2

Assessment and Literature Review

Small papillary thyroid carcinomas are very common and rarely threaten long-term survival, especially in young people, unless associated with some poor prognostic features. The management strategy for this common tumor requires coordination of the plan prior to operation, in order to ensure that the procedure performed supports the intended adjuvant therapies and follow-up surveillance.

Prognostic Features

The 2009 version of the ATA thyroid cancer guidelines proposed a three-tiered *recurrence risk* stratification system that classified patients as low, intermediate, or high risk; this system is being modified in the proposed update to the ATA thyroid cancer guidelines that is in current development [1]. The pathological features that increase the risk of recurrence include vascular invasion by the tumor, invasion of tumor into tissues outside of the thyroid capsule, clinically apparent lymph node metastases, or aggressive histologic features. The implications of V600E BRAF mutation in the tumor are not yet clear, especially for small primary tumors [2]. The findings during treatment that increase the patient's risk of recurrence include the presence of local or distant metastases on postoperative radioiodine scan or other imaging modalities and a persistently elevated serum thyroglobulin. High-risk pathological features include gross extrathyroidal extension or incomplete tumor resection; distant metastases, thyroglobulin levels that suggest distant metastases, large node metastases (>3 cm), and extranodal extension are other high-risk findings. These features have been shown to predict recurrence risk and can therefore be used to inform patients and clinicians who are choosing treatment and follow-up plans, rather than basing those plans solely on predictions of survival [3], which is typically unaffected in low-risk patients.

The ATA initial risk stratification also predicts the type of persistent or recurrent disease pattern observed; most persistent disease in low-risk patients is solely an abnormal serum thyroglobulin level without structurally identifiable disease which is unlikely to lead to disease-related morbidity. Greater proportions of intermediate- and high-risk patients who have persistent or recurrent disease have clinically or radiologically identifiable structural disease and have a greater likelihood of disease-related morbidity or mortality.

Management Strategies

The operation for thyroid cancer is the initial step in the treatment strategy and follow-up plan established by the managing team. In the past, total thyroidectomy has been promoted as the optimal option for papillary thyroid cancers greater than 1 cm. There are data showing that total thyroidectomy leads to decreased recurrence rates and improved survival [4], as well as optimally positioning the patient for subsequent follow-up using serum thyroglobulin measurements. However, there are also data to support more limited thyroid resection as an equivalent strategy for patients with low-risk disease [5]. As a selective approach to RAI ablation has become more favored in low-risk patients, the utilization of total thyroidectomy specifically as preparation for the use of RAI in treatment or follow-up has become a less important rationale. If a patient population can be identified that has equivalent long-term disease outcomes with thyroid lobectomy, without radioiodine therapy or TSH suppression, then they would best be served by limiting the aggressiveness of treatment, minimizing adverse events, and maximizing quality of life. This is a very important clinical issue, since patients with very low-risk thyroid cancer comprise a very large proportion of the thyroid cancer population [6].

A bilateral thyroidectomy (total or near-total) is preferred if the treatment strategy is to include RAI scanning or therapy postoperatively. This is most clearly applicable to the high-risk groups. For patients at intermediate risk, either a bilateral or unilateral thyroidectomy may serve as the surgical platform for an overall treatment plan. Features that place the patient at increased risk of recurrent disease or of concomitant contralateral disease, such as age >45 years, contralateral thyroid nodules, known multifocal cancer in the lobe to be operated upon, a personal history of radiation therapy to the head and neck, or a family history of differentiated thyroid cancer, may inform the decision to employ a bilateral procedure to preserve the option of RAI scanning or therapy or to resolve questions of bilateral disease. It is clearly in the patient's best interest to work with a treatment team that can coordinate this decision-making prior to the initial operation, to avoid awkward planning compromises at later points in the treatment course [7].

Complications of Total Thyroidectomy

Though both are quite safe operations, total thyroidectomy carries a significantly greater risk of complications than thyroid lobectomy. A 2013 meta-analysis showed a relative risk (RR) that was greater for total thyroidectomy for all significant complications [8]. These included permanent recurrent laryngeal nerve injury ($RR = 1.9$), permanent hypocalcemia ($RR = 3.2$), and hemorrhage/hematoma ($RR = 2.6$). Most importantly, thyroid lobectomy has a negligible risk of permanent hypoparathyroidism because the parathyroid glands near the contralateral lobe are not dissected, making it impossible to cause permanent hypoparathyroidism.

There is a relationship between surgeon volume and patient outcomes for thyroid surgery that may inform the choice of approach in some instances. Differences have been identified in studies evaluating data at the state and national levels in the USA and in other countries [9, 10]. These studies have consistently shown that patients operated on by low-volume surgeons (as variably defined) have more complications than those operated on by intermediate- or high-volume surgeons. Furthermore, the majority of thyroid surgery is performed by low-volume surgeons. These data suggest that patients should ideally receive care from high-volume thyroid surgeons where, overall, they are more likely to have good results. However, the distribution and limited number of high-volume surgeons make this impractical in the USA. The ATA guidelines do support a policy of sending patients with more extensive disease and concern for grossly invasive disease to high-volume centers that have experience in the management of advanced thyroid cancer.

For an individual patient, the decision regarding the extent of surgery should depend upon the clinical status, preoperative risk group, and treatment team plans for adjuvant therapy and follow-up. Since even high-volume surgeons have a higher risk of complications with bilateral procedures, the decision is more dependent upon the clinical scenario than upon the available surgeon.

Indications for Adjuvant Radioiodine Therapy

The patient risk category as informed by the preoperative, intraoperative, and postoperative findings can be used to determine the utility of thyroid remnant ablation of adjuvant radioiodine therapy for papillary thyroid cancer. The use of postoperative administration of radioactive iodine after total thyroidectomy is to further some combination of these goals:

- Remnant ablation is intended to destroy remaining normal thyroid tissue in order to enable detection of persistent and recurrent disease by RAI scan and thyroglobulin measurement.
- Adjuvant therapy is intended to affect disease-free survival by destroying microscopic undetected metastatic disease in lymph nodes or distant sites.
- Radioiodine therapy is intended to improve disease-specific and disease-free survival by treating known persistent disease.

The use of radioiodine in any of these contexts (ablation, adjuvant therapy, or RAI therapy) can also be accompanied by scanning that can provide diagnostic information regarding the presence or absence of RAI avid persistent disease.

For patients with low-risk papillary thyroid cancer, follow-up without RAI ablation, using neck ultrasound and thyroglobulin, is reasonable [11]. Because of the low risk of disease recurrence and the feasibility of follow-up without the use of radioiodine scans, radioiodine ablation or adjuvant therapy is not generally recommended for patients in the ATA low-risk category [12]. However, practices vary widely, with great variation in the use of radioiodine for low-risk patients in the USA [13].

Management of the Case

In this case, the patient's clinical features are all low risk. She is <45 years of age, with BRAF mutation-negative papillary thyroid cancer confined to the thyroid. There are no features (contralateral nodules, radiation exposure history, family history) to suggest a significant current or future risk of contralateral disease. Her formal node survey done with ultrasound does not show evidence of clinically significant metastases in the central or lateral neck.

Her preoperative discussion focused on the likelihood that in her clinical scenario she would not benefit from adjuvant therapy with radioiodine. The main risk factor that could be discovered at operation without being evident preoperatively is small but grossly identifiable central neck (level 6) lymphadenopathy. With her preoperative assent, the plan for intraoperative decision-making could have led to a bilateral thyroid procedure to facilitate postoperative radioiodine treatment and scanning if there were confirmed central neck metastases (clinical N1 disease). This would have placed her into the intermediate-risk group, where the benefit of this strategy is still somewhat uncertain, but was recommended and agreed upon by the patient and treatment team. Whether RAI therapy in this setting is done for remnant ablation to make follow-up easier or as adjuvant therapy is a matter of clinical viewpoint, but in any case was not indicated for her management.

Clinical Pearls/Pitfalls

- The treatment should be based upon the defined risk category of the patient.
- The "doses" of therapy, including surgery, radioiodine administration, and TSH suppression, can each be altered in response to the risk of the disease and the therapy for that individual patient.
- The current trend in the management of low-risk differentiated thyroid cancer is toward more conservative therapy (lower doses of surgery and radioiodine in particular) based upon patient risk group.

References

1. Cooper DS, Doherty GM, Haugen BR, Kloos RT, Lee SL, Mandel SJ, et al. Revised American Thyroid Association management guidelines for patients with thyroid nodules and differentiated thyroid cancer. Thyroid. 2009;19(11):1167–214.
2. Niemeier LA, Kuffner Akatsu H, Song C, Carty SE, Hodak SP, Yip L, et al. A combined molecular-pathologic score improves risk stratification of thyroid papillary microcarcinoma. Cancer. 2012;118(8):2069–77.
3. Tuttle RM, Tala H, Shah J, Leboeuf R, Ghossein R, Gonen M, et al. Estimating risk of recurrence in differentiated thyroid cancer after total thyroidectomy and radioactive iodine remnant ablation: using response to therapy variables to modify the initial risk estimates predicted by the new American Thyroid Association staging system. Thyroid. 2010;20(12):1341–9.
4. Bilimoria KY, Bentrem DJ, Ko CY, Stewart AK, Winchester DP, Talamonti MS, et al. Extent of surgery affects survival for papillary thyroid cancer. Ann Surg. 2007;246(3):375–81, discussion: 81–4.
5. Matsuzu K, Sugino K, Masudo K, Nagahama M, Kitagawa W, Shibuya H, et al. Thyroid lobectomy for papillary thyroid cancer: long-term follow-up study of 1088 cases. World J Surg. 2014;38(1):68–79.

6. Davies L, Welch HG. Current thyroid cancer trends in the United States. JAMA Otolaryngol Head Neck Surg. 2014;140(4):317–22.
7. Carty SE, Doherty GM, Inabnet 3rd WB, Pasieka JL, Randolph GW, Shaha AR, et al. American Thyroid Association statement on the essential elements of interdisciplinary communication of perioperative information for patients undergoing thyroid cancer surgery. Thyroid. 2012;22(4):395–9.
8. Kandil E, Krishnan B, Noureldine SI, Yao L, Tufano RP. Hemithyroidectomy: a meta-analysis of postoperative need for hormone replacement and complications. ORL J Otorhinolaryngol Relat Spec. 2013;75(1):6–17.
9. Sosa JA, Bowman HM, Tielsch JM, Powe NR, Gordon TA, Udelsman R. The importance of surgeon experience for clinical and economic outcomes from thyroidectomy. Ann Surg. 1998;228(3):320–30.
10. Dralle H, Sekulla C, Haerting J, Timmermann W, Neumann HJ, Kruse E, et al. Risk factors of paralysis and functional outcome after recurrent laryngeal nerve monitoring in thyroid surgery. Surgery. 2004;136(6):1310–22.
11. Ibrahimpasic T, Nixon IJ, Palmer FL, Whitcher MM, Tuttle RM, Shaha A, et al. Undetectable thyroglobulin after total thyroidectomy in patients with low- and intermediate-risk papillary thyroid cancer—is there a need for radioactive iodine therapy? Surgery. 2012;152(6):1096–105.
12. Schvartz C, Bonnetain F, Dabakuyo S, Gauthier M, Cueff A, Fieffe S, et al. Impact on overall survival of radioactive iodine in low-risk differentiated thyroid cancer patients. J Clin Endocrinol Metab. 2012;97(5):1526–35.
13. Haymart MR, Banerjee M, Stewart AK, Koenig RJ, Birkmeyer JD, Griggs JJ. Use of radioactive iodine for thyroid cancer. JAMA. 2011;306(7):721–8.

Chapter 3
The Decision-Making Process for Prophylactic Central Neck Dissection in a Patient Presenting with an Indeterminate Thyroid Nodule on Cytology Assessment: Role of Preoperative Ultrasound and Molecular Marker Testing

Salem I. Noureldine and Ralph P. Tufano

Case Presentation

A 62-year-old woman presented with a thyroid nodule that was identified during a routine physical examination. A thyroid ultrasound (US) was performed and a 2.8 cm cystic nodule with a mural component was identified in the isthmus. An US-guided fine-needle aspiration (FNA) biopsy was performed, and the nodule was interpreted to be suspicious for papillary thyroid cancer (PTC) (Bethesda category V). A Quest (Quest Diagnostics, Lyndhurst, NJ) diagnostic study was also performed for the molecular analysis of *BRAF V600E, RAS (including HRAS, KRAS, and NRAS), RET/PTC,* and *PAX8/PPARγ*, all of which were negative except for *KRAS*. A comprehensive US of the neck was performed and no lymphadenopathy was appreciated. The patient underwent total thyroidectomy, and no lymphadenopathy was also appreciated intraoperatively. On surgical pathology, a single focus of an encapsulated, follicular variant of PTC was identified that was 1.6 cm in greatest dimension. The patient was started on thyroid hormone replacement and did not require postoperative radioactive iodine treatment as determined by her

S.I. Noureldine, MD • R.P. Tufano, MD, MBA, FACS
Division of Head and Neck Endocrine Surgery, Department of Otolaryngology-Head and Neck Surgery, Johns Hopkins University School of Medicine, 601 N. Caroline Street, 6th floor (6242), Baltimore, MD, 21287, USA
e-mail: snourel1@jhmi.edu; rtufano@jhmi.edu

D.S. Cooper, C. Durante (eds.), *Thyroid Cancer*,
DOI 10.1007/978-3-319-22401-5_3

multidisciplinary caregivers. At the 6-month follow-up, US of the neck did not show any lymphadenopathy and serum thyroglobulin (Tg) levels were undetectable with negative Tg antibodies.

Background

Thyroid nodules are quite prevalent in the United States and are often discovered on a routine physical exam or incidentally through radiographic studies. The clinical importance of thyroid nodules rests with the need to exclude those that are malignant. This is usually accomplished by obtaining a detailed history, physical exam, and thyroid function tests, in addition to a thyroid and neck US. The information that is obtained will then direct subsequent evaluation, including the need for FNA biopsy assessment [1]. Biopsy yields a final diagnosis in 70–80 % of cases, and the remaining 20–30 % of samples are characterized as "indeterminate".

The Bethesda System for Reporting Thyroid Cytopathology (BSRTC) identifies six diagnostic categories on thyroid nodule cytopathology [2]: (I) nondiagnostic or unsatisfactory, (II) benign, (III) atypia of undetermined significance (AUS) or follicular lesion of undetermined significance (FLUS), (IV) suspicious for a follicular neoplasm or suspicious for a Hürthle cell neoplasm, (V) suspicious for malignancy, and (VI) malignant. Categories III, IV, and V together represent the indeterminate or suspicious classification and have an approximate cancer risk of 5–15, 15–30, and 60–75 %, respectively, allowing for variability between cytopathologists (Table 3.1). These indeterminate nodules may show a follicular growth pattern and/or follicular cell atypia, but the degree of abnormality is not sufficient to distinguish between benign and malignant lesions, since diagnostic hallmarks of thyroid cancer (i.e., vascular and capsular invasion) are not detected by cytopathology or the nuclear features of PTC are not adequately apparent to make a diagnosis of cancer. Therefore, thyroid nodules with indeterminate features on FNA cause a significant problem for the clinician and the patient, and currently, only surgical excision with histopathological analysis is able to provide a final diagnosis [3].

Table 3.1 The Bethesda system for reporting thyroid cytopathology [2]: risk of malignancy

Category	Cytology diagnostic category	Malignancy risk (%)
I	Nondiagnostic or unsatisfactory	1–4
II	Benign	0–3
III	AUS/FLUS	5–15
IV	FN/SFN or SHCN	15–30
V	Suspicious for malignancy	60–75
VI	Malignant	97–99

Abbreviations: *AUS* atypia of undetermined significance, *FLUS* follicular lesion of undetermined significance, *FN* follicular neoplasm, *SFN* suspicious for follicular neoplasm, *SHCN* suspicious for Hürthle cell neoplasm

Preoperative Evaluation

Ultrasound Evaluation

High-resolution ultrasound is generally considered to be the first-line imaging modality to assess the primary tumor and identify lymph node metastases at the initial evaluation of a suspected thyroid malignancy [1]. Ultrasound is widely available and inexpensive, provides detailed high-resolution anatomic information, avoids ionizing radiation, and facilitates ultrasound-guided FNA of suspicious lesions [4]. Ultrasound evaluation of bilateral cervical lymph node compartments (levels I–VI) should be performed routinely in the evaluation of patients with lesions suspicious for thyroid malignancy to guide a complete resection of the primary tumor as well as a compartment-oriented dissection of affected lymph node basins as necessary [1]. This will also facilitate patient counseling regarding surgical risks, since the addition of central or lateral neck dissection to total thyroidectomy is accompanied by a different or increased morbidity risk profile.

There have been many studies examining the utility of US to predict the risk of malignancy in patients with indeterminate FNA cytology, and several findings are commonly used to help guide preoperative surgical planning [5, 6]. Hypoechogenicity, increased nodular vascularity, irregular margins, the presence of microcalcifications, and taller-than-wide shape all correlate with an increased risk of malignancy [3]. These US findings may be used in a supplementary fashion to predict increased malignant potential in cytologically indeterminate nodules [5, 6].

Thyroid cancer lymph node metastases are common, especially in the central compartment, and are reported to occur in 12–81 % of patients with PTC overall and in a smaller proportion of patients with other histotypes (i.e., follicular thyroid cancer and Hürthle cell carcinoma) [7–9]. Lymph node metastases apparent preoperatively or intraoperatively (cN1) can be present in approximately 21–35 % of patients with differentiated thyroid cancer [10–12]. Microscopically positive lymph node metastases are far more prevalent, occurring in 38–62 % of patients with clinically negative (cN0) preoperative and intraoperative nodal assessments [13–15]. Not all lymph node metastases are the same in terms of their implications for recurrence and mortality. Macroscopic lymph node metastases (gross nodal disease) in patients with PTC are associated with higher recurrence rates, and an increased mortality rate has been observed in older patients with lymph node metastases [16–18]. In contrast, microscopic lymph node metastases do not affect patient survival and are associated with much lower rates of recurrence [19–21]. Clearly, the prognostic importance of nodal disease in PTC seems to be centered on detection and treatment of gross lymph node metastases. Despite occult lymph node micrometastases being found in the central compartment of the neck in 38–80 % of patients with PTC, the median rate of recurrence for patients with clinically node-negative disease is 2 %, whether or not a central neck dissection (CND) is performed [22, 23]. This finding suggests that most micrometastases remain dormant and infrequently evolve into clinically significant disease or alternatively that radioiodine ablation is adequate for the treatment of micrometastatic disease.

Ultrasound features predictive of malignant lymph node involvement include size greater than 1 cm, round shape, loss of hilum, cystic appearance, the presence of punctate calcification, and peripheral hypervascularity [1]. The sensitivity of US in detecting abnormal lymph nodes ranges from 25 to 60 % for the central neck and from 70 to 95 % for the lateral neck [1]. The sensitivity of US of the central neck is lower because the presence of the thyroid gland may prevent small central neck nodes from being detected. The specificity of US in detecting lymph nodes affected by metastatic PTC is high, ranging from 80 to 95 % in both the central neck and the lateral neck [24].

Ultrasound interrogation of the central and lateral neck lymph nodes may inform the clinician in the planning of surgery for cytologically indeterminate nodules. The discovery of lymph node metastases in this setting affords the opportunity to move forward with complete initial resection of all tumor tissue. Patients found to have abnormal central or lateral neck lymph nodes on US should undergo FNA biopsy of at least one of these nodes. The finding of cells of thyroid origin within lymph nodes or the presence of an elevated Tg in the needle washout, (taking into account the fact that serum Tg is normal or high because of the presence of the thyroid gland) confirms the diagnosis of metastatic thyroid cancer and may significantly alter surgical management in the patient with indeterminate thyroid cytology.

Molecular Marker Testing

Because about 25 % of thyroid nodules are "indeterminate" on FNA, a large number of diagnostic surgeries are performed every year in the United States and result in morbidity and higher health-care costs. Moreover, patients who are ultimately found to have malignant tumors, but who had indeterminate or suspicious FNA lesions, may require a completion thyroidectomy, especially if postoperative radioiodine is being considered. This challenge has led many scientists to investigate the utility of molecular markers in predicting the actual pathology of cytologically indeterminate thyroid nodules, in order to improve the sensitivity and specificity of FNA cytology. Owing to the overlap between follicular adenomas and follicular thyroid cancer, as well as the relatively low prevalence of known mutations in indeterminate FNA lesions, only a few molecular diagnostic tests with their own limitations have become commercially available.

Diagnostic molecular testing can detect mutations and translocations commonly seen in differentiated thyroid cancer including BRAF, RAS, RET/PTC, and PAX8/PPARγ and can be applied to FNA specimens. Another test, the gene expression classifier, analyzes the expression of over 140 genes and has a high negative predictive value if the result is benign. Recent large prospective studies have confirmed the ability of genetic markers (BRAF, RAS, RET/PTC, and PAX8/PPARγ), the gene expression classifier, and protein markers (galectin-3) to improve the preoperative diagnostic accuracy for patients with indeterminate thyroid nodules [25–27] and may become a more commonly utilized component of FNA evaluation in the future (Table 3.2).

Table 3.2 The performance of currently available molecular tests used when FNA biopsy yields indeterminate results

Test (reference)	Sensitivity (%)	Specificity (%)	PPV (%)	NPV (%)	Malignancy rate (%)
Mutation panel [25]	61	89	89	89	24
GEC [26]	92	52	47	93	32
Galectin-3 [27]	78	93	82	91	30

Abbreviations: *GEC* gene expression classifier (Afirma), *PPV* positive predictive value, *NPV* negative predictive value

In addition, reverse transcription-polymerase chain reaction to detect thyroglobulin mRNA and thyrotropin-receptor mRNA from a lymph node is accurate for diagnosing metastatic thyroid cancer [28]. The current ATA management guidelines state that the use of molecular markers might be considered for specific patients with indeterminate thyroid nodules, rather than proceeding to surgery [3]. However, their utility in guiding preoperative surgical decision-making is yet to be proven. In addition, a recent study indicates these tests may be overused in patients for whom the results would not change surgical management [29].

Management

For patients with lesions suspicious for PTC or diagnostic of PTC (Bethesda category V or VI), total thyroidectomy should be performed and compartment-oriented neck dissection reserved for clinically apparent lymph node metastases to the central and lateral neck compartments [3]. CND plays an important role in the management of clinically apparent nodal disease. Completeness of surgical resection is an important determinant of outcome in patients with gross lymph node metastases, as residual metastatic lymph nodes represent the most common reason for disease persistence or recurrence, therefore influencing prognosis [3].

An area of major controversy in the management of DTC is whether patients with clinically negative lymph nodes (cN0) should undergo elective central neck dissection. This controversy largely came about following the 2006 ATA guidelines, which stated under recommendation 27, "Routine central compartment (level VI) neck dissection should be considered for patients with PTC" [30]. The strength of the recommendation was given a rating of B, indicating it was based on fair evidence that CND may improve health outcomes. At the same time, a European consensus statement on elective CND was endorsed by the European Thyroid Association and read: "there is no evidence that elective CND improves recurrence or mortality rates, but it does allow an accurate staging of the disease that may guide subsequent treatment and follow-up" [31]. In 2009, the revised ATA guidelines were published with a modification in the recommendation for CND. Recommendation 27B was modified to read "prophylactic CND (ipsilateral or bilateral) may be performed in patients with PTC with clinically uninvolved central neck lymph nodes, especially for advanced primary tumors (T3 or T4)." The strength of the recommendation was lowered to C, meaning that this was based on expert opinion [3]. In the new 2015 ATA guidelines [32], this recommendation is "weak, based on low quality evidence." On the other hand, the 2009 and 2015 ATA guidelines state: "Thyroidectomy without prophylactic central neck dissection may be appropriate for small (T1 or T2), noninvasive, clinically node-negative PTC (cN0)."

This controversy is further compounded by fact that no randomized controlled trial exists to evaluate prophylactic CND for the treatment of DTC. A feasibility study completed by the ATA estimated that a randomized trial would require 5840 patients and would cost approximately $15 million [33]. The controversy over whether to perform prophylactic CND also relates to the differing interpretations of existing data. Nevertheless, a meta-analysis involving 1,264 patients found no significant difference in locoregional recurrence rates overall (2 % vs. 3.9 %) or within the central (1.9 % vs. 1.7 %) or lateral (3.7 % vs. 3.8 %) neck compartment with or without prophylactic CND [34].

Those who advocate prophylactic CND do so for its theoretical potential benefits, including reduced rates of recurrence [35, 36], lower postoperative serum Tg levels [14, 35], accurate staging to help modify indication for radioactive iodine ablation and dosing [37–40], and reduced reoperation in the central neck with its potential for higher morbidity [14, 19, 20, 41]. Those who oppose prophylactic CND do so because there is no proven oncologic benefit, primarily in terms of disease-specific mortality, and there is concern for an increased risk of recurrent laryngeal nerve injury and hypoparathyroidism [13, 38, 41–43].

Prophylactic CND for Small-Volume Microscopic Lymph Node Metastasis (cN0)

Small-volume microscopic LN metastases, not apparent on preoperative US exam, appear to be present in up to 80 % of patients diagnosed with papillary thyroid microcarcinomas. The locoregional recurrence rates in treated patients range from 2 to 6 %, regardless of the extent of lymph node dissection and whether or not radioactive iodine was given as adjuvant therapy after surgical resection [9].

Patients with macroscopic PTC (primary tumor >1 cm) have rates of microscopic nodal disease in up to 62 % of cN0 central neck compartments even though recurrence rates are only 1–6 % if CND was not performed [13, 14]. It appears that both microscopic and macroscopic PTCs are often associated with subclinical microscopic lymph node metastases that usually do not progress and become clinically relevant even if untreated [9]. A recent retrospective study by Bardet et al. [44] has shown that patients referred for radioactive iodine ablation between 2006 and 2011 with small lymph node metastasis (0.2 to <1 cm), and not micrometastases as defined by Randolph et al. [9], presented an intermediate outcome for persistence/recurrence between that observed in pN0-pNx patients and pN1 macroscopic patients.

Moreover, many researchers have reported the identification of various factors (i.e., larger tumors, extrathyroidal extension, and aggressive histological subtypes) that might favor prophylactic CND [45]. However, some of these factors such as extrathyroidal extension and aggressive histological subtypes cannot help in the decision to perform prophylactic CND because they are determined primarily by postsurgical histopathology.

Molecular Markers as a Guide for Surgical Extent

The presence of a BRAF V600E mutation has been associated in many studies with the aggressiveness of PTC (extrathyroidal invasion, lymph node metastasis, and advanced stage) and also with disease-specific mortality when associated with other aggressive features, such as extrathyroidal extension [46, 47]. However, BRAF V600E mutation analysis offers a limited positive predictive value (28 %) for disease recurrence [48], therefore suggesting that preoperative knowledge of BRAF V600E mutation status in the primary tumor should not impact on the decision for prophylactic CND.

RAS mutations are associated with a follicular pattern of thyroid neoplasms and have also been reported in poorly differentiated PTC [49]. The clinical significance of RAS mutations in thyroid cancer is controversial; some reports show that RAS mutations are associated with tumor aggressive phenotypes and poor prognosis [50, 51], while others could not confirm this association [52]. Similarly, RET/PTC rearrangements are associated in some reports with lymph node metastasis and extrathyroidal extension [53] and with a better prognosis in other studies [54, 55]. PAX8/PPARγ rearrangements have been associated with multifocality of the tumors and vascular invasion, conferring an invasive potential [56–58]. Others have found that PAX8/PPARγ rearrangement in thyroid nodules predicts follicular-pattern carcinomas, in particular the encapsulated follicular variant of PTC [59]. Despite this, the consistent detection of PAX8/PPARγ rearrangements in benign tumors hinders its value as a diagnostic and prognostic molecular marker [60]. In the above-presented case, the patient underwent molecular analysis for *BRAF V600E, RAS, RET/PTC,* and *PAX8/PPARγ*, all of which were negative except for *KRAS*. However, because none of these markers have been demonstrated to be clear independent prognostic indicators, the information obtained from the mutation panel did not influence our decision to whether or not perform a prophylactic CND. As with any predictor of recurrence or mortality, interventional studies are required to determine which at-risk patients may benefit from additional therapies, prior to the widespread utilization of these molecular studies in clinical practice to determine the extent of treatment.

Recently, however, two more markers have been identified and appear to confer an increased risk of tumor recurrence and tumor-related mortality: the TP53 and TERT mutations. These markers are currently being tested for in cytology specimens in an effort to provide more accurate tumor prognostication preoperatively. Nonetheless, TP53 mutations have been known to occur mostly in poorly differentiated and anaplastic thyroid cancers. More recent broad genotypic analyses identified TP53 mutations in 3.5 % of well-differentiated PTC and 11 % of well-differentiated follicular thyroid carcinomas [61]. PTCs in this series that were positive for TP53 mutation also showed mutation in BRAF and developed lung metastases. All of the TP53-positive follicular thyroid carcinomas showed no other coexisting mutations and were oncocytic, while 75 % were widely invasive.

TERT mutations are found in 7–22 % of PTC and 14–17 % of FTC. There is a significantly higher prevalence in dedifferentiated thyroid cancer [62–65], in addition to PTC carrying the BRAF mutation [62, 63]. In the largest reported series by Melo et al. [62], TERT mutation was found to be an independent predictor of disease-free survival and mortality for DTC. Furthermore, the combination of a TERT mutation and a BRAF mutation within the same tumor was associated with a high risk of structural disease recurrence [66]. These results suggest that these molecular markers may be helpful for risk stratification of thyroid cancer and will provide a significantly more accurate risk assessment than BRAF mutational status taken in isolation. However, the identification of a molecular marker that is predictive of aggressive behavior does not necessarily mean that more extensive surgery, such as a prophylactic CND, or other aggressive therapy (e.g., radioiodine remnant ablation) will have a significant impact on clinical outcomes.

Summary

Ultrasound is a reliable assessment tool for the preoperative central and lateral neck compartments that helps inform the planning of surgery for cytologically indeterminate nodules. The discovery of lymph node metastases in this setting affords the opportunity for complete initial resection of all tumor tissue, that is, thyroidectomy and therapeutic CND (and lateral neck dissection when those compartments are involved). Despite occult metastases being found in the central neck compartment in 28–80 % of patients with PTC, the median rate of recurrence for clinically node-negative disease is 2 %, whether or not a CND is performed.

The role of commercially available molecular markers to assist in determining the optimal surgical extent in this patient population remains controversial and should not impact the decision for prophylactic CND.

Conflicts of Interest Disclosures All authors report no conflicts of interest.

References

1. Yeh MW, Bauer AJ, Bernet V, Ferris RL, Loevner LA, Mandel SJ, et al. American Thyroid Association statement on preoperative imaging for thyroid cancer surgery. Thyroid. 2014;25(1):3–14.

2. Cibas ES, Ali SZ. The Bethesda system for reporting thyroid cytopathology. Am J Clin Pathol. 2009;132(5):658–65.
3. Cooper DS, Doherty GM, Haugen BR, Kloos RT, Lee SL, Mandel SJ, et al. Revised American Thyroid Association management guidelines for patients with thyroid nodules and differentiated thyroid cancer. Thyroid. 2009;19(11):1167–214.
4. Carty SE, Cooper DS, Doherty GM, Duh QY, Kloos RT, Mandel SJ, et al. Consensus statement on the terminology and classification of central neck dissection for thyroid cancer. Thyroid. 2009;19(11):1153–8.
5. Roy R, Kouniavsky G, Venkat R, Felger EA, Shiue Z, Schneider E, et al. The role of preoperative neck ultrasounds to assess lymph nodes in patients with suspicious or indeterminate thyroid nodules. J Surg Oncol. 2012;105(6):601–5.
6. Yoon JH, Kwak JY, Kim EK, Moon HJ, Kim MJ, Kim JY, et al. How to approach thyroid nodules with indeterminate cytology. Ann Surg Oncol. 2010;17(8):2147–55.
7. Grebe SK, Hay ID. Thyroid cancer nodal metastases: biologic significance and therapeutic considerations. Surg Oncol Clin N Am. 1996;5(1):43–63.
8. Kouvaraki MA, Shapiro SE, Fornage BD, Edeiken-Monro BS, Sherman SI, Vassilopoulou-Sellin R, et al. Role of preoperative ultrasonography in the surgical management of patients with thyroid cancer. Surgery. 2003;134:946–54, discussion 54–5.
9. Randolph GW, Duh QY, Heller KS, LiVolsi VA, Mandel SJ, Steward DL, et al. The prognostic significance of nodal metastases from papillary thyroid carcinoma can be stratified based on the size and number of metastatic lymph nodes, as well as the presence of extranodal extension. Thyroid. 2012;22(11):1144–52.
10. Bardet S, Malville E, Rame JP, Babin E, Samama G, De Raucourt D, et al. Macroscopic lymph-node involvement and neck dissection predict lymph-node recurrence in papillary thyroid carcinoma. Eur J Endocrinol. 2008;158(4):551–60.
11. Cranshaw IM, Carnaille B. Micrometastases in thyroid cancer. An important finding? Surg Oncol. 2008;17(3):253–8.
12. Gemsenjager E, Perren A, Seifert B, Schuler G, Schweizer I, Heitz PU. Lymph node surgery in papillary thyroid carcinoma. J Am Coll Surg. 2003;197:182–90.
13. Hughes DT, White ML, Miller BS, Gauger PG, Burney RE, Doherty GM. Influence of prophylactic central lymph node dissection on postoperative thyroglobulin levels and radioiodine treatment in papillary thyroid cancer. Surgery. 2010;148:1100–6, discussion 006–7.
14. Sywak M, Cornford L, Roach P, Stalberg P, Sidhu S, Delbridge L. Routine ipsilateral level VI lymphadenectomy reduces postoperative thyroglobulin. Surgery. 2006;140(6):1000–5, discussion 5–7.
15. Qubain SW, Nakano S, Baba M, Takao S, Aikou T. Distribution of lymph node micrometastasis in pN0 well-differentiated thyroid carcinoma. Surgery. 2002;131(3):249–56.
16. Lundgren CI, Hall P, Dickman PW, Zedenius J. Clinically significant prognostic factors for differentiated thyroid carcinoma: a population-based, nested case-control study. Cancer. 2006;106(3):524–31.
17. Zaydfudim V, Feurer ID, Griffin MR, Phay JE. The impact of lymph node involvement on survival in patients with papillary and follicular thyroid carcinoma. Surgery. 2008; 144(6):1070–7, discussion 7–8.
18. Sugitani I, Kasai N, Fujimoto Y, Yanagisawa A. A novel classification system for patients with PTC: addition of the new variables of large (3 cm or greater) nodal metastases and reclassification during the follow-up period. Surgery. 2004;135(2):139–48.
19. Tisell LE, Nilsson B, Molne J, Hansson G, Fjalling M, Jansson S, et al. Improved survival of patients with papillary thyroid cancer after surgical microdissection. World J Surg. 1996;20(7):854–9.
20. Scheumann GF, Gimm O, Wegener G, Hundeshagen H, Dralle H. Prognostic significance and surgical management of locoregional lymph node metastases in papillary thyroid cancer. World J Surg. 1994;18(4):559–67, discussion 67–8.
21. Ito Y, Tomoda C, Uruno T, Takamura Y, Miya A, Kobayashi K, et al. Preoperative ultrasonographic examination for lymph node metastasis: usefulness when designing lymph node dissection for papillary microcarcinoma of the thyroid. World J Surg. 2004;28(5):498–501.

22. Wang TS, Cheung K, Farrokhyar F, Roman SA, Sosa JA. A meta-analysis of the effect of prophylactic central compartment neck dissection on locoregional recurrence rates in patients with papillary thyroid cancer. Ann Surg Oncol. 2013;20(11):3477–83.
23. Shan CX, Zhang W, Jiang DZ, Zheng XM, Liu S, Qiu M. Routine central neck dissection in differentiated thyroid carcinoma: a systematic review and meta-analysis. Laryngoscope. 2012;122(4):797–804.
24. Kim E, Park JS, Son KR, Kim JH, Jeon SJ, Na DG. Preoperative diagnosis of cervical metastatic lymph nodes in papillary thyroid carcinoma: comparison of ultrasound, computed tomography, and combined ultrasound with computed tomography. Thyroid. 2008;18(4):411–8.
25. Nikiforov YE, Ohori NP, Hodak SP, Carty SE, LeBeau SO, Ferris RL, et al. Impact of mutational testing on the diagnosis and management of patients with cytologically indeterminate thyroid nodules: a prospective analysis of 1056 FNA samples. J Clin Endocrinol Metab. 2011;96(11):3390–7.
26. Alexander EK, Kennedy GC, Baloch ZW, Cibas ES, Chudova D, Diggans J, et al. Preoperative diagnosis of benign thyroid nodules with indeterminate cytology. N Engl J Med. 2012;367(8):705–15.
27. Bartolazzi A, Orlandi F, Saggiorato E, Volante M, Arecco F, Rossetto R, et al. Galectin-3-expression analysis in the surgical selection of follicular thyroid nodules with indeterminate fine-needle aspiration cytology: a prospective multicentre study. Lancet Oncol. 2008; 9(6):543–9.
28. Belfiore A, La Rosa GL. Fine-needle aspiration biopsy of the thyroid. Endocrinol Metab Clin N Am. 2001;30(2):361–400.
29. Aragon Han P, Olson MT, Fazeli R, Prescott JD, Pai SI, Schneider EB, et al. The impact of molecular testing on the surgical management of patients with thyroid nodules. Ann Surg Oncol. 2014;21:1862–9.
30. Cooper DS, Doherty GM, Haugen BR, Kloos RT, Lee SL, Mandel SJ, et al. Management guidelines for patients with thyroid nodules and differentiated thyroid cancer. Thyroid. 2006;16(2):109–42.
31. Pacini F, Schlumberger M, Dralle H, Elisei R, Smit JW, Wiersinga W. European consensus for the management of patients with differentiated thyroid carcinoma of the follicular epithelium. Eur J Endocrinol. 2006;154(6):787–803.
32. Haugen BR, Alexander EK, Bible KC, Doherty GM, Mandel SJ, Nikiforov YE, et al. The American Thyroid Association (ATA) guidelines taskforce on thyroid nodules and differentiated thyroid cancer. Thyroid. 2015.
33. Carling T, Carty SE, Ciarleglio MM, Cooper DS, Doherty GM, Kim LT, et al. American Thyroid Association design and feasibility of a prospective randomized controlled trial of prophylactic central lymph node dissection for papillary thyroid carcinoma. Thyroid. 2012;22(3):237–44.
34. Zetoune T, Keutgen X, Buitrago D, Aldailami H, Shao H, Mazumdar M, et al. Prophylactic central neck dissection and local recurrence in papillary thyroid cancer: a meta-analysis. Ann Surg Oncol. 2010;17(12):3287–93.
35. Popadich A, Levin O, Lee JC, Smooke-Praw S, Ro K, Fazel M, et al. A multicenter cohort study of total thyroidectomy and routine central lymph node dissection for cN0 papillary thyroid cancer. Surgery. 2011;150(6):1048–57.
36. Hartl DM, Mamelle E, Borget I, Leboulleux S, Mirghani H, Schlumberger M. Influence of prophylactic neck dissection on rate of retreatment for papillary thyroid carcinoma. World J Surg. 2013;37(8):1951–8.
37. Hartl DM, Leboulleux S, Al Ghuzlan A, Baudin E, Chami L, Schlumberger M, et al. Optimization of staging of the neck with prophylactic central and lateral neck dissection for papillary thyroid carcinoma. Ann Surg. 2012;255(4):777–83.
38. Wang TS, Evans DB, Fareau GG, Carroll T, Yen TW. Effect of prophylactic central compartment neck dissection on serum thyroglobulin and recommendations for adjuvant radioactive iodine in patients with differentiated thyroid cancer. Ann Surg Oncol. 2012;19(13):4217–22.

39. Bonnet S, Hartl D, Leboulleux S, Baudin E, Lumbroso JD, Al Ghuzlan A, et al. Prophylactic lymph node dissection for papillary thyroid cancer less than 2 cm: implications for radioiodine treatment. J Clin Endocrinol Metab. 2009;94:1162–7.
40. Laird AM, Gauger PG, Miller BS, Doherty GM. Evaluation of postoperative radioactive iodine scans in patients who underwent prophylactic central lymph node dissection. World J Surg. 2012;36(6):1268–73.
41. Roh JL, Park JY, Park CI. Total thyroidectomy plus neck dissection in differentiated papillary thyroid carcinoma patients: pattern of nodal metastasis, morbidity, recurrence, and postoperative levels of serum parathyroid hormone. Ann Surg. 2007;245:604–10.
42. Lang BH, Wong KP, Wan KY, Lo CY. Impact of routine unilateral central neck dissection on preablative and postablative stimulated thyroglobulin levels after total thyroidectomy in papillary thyroid carcinoma. Ann Surg Oncol. 2012;19(1):60–7.
43. Chisholm EJ, Kulinskaya E, Tolley NS. Systematic review and meta-analysis of the adverse effects of thyroidectomy combined with central neck dissection as compared with thyroidectomy alone. Laryngoscope. 2009;119(6):1135–9.
44. Bardet S, Ciappuccini R, Quak E, Rame JP, Blanchard D, de Raucourt D, et al. Prognostic value of microscopic lymph node involvement in patients with papillary thyroid cancer. J Clin Endocrinol Metab. 2015;100(1):132–40.
45. Iyer NG, Shaha AR. Central compartment dissection for well differentiated thyroid cancer … and the band plays on. Curr Opin Otolaryngol Head Neck Surg. 2011;19(2):106–12.
46. Xing M, Alzahrani AS, Carson KA, Viola D, Elisei R, Bendlova B, et al. Association between BRAF V600E mutation and mortality in patients with papillary thyroid cancer. JAMA. 2013;309(14):1493–501.
47. Kim TH, Park YJ, Lim JA, Ahn HY, Lee EK, Lee YJ, et al. The association of the BRAF(V600E) mutation with prognostic factors and poor clinical outcome in papillary thyroid cancer: a meta-analysis. Cancer. 2012;118(7):1764–73.
48. Xing M. Prognostic utility of BRAF mutation in papillary thyroid cancer. Mol Cell Endocrinol. 2010;321(1):86–93.
49. Kondo T, Ezzat S, Asa SL. Pathogenetic mechanisms in thyroid follicular-cell neoplasia. Nat Rev Cancer. 2006;6(4):292–306.
50. Volante M, Rapa I, Gandhi M, Bussolati G, Giachino D, Papotti M, et al. RAS mutations are the predominant molecular alteration in poorly differentiated thyroid carcinomas and bear prognostic impact. J Clin Endocrinol Metab. 2009;94(12):4735–41.
51. Garcia-Rostan G, Zhao H, Camp RL, Pollan M, Herrero A, Pardo J, et al. ras mutations are associated with aggressive tumor phenotypes and poor prognosis in thyroid cancer. J Clin Oncol. 2003;21(17):3226–35.
52. Ricarte-Filho JC, Ryder M, Chitale DA, Rivera M, Heguy A, Ladanyi M, et al. Mutational profile of advanced primary and metastatic radioactive iodine-refractory thyroid cancers reveals distinct pathogenetic roles for BRAF, PIK3CA, and AKT1. Cancer Res. 2009; 69(11):4885–93.
53. Sassolas G, Hafdi-Nejjari Z, Ferraro A, Decaussin-Petrucci M, Rousset B, Borson-Chazot F, et al. Oncogenic alterations in papillary thyroid cancers of young patients. Thyroid. 2012;22(1):17–26.
54. Adeniran AJ, Zhu Z, Gandhi M, Steward DL, Fidler JP, Giordano TJ, et al. Correlation between genetic alterations and microscopic features, clinical manifestations, and prognostic characteristics of thyroid papillary carcinomas. Am J Surg Pathol. 2006;30(2):216–22.
55. Santoro M, Melillo RM, Fusco A. RET/PTC activation in papillary thyroid carcinoma: European Journal of Endocrinology Prize Lecture. Eur J Endocrinol. 2006;155:645–53.
56. Castro P, Rebocho AP, Soares RJ, Magalhaes J, Roque L, Trovisco V, et al. PAX8-PPARgamma rearrangement is frequently detected in the follicular variant of papillary thyroid carcinoma. J Clin Endocrinol Metab. 2006;91:213–20.
57. Nikiforova MN, Biddinger PW, Caudill CM, Kroll TG, Nikiforov YE. PAX8-PPARgamma rearrangement in thyroid tumors: RT-PCR and immunohistochemical analyses. Am J Surg Pathol. 2002;26(8):1016–23.

58. Nikiforova MN, Lynch RA, Biddinger PW, Alexander EK, Dorn 2nd GW, Tallini G, et al. RAS point mutations and PAX8-PPAR gamma rearrangement in thyroid tumors: evidence for distinct molecular pathways in thyroid follicular carcinoma. J Clin Endocrinol Metab. 2003;88(5):2318–26.
59. Armstrong MJ, Yang H, Yip L, Ohori NP, McCoy KL, Stang MT, et al. PAX8/PPARgamma rearrangement in thyroid nodules predicts follicular-pattern carcinomas, in particular the encapsulated follicular variant of papillary carcinoma. Thyroid. 2014;24(9):1369–74.
60. Soares P, Celestino R, Melo M, Fonseca E, Sobrinho-Simoes M. Prognostic biomarkers in thyroid cancer. Virchows Arch. 2014;464:333–46.
61. Nikiforova MN, Wald AI, Roy S, Durso MB, Nikiforov YE. Targeted next-generation sequencing panel (ThyroSeq) for detection of mutations in thyroid cancer. J Clin Endocrinol Metab. 2013;98(11):E1852–60.
62. Melo M, da Rocha AG, Vinagre J, Batista R, Peixoto J, Tavares C, et al. TERT promoter mutations are a major indicator of poor outcome in differentiated thyroid carcinomas. J Clin Endocrinol Metab. 2014;99(5):E754–65.
63. Liu X, Bishop J, Shan Y, Pai S, Liu D, Murugan AK, et al. Highly prevalent TERT promoter mutations in aggressive thyroid cancers. Endocr Relat Cancer. 2013;20(4):603–10.
64. Landa I, Ganly I, Chan TA, Mitsutake N, Matsuse M, Ibrahimpasic T, et al. Frequent somatic TERT promoter mutations in thyroid cancer: higher prevalence in advanced forms of the disease. J Clin Endocrinol Metab. 2013;98(9):E1562–6.
65. Liu X, Qu S, Liu R, Sheng C, Shi X, Zhu G, et al. TERT promoter mutations and their association with BRAF V600E mutation and aggressive clinicopathological characteristics of thyroid cancer. J Clin Endocrinol Metab. 2014;99(6):E1130–6.
66. Xing M, Liu R, Liu X, Murugan AK, Zhu G, Zeiger MA, et al. BRAF V600E and TERT promoter mutations cooperatively identify the most aggressive papillary thyroid cancer with highest recurrence. J Clin Oncol. 2014;32(25):2718–26.

Chapter 4
Incidentally Discovered Micropapillary Thyroid Cancer

Douglas S. Ross

Case Presentation

A 49-year-old woman presented to her primary care physician with a chronic nonproductive cough of 3-month duration. A chest CT scan showed a 12 mm right thyroid nodule. Thyroid ultrasound showed a right 15×8×7 mm hypoechoic nodule with mild central vascularity but no microcalcifications. Several other 3–5 mm nodules were noted in both lobes, none with suspicious ultrasonographic characteristics. Fine-needle aspiration cytology of the dominant nodule was read as follicular lesion of uncertain significance. The sample was composed of approximately equal numbers of micro- and macrofollicles. There was no nuclear atypia. Three months later, the nodule measured 16×7×7 mm. Repeat fine-needle aspiration cytology was again read as a follicular lesion of uncertain significance. The sample was assessed by a gene expression classifier and was felt to be suspicious. The patient had a right hemithyroidectomy. The pathology revealed a 12 mm follicular adenoma composed of mixed micro- and macrofollicular tissue. There was an incidental 5 mm intrathyroidal micropapillary thyroid cancer. Six weeks after her surgery, the patient had a serum TSH of 1.6 mIU/L.

Assessment and Literature Review

Micropapillary thyroid cancer is an extremely common neoplasm associated with an excellent prognosis. Our knowledge of this tumor comes from both retrospective clinical series and prospective observational trials. Both argue for conservative management.

D.S. Ross, MD (✉)
Thyroid Unit WAC 730 S, Massachusetts General Hospital, Boston, MA 02114, USA
e-mail: dross@partners.org

D.S. Cooper, C. Durante (eds.), *Thyroid Cancer*,
DOI 10.1007/978-3-319-22401-5_4

Definition

Thyroid micropapillary cancers are defined by the World Health Organization as papillary cancers that measure 10 mm or less in their largest diameter. The increasing incidence of thyroid cancers of all sizes has been attributed in part to both the increased use and increased sensitivity of imaging used for assessing non-thyroid-related problems. The incidental findings of a thyroid nodule on chest CT, carotid Doppler study, or neck MRI are common examples of the incidental detection of thyroid nodules. Since microcarcinomas are rarely palpable, they are usually discovered in this manner or on a neck ultrasound ordered to assess a palpable nodule or goiter. The term "incidental," when applied to micropapillary cancer, refers to cancers that were *not* identified preoperatively and are found unexpectedly in the postsurgical pathology specimen.

Prevalence

Prevalence data for micropapillary cancer come from autopsy data. In the United States 6–13 % of the population are found to have micropapillary cancers [1], while percentages as high as 36 % have been reported in Finland [2]. In a series from Sweden, the prevalence was 7 % for patients under age 50 or over age 80 [3]. In a series from Wisconsin, 3 % of young adults had micropapillary cancers [4]. It is therefore not surprising that incidental micropapillary cancers are found in 2–24 % of surgical pathology specimens [5].

Retrospective Studies

There are many institutional as well as registry-based reports regarding outcome in patients with micropapillary cancer. A series from the Mayo Clinic of 900 patients has an average follow-up of 17.2 years (range 6–89 years) [6]. At presentation, 23 % were multifocal, 30 % had cervical lymph node involvement, 2 % had extrathyroidal extension, and only 0.3 % had distant metastases. The 40-year cause-specific mortality was 0.7 %. The recurrence rate was 8 %—1.5 % in the thyroid bed and the remainder in cervical nodes. Recurrences were more common in patients with nodes at presentation: 16 vs. 0.8 %. Recurrences were also more common in patients with multifocal disease: 11 vs. 4 %. The recurrence rates were not diminished with postoperative radioiodine therapy.

Similar data have been reported from Japan. The Noguchi Thyroid Clinic series of 2070 patients has an average follow-up of 15 years [7]. The authors report recurrences in only 3.5 % of patients and distant metastases in only 0.2 % of patients.

The National Thyroid Cancer Treatment Cooperative Study Group maintains a registry of thyroid cancer patients from 11 centers in North America. A report of 611 patients with intrathyroidal micropapillary cancer who were disease-free after initial therapy found a recurrence rate of 6.2 %, almost all in the neck [8]. Distant metastases occurred in one patient (0.2 %) and mediastinal nodes in two patients (0.3 %). Half of the recurrences occurred in the first 2.8 years. Recurrence was more common in patients with multifocal disease who had only a hemithyroidectomy (18 vs. 6 %), but as in the Mayo Clinic experience, recurrence was not reduced by adjunctive radioiodine treatment.

Observational Studies

Because micropapillary thyroid cancer has a near-negligible mortality rate and low recurrence rate, and because cervical node recurrences are not life-threatening, two groups of investigators from Japan have published observational data on micropapillary thyroid cancer. Ito et al. have reported on 1235 patients, after excluding those with tumors adjacent to the trachea, those possibly invading the recurrent laryngeal nerve, and those associated with high-grade histology or central or lateral compartment lymph nodes [9, 10]. Twenty eight percent had multifocal tumors. These patients have been observed for an average of 5 years, but some as long as 19 years. After 10 years of observation, only 8 % of the tumors grew by 3 mm or more, and only 3.8 % have developed lateral compartment nodes. Among the 191 patients who had surgery after a period of observation because of tumor growth, the development of lateral nodes, or patient preference, no one has died, no one has developed distant metastases, and one patient has had a recurrence in a thyroid remnant, which is being observed.

In another Japanese study of 230 patients, 7 % of the tumors grew by 3 mm or more, and only 1 % of tumors were associated with new nodal metastases during a mean observation period of 5 years [11].

Incidental Versus Non-incidental Tumors

A meta-analysis of 17 studies that identified tumors as incidental or non-incidental included 854 incidental and 2669 non-incidental micropapillary cancers with an average follow-up of 70 months [12]. At presentation, the non-incidental tumors were larger (6.9 vs. 4.6 mm), were more likely to be multifocal (30 vs. 19 %), and have lymph node metastases (30 vs. 2.6 %). The patients with non-incidental tumors were more likely to have had a total thyroidectomy (59 vs. 51 %) and to have received radioiodine (47 vs. 33 %).

Overall recurrence was 7.9 % in the non-incidental group and 0.45 % in the incidental group. However, a disproportionate number of recurrences were recorded in two small studies (including 129 patients); exclusion of these reduced the recurrence rate in the non-incidental group to 4 %. All four recurrences in the incidental group were in cervical lymph nodes. Mortality was 0.1 % in the non-incidental group; no one died in the incidental group. Thus, incidentally discovered micropapillary cancer has an even better prognosis than that of non-incidental tumors.

BRAF

BRAF mutations have recently been associated with increased aggressiveness in papillary thyroid cancers. The V600E mutation was found in 53 % of papillary cancers in a South Korean study [13]. Cancers that had the mutation were more likely to have extracapsular invasion, cervical nodes, or advanced stage. In an Italian study of 134 patients with micropapillary cancers, disease persistence was found in 12 % of patients who had the BRAF mutation vs. 2 % with wild-type BRAF [14]. In a multicenter study, the BRAF mutation was associated with increased mortality, but after adjusting for extracapsular invasion, and nodal and distant metastases, the BRAF mutation did not add any additional risk [15]. In that study, 435 patients had micropapillary cancers, and while their presenting characteristics are not separately reported, overall mortality for patients with micropapillary cancer was 0.9 %, but all patients who died had the BRAF mutation (2.4 % of those with the mutation).

Management of the Case

It should be evident from the forgoing discussion that micropapillary thyroid cancer is associated with an excellent prognosis. While rare patients do present with or develop distant metastases, or die, these unusual patients can frequently be identified as high-risk at presentation, and this information is hard to extract from published series. For example, in the Mayo Clinic series [6], of the three patients who died, all had lymphadenopathy at presentation (massive in one patient), and one had pulmonary metastases at presentation. In the National Thyroid Cancer Treatment Cooperative Study Group report [8], one death occurred in a patient who had anaplastic transformation of the tumor.

The patient under discussion had a 5 mm intrathyroidal papillary cancer. No lymph nodes were excised, but none were seen on preoperative ultrasonography or at the time of surgery. There was no indication of extrathyroidal spread. Possible management options are measurement of BRAF, excision of the contralateral lobe (completion thyroidectomy) or biopsy of the remaining subcentimetric thyroid nodules, radioiodine ablation, and thyroid hormone-suppressive therapy. None of these are necessary in this case.

BRAF

We know from recent reports that many papillary cancers have the BRAF mutation: 53 % in the South Korean study discussed previously [13]. The meta-analysis and the clinical series discussed above were based on data collected before the assessment of BRAF mutations [6–8, 12]. Presumably approximately half of the patients in those series were BRAF positive, yet the recurrence rate for incidental micropapillary cancer was 0.45 % [12], and no one died. As noted above, while the presence of a BRAF mutation is associated with a more aggressive tumor, it does not increase the risk of mortality after adjusting for extracapsular invasion and lymph node or distant metastases [15]. Since the patient's incidental tumor does not present with any worrisome histology or other characteristics, measurement of BRAF would not change clinical management and would probably cause unnecessary anxiety for the patient.

Completion Thyroidectomy or Fine-Needle Aspiration of the Remaining Nodules

There are no data regarding the use of completion thyroidectomy for micropapillary cancer. The rationale for completion thyroidectomy is that papillary cancer is frequently multifocal and that it facilitates radioiodine therapy. A completion thyroidectomy is associated with a 1–2 % risk of complications in even the best surgical hands, including damage to a recurrent laryngeal nerve or permanent hypoparathyroidism. The patient's ultrasound shows only non-suspicious subcentimetric nodules in the contralateral lobe. In view of the reassuring results from observational studies of micropapillary cancer, observation of these nodules for growth seems most appropriate. Should one of these nodules grow by 3 mm, or exceed 10 mm, or if lymphadenopathy should develop, then a fine-needle aspiration biopsy should be obtained, and if positive, the lobe should be excised.

Radioiodine

In the Mayo Clinic and National Thyroid Cancer Treatment Cooperative Study Group reports, there was no benefit of giving radioiodine to micropapillary cancer whether multifocal or associated with lymphadenopathy [6, 8]. An analysis of the SEER database demonstrated a 99.9 % 15-year disease-specific survival whether or not patients received radioiodine [16]. Professional society guidelines recommend radioiodine only for stage 1 tumors with concerning clinical features [17].

Thyroid Hormone Suppression

Thyroid hormone-suppressive therapy has been the standard treatment for thyroid cancer for decades, yet its efficacy remains controversial. Suppressive therapy is associated with adverse effects on the cardiovascular and skeletal systems. There is a threefold increased risk of atrial fibrillation in older patients, as well as reduced bone density and increased fracture risk in postmenopausal women [18]. On the other hand, serum TSH levels positively correlate with malignancy in patients with thyroid nodules [19] and correlate with initial stage in patients with thyroid cancer [20]. In one of the observational studies of micropapillary cancer, however, higher TSH levels were not associated with tumor growth [21]. While the effects of thyroid hormone suppression on the outcome of micropapillary cancers per se have not been reported, several reports of its efficacy in all sizes and stages of papillary thyroid cancer have been contradictory. Pujol et al. demonstrated longer relapse-free survival in thyroid cancer patients with constantly suppressed TSH [22], while Sugitani and Fujimoto found no difference in disease-free survival in a randomized control trial [23]. Data from the National Thyroid Cancer Treatment Cooperative Study Group have evolved as the registry has matured. The analysis published in 2006 failed to show a benefit of suppressive therapy in stage 1 patients [24], but current data (personal communication) suggest that moderate TSH suppression (subnormal to normal levels) may improve outcome in stage 1 disease.

The patient under discussion has a TSH in the middle of the normal range, and she will soon be postmenopausal if she is not already. In view of her excellent thyroid cancer prognosis, further suppression of her TSH is unlikely to provide a benefit and might well be detrimental to her bone health. Given the uncertainty, the goal for her TSH is a low normal value (or avoidance of high levels). Her current TSH level is satisfactory, although reducing it into the lower portion of the normal range could be considered.

Clinical Pearls/Pitfalls

- The treatment should not be worse than the disease.
- It is difficult to improve mortality when the risk of dying is 0.45 % (less than accidental death).
- Most recurrences in patients with micropapillary cancer are in cervical lymph nodes and are not life-threatening. Therefore, most patients do not require surgery (completion thyroidectomy or node dissection) to potentially prevent the need for surgery in a few patients.

References

1. Wang C, Crapo LM. The epidemiology of thyroid disease and implications for screening. Endocrinol Metab Clin N Am. 1997;26:189–218.
2. Harach HR, Franssila KO, Wasenius VM. Occult papillary cancer of the thyroid. A "normal" finding in Finland. A systematic autopsy study. Cancer. 1985;56:531–8.
3. Bondenson L, Ljungberg O. Occult papillary thyroid carcinoma in the young and the aged. Cancer. 1984;53:1790–2.
4. Komorowski RA, Hanson GA. Occult thyroid pathology in the young adult: an autopsy study of 138 patients without clinical thyroid disease. Hum Pathol. 1988;19:689–96.
5. Sakorafas GH, Giotakis J, Stafyla V. Papillary thyroid microcarcinoma: a surgical perspective. Cancer Treat Rev. 2005;31:423–38.

6. Hay ID, Hutchinson ME, Gonzalez-Losada T, McIver B, Reinalda ME, Grant CS, et al. Papillary thyroid microcarcinoma: a study of 900 cases observed in a 60-year period. Surgery. 2008;144:980–8.
7. Noguchi S, Yamashita H, Uchino S, Watanabe S. Papillary microcarcinoma. World J Surg. 2008;32:747–53.
8. Ross DS, Litofsky D, Ain KB, Bigos T, Brierley JD, Cooper DS, et al. Recurrence after treatment of micropapillary thyroid cancer. Thyroid. 2009;19:1043–8.
9. Ito Y, Miyauchi A, Inoue H, Fukushima M, Kihara M, Higashiyama T, et al. An observational trial for papillary thyroid microcarcinoma in Japanese patients. World J Surg. 2010;34: 28–35.
10. Ito Y, Miyauchi A, Kihara M, Higashiyama T, Kobayashi K, Miya A. Patient age is significantly related to the progression of papillary microcarcinoma of the thyroid under observation. Thyroid. 2014;24:27–34.
11. Sugitani I, Toda K, Yamada K, Yamamoto N, Ikenaga M, Fujimoto Y. Three distinctly different kinds of papillary thyroid microcarcinoma should be recognized: our treatment strategies and outcomes. World J Surg. 2010;34:1222–31.
12. Mehanna H, Al-maqbili T, Carter B, Martin E, Campain N, Watkinson J, et al. Differences in the recurrence and mortality outcome rates of incidental and nonincidental papillary thyroid microcarcinoma: a systematic review and meta-analysis of 21,329 person-years of follow-up. J Clin Endocrinol Metab. 2014;99:2834–43.
13. Joo JY, Park JY, Yoon YH, Choi B, Kim JM, Jo YS, et al. Prediction of occult central lymph node metastasis in papillary thyroid carcinoma by preoperative BRAF analysis using fine-needle aspiration biopsy: a prospective study. J Clin Endocrinol Metab. 2012;97:3996–4003.
14. Elisei R, Viola D, Torregrossa L, Giannini R, Romei C, Ugolini C, et al. The BRAF(V600E) mutation is an independent, poor prognostic factor for the outcome of patients with low-risk intrathyroidal papillary thryoid carcinoma: single institution results from a large cohort study. J Clin Endocrinol Metab. 2012;97:4390–8.
15. Xing M, Alzahrani AS, Carson KA, Viola D, Elisei R, Bendlova B, et al. Association between BRAF V600E mutation and mortality in patients with papillary thyroid cancer. JAMA. 2013;309:1493–501.
16. Lin HW, Bhattacharyya N. Survival impact of treatment options for papillary microcarcinoma of the thyroid. Laryngoscope. 2009;119:1983–7.
17. Cooper DS, Doherty GM, Haugen B, Kloos RJ, Lee SL, Mandel SJ, et al. Revised American Thyroid Association management guidelines for patients with thyroid nodules and differentiated thyroid cancer. Thyroid. 2009;19:1167–214.
18. Ross DS. Subclinical hyperthyroidism. UpToDate, http://www.uptodate.com. Accessed 24 Aug 2014.
19. Boelaert K, Horacek J, Holder RL, Watkinson JC, Sheppard MC, Franklyn JA. Serum thyrotropin concentration as a novel predictor of malignancy in thyroid nodules investigated by fine-needle aspiration. J Clin Endocrinol Metab. 2006;91:4295–301.
20. McLeod DSA, Cooper DS, Ladenson PW, Ain KB, Brierley JD, Fein HG, et al. Prognosis in differentiated thyroid cancer in relation to serum thyrotropin and thyroglobulin antibody status at time of diagnosis. Thyroid. 2014;24:35–42.
21. Sugitani I, Fujimoto Y, Yamada K. Association between serum thyrotropin concentration and growth of asymptomatic papillary thyroid microcarcinoma. World J Surg. 2014;38:673–8.
22. Pujol P, Daures JP, Nsakala N, Baldet L, Bringer J, Jaffiol C. Degree of thyrotropin suppression as a prognostic determinant in differentiated thyroid cancer. J Clin Endocrinol Metab. 1996;81:4318–23.
23. Sugitani I, Fujimoto Y. Does postoperative thyrotropin suppression therapy truly decrease recurrence in papillary thyroid carcinoma? A randomized controlled trial. J Clin Endocrinol Metab. 2010;95:4576–83.
24. Jonklaas J, Sarlis NJ, Litofsky D, Ain KB, Bigos ST, Brierly JD, et al. Outcomes of patients with differentiated thyroid carcinoma following initial therapy. Thyroid. 2006;16:1229–42.

Chapter 5
Completion Thyroidectomy in a Patient with Low-Risk Papillary Cancer

David S. Cooper

The Case

The patient is a 25-year-old woman who was found to have a 2 cm right thyroid nodule on routine physical examination by her gynecologist. Thyroid ultrasound revealed a 2 cm nodule that was mildly hypoechoic with a sonolucent rim and internal vascularity. The contralateral lobe looked normal sonographically. FNA showed a "follicular lesion of undetermined significance" (Bethesda class III). After discussing the pros and cons of lobectomy versus total thyroidectomy, she underwent a right hemithyroidectomy. The final pathology revealed a 1.5 cm unifocal follicular variant papillary cancer with no extrathyroidal extension, negative margins, and no evidence of venous or lymphatic invasion. No lymph nodes were removed at the time of surgery. Her surgeon recommended a completion thyroidectomy in the near future, and she comes to discuss whether this is really necessary.

Assessment and Literature Review

Many patients undergo thyroid lobectomy because of indeterminate thyroid nodules. Anywhere from 15 to 40 % of these patients prove to have thyroid cancer [1], and the question of completion thyroidectomy is often raised. But, it remains unsettled whether completion thyroidectomy is necessary in all patients who are found to have low-risk papillary cancer in the operated lobe. Theoretically, there are two reasons to consider completion thyroidectomy: (1) the contralateral lobe may

D.S. Cooper, MD (✉)
Division of Endocrinology, Diabetes, and Metabolism, The Johns Hopkins University School of Medicine, 1830 E. Monument St., Suite 333, Baltimore, MD 21287, USA
e-mail: dscooper@jhmi.edu

D.S. Cooper, C. Durante (eds.), *Thyroid Cancer*,
DOI 10.1007/978-3-319-22401-5_5

harbor occult disease which could be the source of recurrence in the future, and (2) in order to enable the patient to receive radioiodine ablative therapy, a total thyroidectomy is generally required. A third, less compelling reason may be that follow-up with thyroglobulin measurements may be less ambiguous in patients who have been thyroidectomized.

With regard to the first potential indication, numerous studies have shown that there is 30–80 % prevalence of contralateral thyroid cancer [2]. This is typically micropapillary thyroid cancer (foci <10 mm), with a higher frequency in patients who have multifocal disease in the removed lobe and possibly also in patients who are older or who have larger primary tumors (e.g., [2]). However, despite this high frequency of residual malignant foci, the clinical recurrence rates in the contralateral lobe are very low, in the 1–4 % range, consistent with the concept that these small thyroid cancer foci are relatively innocuous [3]. This observation is similar to what is known about small subclinical central lymph node metastases that are found after a prophylactic central neck dissection, which have a similar prevalence (30–80 %), but which also have a very low rate of clinical recurrence, in the 1–2 % range [4].

In the 2009 American Thyroid Association guidelines for the management of thyroid cancer, completion thyroidectomy was recommended for patients with primary tumors ≥1 cm in diameter [5]. This recommendation was based on two studies. The first was an older study by Hay et al. showing that while completion thyroidectomy did not improve cause-specific mortality, it did decrease the risk of locoregional recurrence [19 % nodal metastasis rate at 20 years for lobectomy versus a 6 % recurrence rate for "bilateral lobar resection" ($P=0.0001$)] [6]. However, it was the large study by Bilimoria et al. [7] which used data from the National Cancer Data Base that included over 52,000 patients that was the main driver of the 2009 ATA recommendation. These authors found that recurrence rates were higher [hazard ratio 1.24 (95 % confidence interval 1.01–1.54, $P=0.04$)] and overall survival was lower [hazard ratio 1.49 (95 % CI 1.02–2.17, $P=0.04$)] when patients underwent less than a total thyroidectomy for tumors 1–2 cm in diameter, compared to no difference in outcomes in patients with tumors <1 cm in diameter. However, this study has been faulted because only "overall survival" and not "disease-specific survival" was reported [8]. Since the mortality rates for differential thyroid cancer are extremely low, disease-specific survival is a much more important indicator of treatment efficacy. Also, information on extrathyroidal extension and completeness of tumor removal was not available, and if lobectomy was performed in some patients because of other comorbid conditions, or because of a compromised contralateral recurrent nerve, then these factors may have biased the results. Furthermore, the paper reported that 18 % of patients who underwent lobectomy received radioiodine therapy postoperatively, suggesting the possibility that some of the patients were misclassified and actually had undergone completion thyroidectomy.

In addition to the study cited above [3], there have now been other studies also showing no advantage of total thyroidectomy over lobectomy. For example, in a paper using data extracted from the Surveillance, Epidemiology, and End Results (SEER) database involving almost 23,000 patients, of whom almost 6000 patients underwent lobectomy, there were no differences in disease-specific survival between patients who underwent total thyroidectomy versus lobectomy in multivariate analyses, and this was true for all tumor sizes up to 4 cm [9]. Similarly, in another study from Memorial Sloan Kettering Cancer Center involving a retrospective analysis of almost 900 patients with low-risk papillary thyroid cancer followed for an average of 10 years, there were no differences in disease-specific survival and in recurrence-free survival between patients who received a total thyroidectomy versus lobectomy (10-year disease-specific survival was 100 % for the lobectomy group versus 98.5 % for the total thyroidectomy group) [10]. Similarly, local recurrence rates were 0 % for both groups, and regional recurrence rates were 0 % versus 0.8 % in the lobectomy versus total thyroidectomy groups, respectively. In multivariate analyses, only age >45 years and male gender were predictors of worse outcome, whereas the T stage and type of surgery were not predictive [10]. Thus, data showing better outcomes after total thyroidectomy (or completion thyroidectomy) have been questioned in more recent studies. And while completion thyroidectomy does not have greater morbidity than an initial total thyroidectomy, the morbidity of a total thyroidectomy is higher than that of a lobectomy even in the hands of high-volume surgeons [11].

The need for radioiodine remnant ablation is the second major reason to recommend completion thyroidectomy in some patients in whom the diagnosis of thyroid cancer is not known preoperatively. In this scenario, the decision to recommend completion thyroidectomy would depend on whether postoperative radioiodine therapy was deemed to be appropriate for the patient's risk of recurrence and death. Since the indications for remnant ablation have been made more stringent [5], and is now typically reserved for patients considered to be at intermediate risk rather than at low risk for recurrence, many patients would not be considered for postoperative radioactive iodine therapy, even if they had undergone a total thyroidectomy at the first surgery.

Based on these newer data, the 2015 American Thyroid Association guidelines state that "Completion thyroidectomy should be offered to those patients for whom a bilateral thyroidectomy would have been recommended had the diagnosis been available before the initial surgery" [12]. This decision would be based on the size of the tumor, the presence of clinical nodal metastases, or other high-risk histologic features that may have been known about preoperatively. Indeed, in a recent report, completion thyroidectomy was performed more frequently in patients with higher-risk tumors (T3) or other higher-risk features [13]. These clinical, radiologic, and pathologic features would also likely inform the decision to administer radioiodine postoperatively. Thus, in those patients who are not known to have thyroid cancer preoperatively, it makes sense to do a lobectomy in those patients in whom a total thyroidectomy would not have been done, even if the diagnosis of thyroid cancer had been known preoperatively. Indeed, the new ATA guidelines recommend lobectomy as an acceptable procedure in patients with tumors ≤4 cm without any other high-risk features preoperatively [12]. One might anticipate that the question of completion thyroidectomy will continue to be raised if lobectomy becomes a more common primary surgical treatment in the future, given the new ATA guidelines recommendations. Patient preference is another factor which will always need to be considered.

Back to the Patient

It was explained to the patient that her cancer was very low risk and that, as a stage 1 patient, her risk of cancer-related mortality was 0 %. Furthermore, the rate of recurrence was also extremely low, even without additional surgery or radioiodine therapy. We recommended annual monitoring of serum thyroglobulin and neck ultrasound for the next 3–5 years with maintenance of serum TSH in the low normal range. Following surgery, her serum TSH was in the 2–3 mU/L range, so she was started on 50 μg of levothyroxine per day. She has now been followed for 5 years without any evidence of recurrent disease.

Clinical Pearls

1. In patients with indeterminate thyroid nodules, lobectomy is reasonable since the risk of cancer is <50 %. Lobectomy should be offered to those patients in whom lobectomy would have been reasonable even if the diagnosis of thyroid cancer had been known preoperatively.
2. Recent studies suggest that patients with low-risk thyroid cancer do not benefit from completion thyroidectomy.
3. Similarly, since total thyroidectomy is often recommended for patients with more advanced disease, with postoperative radioiodine remnant ablation in mind, the typical patient for whom lobectomy would be recommended would not be a candidate for radioiodine, even if thyroid cancer were discovered on final pathology.
4. Patients with low-risk thyroid cancer who have undergone thyroid lobectomy can be followed with serum thyroglobulin and neck ultrasound.

References

1. Bongiovanni M, Spitale A, Faquin WC, Mazzucchelli L, Baloch ZW. The Bethesda system for reporting thyroid cytopathology: a meta-analysis. Acta Cytol. 2012;56:333–9.
2. Kim ES, Kim TY, Koh JM, Kim YI, Hong SJ, Kim WB, Shong YK. Completion thyroidectomy in patients with thyroid cancer who initially underwent unilateral operation. Clin Endocrinol (Oxf). 2004;61:145–8.
3. Vaisman F, Shaha A, Fish S, Tuttle RM. Initial therapy with either thyroid lobectomy or total thyroidectomy without radioactive iodine remnant ablation is associated with very low rates of structural disease recurrence in properly selected patients with differentiated thyroid cancer. Clin Endocrinol (Oxf). 2011;75:112–9.
4. Randolph GW, Duh QY, Heller KS, LiVolsi VA, Mandel SJ, Steward DL, Tufano RP, Tuttle RM, American Thyroid Association Surgical Affairs Committee's Taskforce on Thyroid Cancer Nodal Surgery. The prognostic significance of nodal metastases from papillary thyroid carcinoma can be stratified based on the size and number of metastatic lymph nodes, as well as the presence of extranodal extension. Thyroid. 2012;22:1144–52.

5. Cooper DS, Doherty GM, Haugen BR, Kloos RT, Lee SL, Mandel SJ, Mazzaferri EL, McIver B, Pacini F, Schlumberger M, Sherman SI, Steward DL, Tuttle RM. Revised American Thyroid Association management guidelines for patients with thyroid nodules and differentiated thyroid cancer. Thyroid. 2009;19:1167–214.
6. Hay ID, Grant CS, Bergstralh EJ, Thompson GB, van Heerden JA, Goellner JR. Unilateral total lobectomy: is it sufficient surgical treatment for patients with AMES low-risk papillary thyroid carcinoma? Surgery. 1998;124:958–64.
7. Bilimoria KY, Bentrem DJ, Ko CY, Stewart AK, Winchester DP, Talamonti MS, Sturgeon C. Extent of surgery affects survival for papillary thyroid cancer. Ann Surg. 2007;246:375–81.
8. Shaha AR. Extent of surgery for papillary thyroid carcinoma: the debate continues: comment on "surgery for papillary thyroid carcinoma". Arch Otolaryngol Head Neck Surg. 2010;136: 1061–3.
9. Mendelsohn AH, Elashoff DA, Abemayor E, St John MA. Surgery for papillary thyroid carcinoma: is lobectomy enough? Arch Otolaryngol Head Neck Surg. 2010;136:1055–61.
10. Nixon IJ, Ganly I, Patel SG, Palmer FL, Whitcher MM, Tuttle RM, Shaha A, Shah JP. Thyroid lobectomy for treatment of well differentiated intrathyroid malignancy. Surgery. 2012;151: 571–9.
11. Hauch A, Al-Qurayshi Z, Randolph G, Kandil E. Total thyroidectomy is associated with increased risk of complications for low- and high-volume surgeons. Ann Surg Oncol. 2014;21:3844–52.
12. Haugen B, Alexander E, Bible K, Doherty G, Mandel S, Nikiforov Y, Pacini F, Randolph G, Sawka A, Schlumberger M, Schuff K, Sherman S, Sosa J, Steward D, Tuttle M, Wartofsky L. 2015 American Thyroid Association Management Guidelines for Adult Patients with Thyroid Nodules and Differentiated Thyroid Cancer. Thyroid 2015 in press.
13. Untch BR, Palmer FL, Ganly I, Patel SG, Tuttle RM, Shah JP, Shaha AA. Oncologic outcomes after completion thyroidectomy for patients with well-differentiated thyroid carcinoma. Ann Surg Oncol. 2014;21:1374–8.

Chapter 6
A Case of Multifocal Papillary Thyroid Microcarcinoma

Victor J. Bernet and Ana-Maria Chindris

Case Presentation

A 68-year-old female reported for evaluation of a 2 cm right thyroid nodule incidentally discovered on an MRI as part of an evaluation for shingles. Thyroid function tests are within normal limits. The patient had no history of radiation exposure involving the head and neck and no family history of thyroid cancer, but there was a family history of lymphocytic thyroiditis. The patient was asymptomatic and physical examination was unremarkable.

Neck ultrasound revealed a diffusely heterogeneous thyroid with a dominant 2.2 × 1.7 × 1.8 cm solid nodule in the right lower pole, a less well-defined 2.0 × 0.8 × 1.6 cm nodule in the right upper pole, a left lower pole 0.3 cm calcification without associated nodule, and a sub-centimeter isthmic nodule.

Fine-needle aspiration (FNA) of the two >1 cm nodules was performed with the cytology for the right lower pole nodule being suspicious for papillary thyroid cancer (PTC) (Bethesda class V).

Diagnosis/Assessment

The patient underwent a total thyroidectomy with central compartment neck dissection. The final pathology reported a 0.3 cm right lobe PTC and a 2.0 cm hyalinizing trabecular adenoma. In the left lobe, there were two foci of PTC measuring 0.2 and 0.4 cm. Margins were uninvolved by carcinoma. Background lymphocytic

V.J. Bernet, MD (✉) • A.-M. Chindris, MD
Division of Endocrinology, Mayo Clinic Florida, Mayo Clinic
College of Medicine, Rochester, Minnesota, USA
e-mail: bernet.victor@mayo.edu

D.S. Cooper, C. Durante (eds.), *Thyroid Cancer*,
DOI 10.1007/978-3-319-22401-5_6

thyroiditis was present. All eleven lymph nodes excised were negative for tumor. The patient was staged T1aN0M0 (AJCC/UICC staging system, seventh edition) and radioactive iodine ablation of the thyroid bed was not recommended.

Postoperative Management

Following surgery the patient was placed on a less than fully suppressive dose of levothyroxine with a target serum thyroid-stimulating hormone (TSH) of 0.1–0.3 mU/L.

Outcome

A 24-month follow-up did not indicate any signs of recurrence by ultrasound. TSH-suppressed thyroglobulin (Tg) remained undetectable, with anti-Tg antibody titer declining from 156 IU/mL at 4 months to 59 IU/mL at two years postsurgery. Serum Tg by HPLC was undetectable.

Literature Review

Epidemiology

Thyroid cancer is the fastest-growing malignancy in incidence within and outside the United States with PTC representing over 85 % of cases [1]. This is at least in part attributable to tumors measuring less than 1 cm in diameter, most of which are diagnosed incidentally through increased use of diagnostic imaging, together with the widespread availability of high-resolution ultrasound that allows FNA of nodules as small as 3–5 mm in diameter.

The World Health Organization defines papillary thyroid microcarcinomas (PTMCs) as tumors measuring less than 1 cm in size [2]. These tumors currently represent about 50 % of all thyroid cancers [3], while their incidence in population, based on autopsy studies, varies between 5.3 and 35.6 % [4, 5].

Diagnosis

There are three common scenarios that can lead to the diagnosis of a PTMC: in the pathology specimen of a thyroid gland removed for benign disease ("incidental" PTMC), by surgery following FNA suspecting PTC, and by diagnosis of PTC in a cervical lymph node or distant metastasis ("occult" PTMC). A few decades ago, over 60 % of PTMCs were diagnosed either incidentally during thyroidectomy performed for benign etiologies or by open biopsy of a cervical lymph node. With the advances in ultrasound techniques and introduction of ultrasound-guided FNA, over the last three decades, almost half of PTMCs are diagnosed preoperatively [6].

An epidemiological review of two national registries reported that 26–33.5 % of PTMCs were multifocal [3], in concordance with other studies [7]; another study reported a frequency of multifocality as high as 42 % [8]. Up to 22 % of these tumors are found to be bilateral [9, 10]. Hay et al. reported multifocality in 20 % and bilaterality in 10 % of a series of 535 PTMCs [7]. The presence of multiple PTC foci in one lobe increases the likelihood that additional foci are present in the contralateral lobe, and by one study, multifocality is also increased in patients over age 45 [10].

Multiple studies have addressed the question whether the multiple foci of PTC arise independently of each other, as opposed to having a unifocal origin followed by intrathyroidal spread. These clonality analyses used various methods including assessment of RET/PTC rearrangement, *X*-chromosome inactivation, and analysis of BRAF mutation. Sugg et al. [11] reported that different synchronous tumor foci in the same thyroid gland exhibited different RET/PTC rearrangements in 15 (88 %) of a series of 17 patients, suggesting that most PTMCs arise in an independent fashion. These findings were later confirmed by Park et al. in a study of 61 cases [12]. Conversely, several other studies found that most multifocal PTMCs arise from intrathyroidal spread [13–16], while in other studies, a similar number of cases appeared to arise from independent foci and intrathyroidal spread [17, 18].

Risk Factors for Aggressive Disease

Several factors have been recognized as influencing the clinical outcome in PTC: the size of the tumor, age at diagnosis, and extrathyroid and extra-nodal extension. Certain histological subtypes such as tall cell, hobnail, and columnar cell variants of PTC are also considered to have a more aggressive behavior [19, 20]. PTMC is generally regarded as a low-risk disease and does not require aggressive treatment or intensive follow-up, with a disease-specific mortality rate less than 1 % [6]. Although the vast majority of thyroid microcarcinomas are low risk, with an excellent long-term outcome [19], a very small subset of these tumors (0.2–1 %) develop distant metastases and subsequent disease-related mortality. Clinical practice is in need of studies to identify biochemical and genetic markers of aggressiveness to assist in identification of this minority of patients, thereby facilitating individualized management [3, 7].

Risk factors for aggressive disease in PTMC have been extensively studied. They include male gender, multifocality [10], and extrathyroidal extension [8]. Hay [7] reported that N1 status at diagnosis increases the risk for locoregional recurrence to 18 % compared to 1 % in N0 patients, similar to findings reported by Wada in a series of 259 PTMCs [21].

Multifocality as a risk factor for recurrence in PTMC has been analyzed by several studies, with conflicting results. In a series of 900 patients with PTMC at the Mayo Clinic, Hay et al. found it as risk factor for recurrence [6]. Similarly, Malandrino et al. found multifocality to be more frequently associated with lymph node involvement, in addition to tumor size >6 mm and extrathyroidal invasion [3]. Conversely, Neuhold et al. did not find a difference with respect to lymph node involvement or increased risk of recurrence compared to unifocal PTMC [22].

Since multifocality is reported in 20–40 % of PTMCs, but these tumors have a significantly lower incidence of recurrence, additional factors must be considered to explain a more aggressive behavior in a small subset. In the recent decades, significant attention has been given to genetic features of PTCs, as predictors for tumor behavior. Among these, the V600E mutation in the BRAF gene has been linked to aggressive histopathologic features of PTC and was reported in a significant percentage of multifocal PTMCs [23]. The presence of V600E mutation in PTMC was found to be associated with higher clinical recurrence in low-risk PTMC, but not confirmed as an independent risk factor [9]. This discrepancy between the number of multifocal PTMCs displaying the V600E mutation and the risk of recurrence indicates that additional factors must contribute to the aggressive nature of some of these cancers. Niemeier et al. proposed a thyroid microcarcinoma predictive risk score comprised of presence of V600E mutation and several histopathological features including anatomic location, tumor size, tumor location with respect to the thyroid capsule, status of surgical margins, presence of infiltrative tumor border, tumor growth pattern, multifocality, extrathyroidal extension, degree of fibrosis, presence of psammoma bodies, and presence of lymphocytic thyroiditis [24]. This scoring system demonstrated 96 % sensitivity and 80 % specificity in differentiating more aggressive PTMC from tumors with less aggressive behavior [24]. Therefore, the management and follow-up of PTMC need to be individualized, taking into account other characteristics in addition to the tumor size alone.

Treatment of Multifocal PTMC

Once PTC is suspected by FNA, the recommended treatment consists of total or near-total thyroidectomy, potentially followed by radioactive iodine ablation of remnant thyroid tissue. These recommendations are endorsed by both the 2009 American Thyroid Association (ATA) guidelines and by the consensus report of the European Society of Endocrine Surgeons [25] and supported by the high incidence of multicentric tumors, with recurrence rates as high as 20 % in the remaining thyroid [26].

While for tumors >1 cm in diameter, total thyroidectomy is generally accepted as standard of care, in management of PTMC, the extent of surgery, the use of radioactive iodine, and TSH suppression are subjects of debate. The challenge consists in choosing the appropriate therapeutic measures so that recurrence-free survival and overall survival benefit exceeds the risks associated with extent of surgery (transient or permanent postoperative hypocalcemia and laryngeal recurrent nerve injury), RAI ablation (xerostomia, xerophtalmia, parotiditis), and prolonged iatrogenic hyperthyroidism (cardiac arrhythmias and loss of bone mass). For a PTMC confined to the thyroid and without lymph node extension, lobectomy is recommended in current ATA guidelines, if there is no definitive indication for removal of the contralateral lobe.

In the case of incidental microcarcinomas diagnosed following a thyroid lobectomy for a benign diagnosis, the lobectomy alone is reasonable in the absence of additional risk factors such as family history of thyroid cancer or a previous history of radiation to the head and neck [19]. Multifocality is associated with a slightly increased risk for structural disease recurrence; however, optimal surgical management is a matter of debate. In a large study on 535 consecutive cases of PTMC treated at the Mayo Clinic, Hay et al. concluded that PTMC has an excellent prognosis if the initial treatment consists of a total or subtotal thyroidectomy, while RAI did not improve the locoregional recurrence rate. The authors however recognize that "hemithyroidectomy as opposed to near-total or total thyroidectomy does not compromise survival," but recommend an initial bilateral lobar resection (near-total thyroidectomy) in order to address the potential risk of cancer in the contralateral thyroid lobes [7]. Studies over the past decade focused on the outcome of patients with PTC who were treated with lobectomy and reported excellent recurrence-free survival rates [27]. A SEER database analysis of 23,605 patients with PTC reported that in low-risk patients, there was no association between lobectomy and poorer cause-specific or overall survival [28], findings confirmed by Mendelsohn et al. who concluded that in properly selected patients, lobectomy alone is associated with excellent disease-free survival [29].

Furthermore, there are proponents of observation rather than intervention in selected patients with unicentric PTMC. Ito et al. studied age as a prognostic factor in PTMC, in a cohort of 1235 cases, and found that in patients over 60 years old with subclinical, low-risk disease, observation with once or twice yearly ultrasonography is a reasonable option. In this study, regardless of age, multifocality was not found to be a significant risk factor for size enlargement, novel lymph node appearance, or risk of clinical disease.

Prophylactic central neck dissection, while recommended by some for larger macro-PTCs, has been another controversial topic in management of PTMC. Several studies indicate that multifocal PTMC is a risk factor for lymph node metastases [6, 30–32], but the controversy with respect to the management continues. In a retrospective study of 1456 patients, Zhao et al. [30] found that PTMCs with a cumulative tumor size of $\geq$1 cm had the same risk of cervical lymph node involvement as macro PTC, therefore recommending prophylactic CND in these cases. Conversely, Hay et al. recommend modified neck dissection only if the cervical lymph nodes are clinically (palpably) abnormal, i.e., clinical N1 disease [7]. Currently, however, there are insufficient data to support prophylactic CND in PTMCs [21].

Role of Remnant Ablation in Treatment of Multifocal PTMC Although PTMCs are in general low-risk tumors with very low mortality, locoregional recurrence is a rather frequent event. Current ATA guidelines do not consider multifocality to be a risk factor requiring remnant ablation as long as each of the cancer foci is less than 1 cm and there is absence of other high-risk factors [rec 32 (d)] [19]. Although multifocality and N1 status were associated with higher recurrence rates in the study by Hay et al. [6], neither more extensive surgery (completion thyroidectomy) nor RAI reduced recurrence rates compared to unilateral lobectomy [6]. Furthermore, in a large prospective study, lack of RAI treatment did not alter the outcome in low-risk (stage I) patients [33].

TSH Suppression has been routinely recommended postoperatively in patients with PTC. While its role in preventing recurrence in high-risk cases has been well demonstrated [33, 34], the same studies indicate no outcome benefit in low-risk patients [33]. As most PTMCs are classified as low risk, current ATA guidelines will recommend initial and long-term TSH goal to be within the low normal range [19].

TSH suppression may be effective in preventing tumor growth in patients with PTMC who did not undergo surgical treatment. Ito et al. reported size enlargement in 1/51 (2 %) patients with PTMC who underwent TSH suppression compared to 57/1184 (4.8 %) patients who did not [35].

Follow-Up

In patients with low-risk PTC, the ATA recommends initial follow-up with TSH-suppressed Tg measurement and neck US every 6–12 months. As the patients remain free of disease, experts recommend that the interval can be lengthened at 1–2 years, although longitudinal studies to provide evidence for this approach are lacking. Ultrasound-guided FNA with Tg washings should be used in suspicious lymph nodes. There are no specific recommendations for long-term follow-up of PTMC currently. As most of these patients are low risk, they should be followed biochemically with Tg and neck US.

Summary

PTMCs are generally considered low-risk tumors with an excellent long-term outcome and do not require either aggressive treatment or intensive follow-up [19]. An extremely small subset of patients with PTMC develops distant metastases or disease-related mortality. Studies to identify markers of aggressiveness in cases of PTMC would facilitate tailoring initial treatment and follow-up intensity. Multifocality, advanced age, and lymph node involvement are factors for more aggressive behavior although some studies were unable to demonstrate this association.

For patients with PTMC diagnosed preoperatively, lobectomy is the standard treatment, although the extent of surgery should be individualized based upon the presence or absence of additional risk factors for poor prognosis.

Clinical Pearls/Pitfalls

1. Multifocal PTMC can arise from either multicentricity or intrathyroidal spread of a single focus.
2. History of neck radiation represents a risk factor for multifocal PTMC, while age and gender have not been proven to be associated with multifocal disease.
3. Studies indicate that multifocal PTMC has not been clearly associated with increased risk of recurrence compared to a single focus of PTMC.
4. Lobectomy is currently recommended for PTMC.
5. Completion thyroidectomy is not routinely recommended unless there is evidence of disease in the remaining lobe.
6. Routine use of RAI in PTMCs is not recommended, and a decision based on patient's individual risk for recurrence should be used instead.
7. TSH suppression is not recommended for patients with uncomplicated PTMC.

References

1. Cramer JD, Fu P, Harth KC, Margevicius S, Wilhelm SM. Analysis of the rising incidence of thyroid cancer using the surveillance, epidemiology and end results national cancer data registry. Surgery. 2010;148:1147–52. discussion 1152–43.
2. Hedinger C, Williams ED, Sobin LH. The WHO histological classification of thyroid tumors: a commentary on the second edition. Cancer. 1989;63:908–11.
3. Malandrino P, Pellegriti G, Attard M, Violi MA, Giordano C, Sciacca L, Regalbuto C, Squatrito S, Vigneri R. Papillary thyroid microcarcinomas: a comparative study of the characteristics and risk factors at presentation in two cancer registries. J Clin Endocrinol Metab. 2013;98:1427–34.
4. Lang W, Borrusch H, Bauer L. Occult carcinomas of the thyroid. Evaluation of 1,020 sequential autopsies. Am J Clin Pathol. 1988;90:72–6.
5. Harach HR, Franssila KO, Wasenius VM. Occult papillary carcinoma of the thyroid. A "normal" finding in Finland. A systematic autopsy study. Cancer. 1985;56:531–8.
6. Hay ID, Hutchinson ME, Gonzalez-Losada T, McIver B, Reinalda ME, Grant CS, Thompson GB, Sebo TJ, Goellner JR. Papillary thyroid microcarcinoma: a study of 900 cases observed in a 60-year period. Surgery. 2008;144:980–7. discussion 987–8.
7. Hay ID, Grant CS, van Heerden JA, Goellner JR, Ebersold JR, Bergstralh EJ. Papillary thyroid microcarcinoma: a study of 535 cases observed in a 50-year period. Surgery. 1992;112:1139–46. discussion 1146–37.
8. Jacquot-Laperriere S, Timoshenko AP, Dumollard JM, Peoc'h M, Estour B, Martin C, Prades JM. Papillary thyroid microcarcinoma: incidence and prognostic factors. Eur Arch Otorhinolaryngol. 2007;264:935–9.
9. Kim TY, Hong SJ, Kim JM, Kim WG, Gong G, Ryu JS, Kim WB, Yun SC, Shong YK. Prognostic parameters for recurrence of papillary thyroid microcarcinoma. BMC Cancer. 2008;8:296.
10. Cho JK, Kim JY, Jeong CY, Jung EJ, Park ST, Jeong SH, Ju YT, Lee YJ, Hong SC, Ha WS, Choi SK. Clinical features and prognostic factors in papillary thyroid microcarcinoma depends on age. J Korean Surg Soc. 2012;82:281–7.
11. Sugg SL, Ezzat S, Rosen IB, Freeman JL, Asa SL. Distinct multiple RET/PTC gene rearrangements in multifocal papillary thyroid neoplasia. J Clin Endocrinol Metab. 1998;83:4116–22.

12. Park SY, Park YJ, Lee YJ, Lee HS, Choi SH, Choe G, Jang HC, Park SH, do Park J, Cho BY. Analysis of differential BRAF(V600E) mutational status in multifocal papillary thyroid carcinoma: evidence of independent clonal origin in distinct tumor foci. Cancer. 2006;107:1831–8.
13. Moniz S, Catarino AL, Marques AR, Cavaco B, Sobrinho L, Leite V. Clonal origin of non-medullary thyroid tumours assessed by non-random X-chromosome inactivation. Eur J Endocrinol. 2002;146:27–33.
14. McCarthy RP, Wang M, Jones TD, Strate RW, Cheng L. Molecular evidence for the same clonal origin of multifocal papillary thyroid carcinomas. Clin Cancer Res. 2006;12:2414–8.
15. Lin X, Finkelstein SD, Zhu B, Silverman JF. Molecular analysis of multifocal papillary thyroid carcinoma. J Mol Endocrinol. 2008;41:195–203.
16. Wang W, Wang H, Teng X, Mao C, Teng R, Zhao W, Cao J, Fahey 3rd TJ, Teng L. Clonal analysis of bilateral, recurrent, and metastatic papillary thyroid carcinomas. Hum Pathol. 2010;41:1299–309.
17. Shattuck TM, Westra WH, Ladenson PW, Arnold A. Independent clonal origins of distinct tumor foci in multifocal papillary thyroid carcinoma. N Engl J Med. 2005;352:2406–12.
18. Kuhn E, Teller L, Piana S, Rosai J, Merino MJ. Different clonal origin of bilateral papillary thyroid carcinoma, with a review of the literature. Endocr Pathol. 2012;23:101–7.
19. Cooper DS, Doherty GM, Haugen BR, Kloos RT, Lee SL, Mandel SJ, Mazzaferri EL, McIver B, Pacini F, Schlumberger M, Sherman SI, Steward DL, Tuttle RM. Revised American Thyroid Association management guidelines for patients with thyroid nodules and differentiated thyroid cancer. Thyroid. 2009;19:1167–214.
20. Ghossein R, Ganly I, Biagini A, Robenshtok E, Rivera M, Tuttle RM. Prognostic factors in papillary microcarcinoma with emphasis on histologic subtyping: a clinicopathologic study of 148 cases. Thyroid. 2014;24:245–53.
21. Wada N, Duh QY, Sugino K, Iwasaki H, Kameyama K, Mimura T, Ito K, Takami H, Takanashi Y. Lymph node metastasis from 259 papillary thyroid microcarcinomas: frequency, pattern of occurrence and recurrence, and optimal strategy for neck dissection. Ann Surg. 2003;237:399–407.
22. Neuhold N, Schultheis A, Hermann M, Krotla G, Koperek O, Birner P. Incidental papillary microcarcinoma of the thyroid--further evidence of a very low malignant potential: a retrospective clinicopathological study with up to 30 years of follow-up. Ann Surg Oncol. 2011;18:3430–6.
23. Lin KL, Wang OC, Zhang XH, Dai XX, Hu XQ, Qu JM. The BRAF mutation is predictive of aggressive clinicopathological characteristics in papillary thyroid microcarcinoma. Ann Surg Oncol. 2010;17:3294–300.
24. Niemeier LA, Kuffner Akatsu H, Song C, Carty SE, Hodak SP, Yip L, Ferris RL, Tseng GC, Seethala RR, Lebeau SO, Stang MT, Coyne C, Johnson JT, Stewart AF, Nikiforov YE. A combined molecular-pathologic score improves risk stratification of thyroid papillary microcarcinoma. Cancer. 2012;118:2069–77.
25. Iacobone M, Jansson S, Barczynski M, Goretzki P. Multifocal papillary thyroid carcinoma—a consensus report of the European Society of Endocrine Surgeons (ESES). Langenbecks Arch Surg. 2014;399:141–54.
26. Mazzaferri EL, Jhiang SM. Differentiated thyroid cancer long-term impact of initial therapy. Trans Am Clin Climatol Assoc. 1995;106:151–68. discussion 168–70.
27. Matsuzu K, Sugino K, Masudo K, Nagahama M, Kitagawa W, Shibuya H, Ohkuwa K, Uruno T, Suzuki A, Magoshi S, Akaishi J, Masaki C, Kawano M, Suganuma N, Rino Y, Masuda M, Kameyama K, Takami H, Ito K. Thyroid lobectomy for papillary thyroid cancer: long-term follow-up study of 1,088 cases. World J Surg. 2014;38:68–79.
28. Barney BM, Hitchcock YJ, Sharma P, Shrieve DC, Tward JD. Overall and cause-specific survival for patients undergoing lobectomy, near-total, or total thyroidectomy for differentiated thyroid cancer. Head Neck. 2011;33:645–9.
29. Mendelsohn AH, Elashoff DA, Abemayor E, St John MA. Surgery for papillary thyroid carcinoma: is lobectomy enough? Arch Otolaryngol Head Neck Surg. 2010;136:1055–61.

30. Zhao Q, Ming J, Liu C, Shi L, Xu X, Nie X, Huang T. Multifocality and total tumor diameter predict central neck lymph node metastases in papillary thyroid microcarcinoma. Ann Surg Oncol. 2013;20:746–52.
31. Chow SM, Law SC, Chan JK, Au SK, Yau S, Lau WH. Papillary microcarcinoma of the thyroid-prognostic significance of lymph node metastasis and multifocality. Cancer. 2003;98:31–40.
32. Lombardi CP, Bellantone R, De Crea C, Paladino NC, Fadda G, Salvatori M, Raffaelli M. Papillary thyroid microcarcinoma: extrathyroidal extension, lymph node metastases, and risk factors for recurrence in a high prevalence of goiter area. World J Surg. 2010;34:1214–21.
33. Jonklaas J, Sarlis NJ, Litofsky D, Ain KB, Bigos ST, Brierley JD, Cooper DS, Haugen BR, Ladenson PW, Magner J, Robbins J, Ross DS, Skarulis M, Maxon HR, Sherman SI. Outcomes of patients with differentiated thyroid carcinoma following initial therapy. Thyroid. 2006;16:1229–42.
34. Pujol P, Daures JP, Nsakala N, Baldet L, Bringer J, Jaffiol C. Degree of thyrotropin suppression as a prognostic determinant in differentiated thyroid cancer. J Clin Endocrinol Metab. 1996;81:4318–23.
35. Ito Y, Miyauchi A, Kihara M, Higashiyama T, Kobayashi K, Miya A. Patient age is significantly related to the progression of papillary microcarcinoma of the thyroid under observation. Thyroid. 2014;24:27–34.

Chapter 7
A Papillary Thyroid Cancer with Minimal Extra-thyroidal Extension

Donald S.A. McLeod

Case Presentation

A 33-year-old woman noticed a right anterior neck lump, prompting presentation to her primary care physician. There were no other symptoms, no family history of thyroid malignancy, and no history of head or neck irradiation. Clinical examination revealed a single 20 mm diameter thyroid nodule. Thyroid ultrasound showed a hypoechoic 21 mm right superficial midpole nodule with microcalcifications. No suspicious lymphadenopathy was seen. Fine needle aspiration was nondiagnostic (Bethesda System I). On the review of the nodule's ultrasound features, her thyroid surgeon recommended diagnostic right hemithyroidectomy. Histopathology revealed a classical 19 mm papillary thyroid carcinoma. Microscopic extra-thyroidal extension was present focally into perithyroidal skeletal muscle. Surgical margins were clear of tumor and there was no lymphovascular invasion. Completion thyroidectomy followed, and the left hemithyroid was free of malignancy. She presents for discussion of further treatment options. Prior to the diagnosis of thyroid cancer, the patient and her husband were attempting pregnancy and wish to conceive as soon as practically possible.

D.S.A. McLeod, MBBS (Hon I), FRACP, MPH, PhD (✉)
Department of Endocrinology and Diabetes, Royal Brisbane and Women's Hospital, Herston, QLD 4029, Australia

Department of Population Health, QIMR Berghofer Medical Research Institute, Herston, QLD 4029, Australia
e-mail: Donald.mcleod@qimrberghofer.edu.au

D.S. Cooper, C. Durante (eds.), *Thyroid Cancer*,
DOI 10.1007/978-3-319-22401-5_7

Assessment and Literature Review

The definition and classification of extra-thyroidal extension have become more precise over time. There is a clear prognostic difference between minimal and major extra-thyroidal extension, which is reflected in modern tumor-node-metastasis (TNM) staging systems. Observational, mostly retrospective, studies help to clarify potential risks of minimal extra-thyroidal extension and the possible utility of treatment approaches. As with almost all thyroid cancer management questions, there is a dearth of prospective and experimental evidence to help inform management decisions.

Definition and Prevalence

Minimal extra-thyroidal extension is defined as thyroid cancer advancing beyond the thyroid capsule into surrounding perithyroid soft tissues of fat and/or skeletal muscle (sternothyroid) [1]. It is often a pathologic diagnosis and thus the term microscopic extra-thyroidal extension is generally synonymous (see below). Minimal extra-thyroidal extension is a precise term that has supplanted descriptions such as "thyroid capsular" extension or invasion; these earlier terms can be confusing on pathology reports because the presence of, and invasion through, the actual thyroid tumors' capsules may also be described.

Minimal extra-thyroidal extension should be distinguished from major (sometimes called extensive) extra-thyroidal extension. Here, the tumor directly invades one or more of the surrounding organs, including larynx, trachea, or esophagus; vascular or neurologic structures including the great vessels or recurrent laryngeal nerve; or the subcutaneous soft tissues [1].

This distinction is now codified in modern TNM staging systems. Before the sixth edition of the American Joint Committee on Cancer/Union for International Cancer Control (AJCC/UICC) staging manuals, any extra-thyroidal extension was classified as T4 [2], but for the two most recent iterations, minimal extra-thyroidal extension has been downstaged to T3, while major extra-thyroidal extension remains T4 (either T4a or T4b) [3, 4].

It is useful to conceptualize minimal extra-thyroidal extension as microscopic extension, because (1) most minimal extra-thyroidal extension is microscopic, (2) many studies assessing minor and major extra-thyroidal extension use the categories of microscopic vs. macroscopic, and (3) the 2009 American Thyroid Association guidelines use the terms microscopic and macroscopic in assigning risk categories for thyroid cancer recurrence [5]. However, tumors classified as T3 using the current TNM system could display macroscopic anterior invasion of perithyroidal tissues [4]. There are inadequate data to determine whether this subgroup of patients is at higher risk of adverse outcome compared with patients showing microscopic extra-thyroidal extension, although the macroscopic growth potentially implies a higher biologic aggressiveness. A reasonable response to the uncertainty is to treat this small subgroup similarly to tumors with major extra-thyroidal extension when considering postoperative treatment options.

Table 7.1 Ranges of minimal extra-thyroidal extension prevalence

Study first author 2006 (References)	% with minimal extra-thyroidal extension
Nixon 2011 [6]	11.6
Radowsky 2014 [7]	14.1
Arora 2008 [8]	22.6
Hotomi 2012 [9]	29.6
Ito 2006 [10]	30.5
Shin 2013 [11]	31.0
Jung 2013 [12]	44.0

Minimal extra-thyroidal extension is common. Estimates vary from series to series, although may be somewhere in the order of 11–44 % (Table 7.1). It is therefore important to have a clear concept of risks related to this pathologic feature, to ensure adequate but not overtreatment of patients.

Comparison of Minimal with Major Extra-thyroidal Extension

Older studies rarely distinguished minimal and major extra-thyroidal extension [13–17]. These classic papers showed that extra-thyroidal extension was associated with poor prognosis. However, other large series gave clues that the most critical factor was major extra-thyroidal extension. The Mayo Clinic and Memorial Sloan Kettering Cancer Center did this by defining extra-thyroidal extension based on visual operative findings (hence classifying patients with microscopic extension as having intrathyroidal tumors) and showed that macroscopic extra-thyroidal extension had markedly impaired prognosis, while patients with only microscopic extra-thyroidal extension had overall very good prognosis [18, 19].

More recent analyses have confirmed large differences in outcome between minimal and major extra-thyroidal extension. Arora and colleagues assessed 212 patients with papillary thyroid cancer for disease-free survival, finding a 6.4 (95 % confidence interval = 1.6–25.9) times increased recurrence risk for patients with major extra-thyroidal extension compared with those who had minimal extension, after taking other prognostic factors into account [8]. The European Multicentre Study Differentiated Thyroid Cancer prospectively recruited 351 patients with extra-thyroidal growth defined using older staging systems, thus giving the opportunity to compare recurrence outcomes in those with minimal vs. major extension [20]. Major extra-thyroidal extension was independently associated with a 3.23 (1.10–9.51)-fold higher risk of progression than minimal extra-thyroidal extension. In 930 patients, Hotomi and colleagues from Japan found that recurrence was 6.76 (4.25–10.76) times more likely and death was 7.97 (4.20–15.14) times more likely for patients with major extra-thyroidal extension than for patients with minimal or no extra-thyroidal extension [9]. Consistent with the clinical outcome data, tumors with more extensive extra-thyroidal extension have been found to harbor higher rates of angioinvasion and are of higher proliferative grade [21].

Given that major extra-thyroidal extension appears to denote more aggressive disease and a significantly poorer prognosis than minor extra-thyroidal extension, it is important to consider whether minor extra-thyroidal extension holds any prognostic influence. We will consider this question for both survival and risk of recurrent disease.

Survival with Minimal Extra-thyroidal Extension

In the absence of other negative prognostic factors, survival of patients with minimal extra-thyroidal extension is excellent. The National Thyroid Cancer Treatment Cooperative Study is a large multicenter registry of thyroid cancer patients from 11 hospitals in North America. For papillary cancer, its unique staging system classifies microscopic extra-thyroidal extension as either stage I (age <45 years) or stage II (≥45 years). Patients can be upstaged in the presence of additional factors (i.e., tumor size >4 cm, positive cervical lymph nodes, or distant metastases). Therefore, in patients aged <45 years, stage I patients with microscopic extra-thyroidal extension also have tumor sizes ≤4 cm and can have positive cervical lymph nodes but not distant metastases. Similarly, in those aged ≥45 years, stage II patients with microscopic extra-thyroidal extension also have tumor sizes ≤4 cm, negative cervical lymph nodes, and no distant metastases [22]. The disease-specific survival for these patients approaches 100 % [22–24], with the most recent published analysis including 3572 patients totally 16,683 person years (2728 patients stage I or II) [24]. Similar excellent survival has been found in 115 otherwise low-risk patients with minimal extra-thyroidal extension treated at Memorial Sloan Kettering Cancer Center [6]. Hotomi and colleagues reported a 97.3 % 10-year disease-specific survival (and similar results out to 15 years) in 275 patients prospectively followed with "minimal" extra-thyroidal extension [9]. These authors' definition of minimal extra-thyroidal extension differed from many other cohorts, being enriched with a substantial number of patients who would otherwise be considered to have major extra-thyroidal extension (i.e., 42.5 % of these patients would be classified as either T4a or T4b on TNM staging, and 14 % of patients had lateral cervical node metastases).

Recurrence Risk with Minimal Extra-thyroidal Extension

Two studies report no increased recurrence risk from minimal extra-thyroidal extension. Ito and colleagues investigated 1167 Japanese patients undergoing curative intent surgery followed for a minimum of 5 years, of whom 356 had minimal extra-thyroidal extension. There was no difference in recurrence in patients with minimal extra-thyroidal extension compared to those without; the recurrence-free survival of patients with minimal extra-thyroidal extension at 15 years post-diagnosis was over 90 % [10]. When considering the 215 patients with minimal extra-thyroidal extension over age 45 years, the overall cohort results were replicated [25]. Nixon and colleagues from Memorial Sloan Kettering assessed 984 patients with clinical T1/T2 N0 well-differentiated disease, of whom 115 had microscopic extra-thyroidal extension [6]. Recurrence at 10 years was no different in those with or without extra-thyroidal extension (95 vs. 98 %; $P=0.188$).

Other investigators have observed higher rates for minimal extra-thyroidal extension, although the differences did not reach statistical significance. Arora and colleagues reported recurrence in 21 % of their 48 patients with minimal extra-thyroidal extension, compared with 13 % of the patients without ($P=0.11$) [8]. Hotomi and colleagues' 265 patients with "minimal" extra-thyroidal extension had a 91.5 % 10-year recurrence-free survival, vs. 96 % for the 412 patients without [9]. Shin and colleagues found that 13.6 % of 103 Korean patients with minimal extra-thyroidal extension had recurrence at 5 years, compared with 7.9 % of 229 patients without ($P=0.153$) [11]. In a small study, Radowsky and colleagues found 9 % of 33 patients with minimal extra-thyroidal extension had recurrent disease, compared with 4 % of 164 patients without ($P=0.178$ using Fisher's exact test of proportions) [7].

Finally, a recent study from Korea found a univariate increase in recurrence risk for patients with minimal extra-thyroidal extension. The authors reported that 5.6 % of 378 patients with minimal extra-thyroidal extension developed recurrence at a median follow-up of 54 months, compared with 1.2 % of 445 patients without ($P=0.012$) [12].

What could account for these results? The most likely explanation is that microscopic extra-thyroidal extension is a marker of slightly more aggressive tumor biology, although, in the presence of careful (pre-)operative evaluation and adequate surgical clearance, it loses importance as an independent prognostic factor. Several lines of evidence support this hypothesis. Firstly, tumors with minimal extra-thyroidal extension are more likely to have other high-risk features that are associated with clinical recurrence (Table 7.2). The one study to report significantly high recurrence risk with minimal extra-thyroidal extension did not perform a multivariate analysis to determine if it independently predicted recurrence [12]. Likewise, the apparent trend in other studies could well be explained by these other prognostic factors. Secondly, the two larger studies showing very low recurrence rates and no increased recurrence risk from minimal extra-thyroidal extension apparently had careful pre- and intraoperative assessment, in addition to surgical clearance of all identified tumor. In particular, meticulous selection of an otherwise low-risk cohort in the Memorial Sloan Kettering study removed these other potential prognostic factors from influencing the study results [6].

Table 7.2 Tumor features more common present in patients with minimal extra-thyroidal extension

Feature
Older age [6, 9]
Tumor size >1 cm [6, 12, 25]
Angioinvasion [8]
Lymph node metastasis [7–9, 11]
Extra-nodal extension [26]
Positive surgical margins [8, 12]

Management of the Case

The above literature review highlights that while major extra-thyroidal extension is an important risk factor for poor outcome, minimal extra-thyroidal extension can have excellent prognosis in the absence of other high-risk features.

Returning to our case, we should therefore ask the following questions:

- Did our patient need completion thyroidectomy?
- Is a postoperative thyroglobulin useful in determining further treatment?
- Will radioiodine ablation be helpful?
- What should the thyrotropin (TSH) target be?
- What do thyroid cancer guidelines suggest?

Did Our Patient Need Completion Thyroidectomy?

Most authorities would recommend total thyroidectomy if minimal extra-thyroidal extension is present [5, 27–30]. This is logical and based on the potential for slightly higher aggressiveness of tumors with minimal extra-thyroidal extension and the ability to more precisely judge small-volume persistent disease based on serum thyroglobulin and to permit radioiodine remnant ablation postoperatively. In addition, there are a number of large single-center studies [16, 18, 31] and a very large population-based analysis that favor total thyroidectomy for recurrence risk [32].

However, not all centers conform to this view, and excellent results have been reported with lobectomy where careful patient selection was performed [33, 34]. Specific to minimal extra-thyroidal extension, Nixon and colleagues reported a 100 % 10-year recurrence-free survival reported in 26 patients treated with lobectomy (who also had tumors <4 cm diameter, without evidence of lymph node metastases) [6]. Further data is required before this approach can be more widely recommended for patients with minimal extra-thyroidal extension.

Is a Postoperative Thyroglobulin Useful in Determining Further Treatment?

The concept of dynamic risk stratification has become essential in the management of differentiated thyroid cancer. Dynamic risk stratification is a biochemical (serum thyroglobulin) and structural (imaging) assessment of response to therapy [35], reflecting that treatment may sometimes clear poor prognosis disease, or in rare cases, seemingly good prognosis tumors can persist and progress. Dynamic risk stratification can be performed whether or not patients have had total thyroidectomy or radioiodine ablation. An undetectable or very low serum thyroglobulin post therapy (i.e., 6–8 weeks after) is associated with very low recurrence risk [35].

Furthermore, a decreasing or stable postoperative serum thyroglobulin is also associated with a very low recurrence risk [36]. In our patient, the postoperative serum thyroglobulin could be especially helpful. As discussed above, minimal extra-thyroidal extension might denote higher biologic aggressiveness but, in the absence of coexisting poor prognostic factors and effective surgical clearance, has excellent prognosis. An undetectable serum thyroglobulin on levothyroxine therapy would not provide absolute proof that microscopic residual disease is absent, but it would suggest significant volume disease has not been left behind and would build a case that recurrence risk will be low.

Will Radioiodine Remnant Ablation Be Helpful?

Given the excellent expected survival of our patient, the major potential rationale for radioiodine remnant ablation is to improve recurrence risk. Unfortunately, few data are available to help guide this decision.

The National Thyroid Cancer Treatment Cooperative Study's data on radioiodine confirm no difference in survival for their stage I patients (our patient's stage) [37]. On univariate analysis, recurrence risk appeared to be higher in patients receiving radioiodine, although this is likely due to patient selection, because on multivariate propensity score analysis, the apparent effect was lost [23]. Stage II patients (including patients aged ≥45 years with microscopic extra-thyroidal extension) had a univariate 71 % (7–74 %) better overall survival than patients not receiving radioiodine, but there were no differences found for disease-specific survival or recurrence, making interpretation of this result difficult.

Two Memorial Sloan Kettering studies assessing overlapping patients, but addressing slightly different clinical questions, also provide some clues [6, 38]. Nixon and colleagues reported that in 23 thyroidectomized patients with minimal extra-thyroidal extension of tumors <4 cm diameter and without evidence of lymph node metastases, recurrence-free survival to 10 years was 100 % [6]. In the corresponding 63 patients who received radioiodine ablation, recurrence-free survival was 90 % (P=0.29). Given the non-randomized nature of the study, it is likely that clinicians selected the lowest risk patients to forgo radioiodine ablation, but the work also highlights the possibility of safely selecting patients for less intensive therapy. Ibrahimpasic and colleagues assessed recurrence in intermediate-risk thyroidectomized patients with undetectable unstimulated serum thyroglobulin, grouped by whether or not they receive radioiodine ablation [38]. Five-year recurrence-free survival in both groups was over 96 %; the one caveat is that most patients with minimal extra-thyroidal extension received radioiodine.

One retrospective Korean study has assessed recurrence in 121 patients with microscopic extra-thyroidal extension receiving radioiodine ablation, compared with 108 patients who did not [39]. Here, Jeon and colleagues found that 13.2 % of patients receiving radioiodine recurred, vs. 9.3 % of those without radioiodine (P=0.441). Radioiodine status remained nonsignificant for recurrence on multivariate analysis.

Finally, radioiodine is rarely used in Japan, yet the Japanese studies of minimal extra-thyroidal extension report excellent recurrence-free survival [9, 10, 25]. Whether these data are possible to generalize to Western countries, where routine central neck dissection is less common, is difficult to discern.

We need better quality data before we reach a definitive conclusion on the role of radioiodine remnant ablation in minimal extra-thyroidal extension. An individualized approach to decision-making, taking into account confidence in available surgical skill, other tumor prognostic features, the postoperative serum thyroglobulin level, patient preference, and availability of quality follow-up, is reasonable.

If radioiodine is to be used for minimal extra-thyroidal extension, low administered activity therapy (i.e., 30 mCi) appears adequate [40].

What Should the Thyrotropin (TSH) Target Be?

TSH suppression has a role in the treatment of high-risk differentiated thyroid cancer [41]. Assuming a low postoperative serum thyroglobulin, the above discussion does not support this label for our patient's thyroid cancer. The National Thyroid Cancer Treatment Cooperative Study did not find any significant differences in survival or recurrence for their stage I patients (our patient's stage) based on serum TSH variations during follow-up [23]. A Dutch study including mostly low-risk patients found that recurrence and death were significantly increased above a serum TSH threshold of 2 mU/L [42]. Therefore, a long-term goal of a low-normal serum TSH that ensures euthyroidism, i.e., 0.5–2.0 mU/L, would be reasonable here. Some authorities recommend commencing treatment with a lower serum TSH target (Table 7.3) before subsequently re-stratifying risk, although an early undetectable postoperative serum thyroglobulin would suggest an "excellent response" using dynamic risk stratification [35] and may allow for earlier arrival at long-term TSH targets.

What Do Thyroid Cancer Guidelines Say About Minimal Extra-thyroidal Extension?

Thyroid cancer guidelines are rapidly evolving as clinicians shift treatment philosophy to one that emphasizes decisions on individual patients' cancer characteristics and treatment risks. In addition, many of the studies specifically dealing with minimal extra-thyroidal extension have been published in the last 5–10 years. Table 7.3 summarizes the published treatment guidelines of representative organizations for patients with minimal extra-thyroidal extension from the last decade.

Table 7.3 Evolution of thyroid cancer treatment guideline recommendations for minimal extra-thyroidal extension

Year and body (References)	Risk classification	Extent of surgery	Radioiodine remnant ablation	Postoperative TSH targets
2014 British Thyroid Association [29]	Intermediate risk Use dynamic risk stratification at 9–12 months	Total thyroidectomy	Selective use /personalized decision-making	If treated with radioiodine remnant ablation, <0.1 mU/L for 9–12 months, then review risk
2014 National Comprehensive Cancer Network [30]	Implies intermediate risk	Total thyroidectomy	Selectively recommended (30 nmCi)	If excellent response to initial therapy, aim near lower limit of reference range
2010 Japanese Society of Thyroid Surgery/Japanese Association of Endocrine Surgeons [43, 44]	Implies intermediate risk	Less than total thyroidectomy	Not recommended	Aim near lower limit of reference range
2009 American Thyroid Association [5]	Intermediate risk	Total thyroidectomy	Selective use	Initially <0.1 mU/L In disease-free patients long term, 0.3–2.0 mU/L
2009 Latin American Thyroid Society [28]	High risk	Total thyroidectomy	Recommended (150–200 mCi)	Initially <0.1 mU/L If disease-free, relax suppression after 3–5 years
2007 British Thyroid Association	No specific recommendation	Total thyroidectomy	Definitely indicated (100 mCi)	<0.1 mU/L
2006 American Thyroid Association [45]	Intermediate risk	Total thyroidectomy	Radioiodine recommended (30–100 mCi)	Not specified (<0.1 mU/L for high risk; 0.1–0.5 mU/L for low risk) In disease-free patients long term, 0.3–2.0 mU/L
2006 European Thyroid Association [27]	High risk	Total thyroidectomy	Definitely indicated (≥100 mCi)	≤0.1 mU/L for 3–5 years, then if disease-free, 0.5–1.0 mU/L

Note: Only the latest version of the National Comprehensive Cancer Network guidelines is included in this table, which is updated at least yearly

Case Progress

The postoperative thyroglobulin on levothyroxine was undetectable (<0.5 ng/mL). Based on this result, the other low-risk clinical and histologic features, and the confidence that an effective pre- and intraoperative assessment of disease burden had been performed, the patient and her clinicians were comfortable to recommend against radioiodine ablation. Avoiding radioiodine also had the advantage in potentially preventing delay in fertility. On 6-month review, the patient was well without clinical or biochemical (serum thyroglobulin <0.5 ng/mL) signs of recurrence disease. Serum TSH was 0.8 mU/L on levothyroxine replacement. She was not yet pregnant.

Clinical Pearls/Pitfalls

- Not all extra-thyroidal extension is equal. Major extra-thyroidal extension has clear prognostic importance. Minimal extra-thyroidal extension more often occurs in tumors with other adverse prognostic features, but its role as an independent prognostic marker is questionable.
- When other high-risk features are absent, survival and probably recurrence-free survival of patients with minimal extra-thyroidal extension is excellent and may approach that of patients without this pathologic feature.
- Most authorities recommend total thyroidectomy in the presence of minimal extra-thyroidal extension, although low recurrence rates have also been reported in small numbers of selected patients undergoing lobectomy.
- Where other high-risk features are absent, a benefit from radioiodine remnant ablation is unclear. An individualized approach to decision-making, taking into account confidence in available surgical skill, other tumor prognostic features, the postoperative serum thyroglobulin level, patient preference, and availability of quality follow-up, is reasonable. Where radioiodine ablation is performed, low activity therapy (i.e., 30 mCi) appears adequate.
- TSH suppression is unlikely to be required for most patients with minimal extra-thyroidal extension, unless other high-risk features are present.

References

1. Ghossein R. Update to the College of American Pathologists reporting on thyroid carcinomas. Head Neck Pathol. 2009;3:86–93.
2. (1997) American Joint Committee on Cancer. Thyroid. In: Fleming ID, Cooper JS, Henson DE, Hutter RVP, Kennedy BJ et al., editors. 5th ed. Philidelphia: Lippincott-Raven. pp. 59–64.
3. American Joint Committee on Cancer. Thyroid. In: Greene FL, Page DL, Fleming ID, Fritz AG, Balch CM et al., editors. AJCC cancer staging manual. 6th ed. New York: Springer. 2002
4. (2010) American Joint Committee on Cancer. Thyroid. In: Edge SB, Byrd DR, Compton CC, Fritz AG, Greene FL et al., editors. AJCC cancer staging manual. 7th ed. New York: Springer. pp. 87–96.

5. Cooper DS, Doherty GM, Haugen BR, Kloos RT, Lee SL, et al. Revised American Thyroid Association management guidelines for patients with thyroid nodules and differentiated thyroid cancer. Thyroid. 2009;19:1167–214.
6. Nixon IJ, Ganly I, Patel S, Palmer FL, Whitcher MM, et al. The impact of microscopic extra-thyroid extension on outcome in patients with clinical T1 and T2 well-differentiated thyroid cancer. Surgery. 2011;150:1242–9.
7. Radowsky JS, Howard RS, Burch HB, Stojadinovic A. Impact of degree of extrathyroidal extension of disease on papillary thyroid cancer outcome. Thyroid. 2014;24:241–4.
8. Arora N, Turbendian HK, Scognamiglio T, Wagner PL, Goldsmith SJ, et al. Extrathyroidal extension is not all equal: implications of macroscopic versus microscopic extent in papillary thyroid carcinoma. Surgery. 2008;144:942–7. discussion 947–948.
9. Hotomi M, Sugitani I, Toda K, Kawabata K, Fujimoto Y. A novel definition of extrathyroidal invasion for patients with papillary thyroid carcinoma for predicting prognosis. World J Surg. 2012;36:1231–40.
10. Ito Y, Tomoda C, Uruno T, Takamura Y, Miya A, et al. Prognostic significance of extrathyroid extension of papillary thyroid carcinoma: massive but not minimal extension affects the relapse-free survival. World J Surg. 2006;30:780–6.
11. Shin JH, Ha TK, Park HK, Ahn MS, Kim KH, et al. Implication of minimal extrathyroidal extension as a prognostic factor in papillary thyroid carcinoma. Int J Surg. 2013;11:944–7.
12. Jung SP, Kim M, Choe JH, Kim JS, Nam SJ, et al. Clinical implication of cancer adhesion in papillary thyroid carcinoma: clinicopathologic characteristics and prognosis analyzed with degree of extrathyroidal extension. World J Surg. 2013;37:1606–13.
13. Carcangiu ML, Zampi G, Pupi A, Castagnoli A, Rosai J. Papillary carcinoma of the thyroid. A clinicopathologic study of 241 cases treated at the University of Florence, Italy. Cancer. 1985;55:805–28.
14. Simpson WJ, McKinney SE, Carruthers JS, Gospodarowicz MK, Sutcliffe SB, et al. Papillary and follicular thyroid cancer. Prognostic factors in 1,578 patients. Am J Med. 1987;83:479–88.
15. Cady B, Rossi R. An expanded view of risk-group definition in differentiated thyroid carcinoma. Surgery. 1988;104:947–53.
16. DeGroot LJ, Kaplan EL, McCormick M, Straus FH. Natural history, treatment, and course of papillary thyroid carcinoma. J Clin Endocrinol Metab. 1990;71:414–24.
17. Mazzaferri EL, Jhiang SM. Long-term impact of initial surgical and medical therapy on papillary and follicular thyroid cancer. Am J Med. 1994;97:418–28.
18. Hay ID, Bergstralh EJ, Goellner JR, Ebersold JR, Grant CS. Predicting outcome in papillary thyroid carcinoma: development of a reliable prognostic scoring system in a cohort of 1779 patients surgically treated at one institution during 1940 through 1989. Surgery. 1993;114:1050–7. discussion 1057–1058.
19. Andersen PE, Kinsella J, Loree TR, Shaha AR, Shah JP. Differentiated carcinoma of the thyroid with extrathyroidal extension. Am J Surg. 1995;170:467–70.
20. Kramer JA, Schmid KW, Dralle H, Dietlein M, Schicha H, et al. Primary tumour size is a prognostic parameter in patients suffering from differentiated thyroid carcinoma with extrathyroidal growth: results of the MSDS trial. Eur J Endocrinol. 2010;163:637–44.
21. Rivera M, Ricarte-Filho J, Tuttle RM, Ganly I, Shaha A, et al. Molecular, morphologic, and outcome analysis of thyroid carcinomas according to degree of extrathyroid extension. Thyroid. 2010;20:1085–93.
22. Sherman SI, Brierley JD, Sperling M, Ain KB, Bigos ST, et al. Prospective multicenter study of thyroiscarcinoma treatment: initial analysis of staging and outcome. National Thyroid Cancer Treatment Cooperative Study Registry Group. Cancer. 1998;83:1012–21.
23. Jonklaas J, Sarlis NJ, Litofsky D, Ain KB, Bigos ST, et al. Outcomes of patients with differentiated thyroid carcinoma following initial therapy. Thyroid. 2006;16:1229–42.
24. Jonklaas J, Nogueras-Gonzalez G, Munsell M, Litofsky D, Ain KB, et al. The impact of age and gender on papillary thyroid cancer survival. J Clin Endocrinol Metab. 2012;97:E878–87.
25. Ito Y, Tomoda C, Uruno T, Takamura Y, Miya A, et al. Minimal extrathyroid extension does not affect the relapse-free survival of patients with papillary thyroid carcinoma measuring 4 cm or less over the age of 45 years. Surg Today. 2006;36:12–8.

26. Clain JB, Scherl S, Dos Reis L, Turk A, Wenig BM, et al. Extrathyroidal extension predicts extranodal extension in patients with positive lymph nodes: an important association that may affect clinical management. Thyroid. 2014;24:951–7.
27. Pacini F, Schlumberger M, Dralle H, Elisei R, Smit JW, et al. European consensus for the management of patients with differentiated thyroid carcinoma of the follicular epithelium. Eur J Endocrinol. 2006;154:787–803.
28. Pitoia F, Ward L, Wohllk N, Friguglietti C, Tomimori E, et al. Recommendations of the Latin American Thyroid Society on diagnosis and management of differentiated thyroid cancer. Arq Bras Endocrinol Metabol. 2009;53:884–97.
29. Perros P, Boelaert K, Colley S, Evans C, Evans RM, et al. Guidelines for the management of thyroid cancer. Clin Endocrinol (Oxf). 2014;81 Suppl 1:1–122.
30. Tuttle RM, Haddad RI, Ball DW, Byrd D, Dickson P, et al. Thyroid carcinoma. Natl Compr Canc Netw. 2014. http://www.nccn.org/professionals/physician_gls/pdf/thyroid.pdf. Accessed 12 Sept 2014.
31. Samaan NA, Schultz PN, Hickey RC, Goepfert H, Haynie TP, et al. The results of various modalities of treatment of well differentiated thyroid carcinomas: a retrospective review of 1599 patients. J Clin Endocrinol Metab. 1992;75:714–20.
32. Bilimoria KY, Bentrem DJ, Ko CY, Stewart AK, Winchester DP, et al. Extent of surgery affects survival for papillary thyroid cancer. Ann Surg. 2007;246:375–81. discussion 381–384.
33. Shaha AR, Shah JP, Loree TR. Low-risk differentiated thyroid cancer: the need for selective treatment. Ann Surg Oncol. 1997;4:328–33.
34. Cross S, Wei JP, Kim S, Brams DM. Selective surgery and adjuvant therapy based on risk classifications of well-differentiated thyroid cancer. J Surg Oncol. 2006;94:678–82.
35. Momesso DP, Tuttle RM. Update on differentiated thyroid cancer staging. Endocrinol Metab Clin North Am. 2014;43:401–21.
36. Durante C, Montesano T, Attard M, Torlontano M, Monzani F, et al. Long-term surveillance of papillary thyroid cancer patients who do not undergo postoperative radioiodine remnant ablation: is there a role for serum thyroglobulin measurement? J Clin Endocrinol Metab. 2012;97:2748–53.
37. Jonklaas J, Cooper DS, Ain KB, Bigos T, Brierley JD, et al. Radioiodine therapy in patients with stage I differentiated thyroid cancer. Thyroid. 2010;20:1423–4.
38. Ibrahimpasic T, Nixon IJ, Palmer FL, Whitcher MM, Tuttle RM, et al. Undetectable thyroglobulin after total thyroidectomy in patients with low- and intermediate-risk papillary thyroid cancer—is there a need for radioactive iodine therapy? Surgery. 2012;152:1096–105.
39. Jeon YW, Ahn YE, Chung WS, Choi HJ, Suh YJ. Radioactive iodine treatment for node negative papillary thyroid cancer with capsular invasion only: results of a large retrospective study. Asia Pac J Clin Oncol. 2013. doi: 10.1111/ajco.12159. [Epub ahead of print]
40. Han JM, Kim WG, Kim TY, Jeon MJ, Ryu JS, et al. Effects of low-dose and high-dose postoperative radioiodine therapy on the clinical outcome in patients with small differentiated thyroid cancer having microscopic extrathyroidal extension. Thyroid. 2014;24:820–5.
41. McLeod DS. Thyrotropin in the development and management of differentiated thyroid cancer. Endocrinol Metab Clin North Am. 2014;43:367–83.
42. Hovens GC, Stokkel MP, Kievit J, Corssmit EP, Pereira AM, et al. Associations of serum thyrotropin concentrations with recurrence and death in differentiated thyroid cancer. J Clin Endocrinol Metab. 2007;92:2610–5.
43. Takami H, Ito Y, Okamoto T, Yoshida A. Therapeutic strategy for differentiated thyroid carcinoma in Japan based on a newly established guideline managed by Japanese Society of Thyroid Surgeons and Japanese Association of Endocrine Surgeons. World J Surg. 2011;35:111–21.
44. Tanaka K, Sonoo H. Current trends in TSH suppression therapy for patients with papillary thyroid carcinoma in Japan: results of a questionnaire distributed to councilors of the Japanese Society of Thyroid Surgery. Surg Today. 2012;42:633–8.
45. Cooper DS, Doherty GM, Haugen BR, Kloos RT, Lee SL, et al. Management guidelines for patients with thyroid nodules and differentiated thyroid cancer. Thyroid. 2006;16:109–42.

Chapter 8
A Case of a Papillary Thyroid Cancer with Lymph Node Metastases Found on Prophylactic Central Neck Dissection (Subclinical Disease, Micrometastases)

Ian D. Hay

Abbreviations

TSH	Thyroid stimulating hormone thyrotropin
US	Ultrasound
PTC	Papillary thyroid carcinoma
cTNM	Clinical tumor node metastasis
pTNM	Postoperative tumor node metastasis
AJCC	American Joint Committee on Cancer
UICC	International Union Against Cancer
CSM	Cause-specific mortality
AGES	Age grade extent size
MACIS	Metastases age completeness invasion size
AMES	Age metastases extrathyroid size
NNM	Neck nodal metastases
TST	Thyroxine-suppressive therapy
Tg	Thyroglobulin
RAI	Radioactive iodine
RRA	Radioiodine remnant ablation
WBS	Whole body scan
CT	Computerized tomographic
OPTC	Occult papillary thyroid carcinoma
DM	Distant metastases
BLR	Bilateral lobar resection
RNR	Regional neck recurrence

I.D. Hay, MD, PhD, FACE, FACP, FRCP (✉)
Division of Endocrinology and Internal Medicine, Mayo Clinic and College of Medicine, 200 First Street SW, Rochester, MN 55905, USA
e-mail: hay.ian@mayo.edu

D.S. Cooper, C. Durante (eds.), *Thyroid Cancer*,
DOI 10.1007/978-3-319-22401-5_8

ATA	American Thyroid Association
ETA	European Thyroid Association
FDA	Food and Drug Administration
BST	Bilateral subtotal thyroidectomy
UL	Unilateral lobectomy
NTT	Near-total thyroidectomy
TT	Total thyroidectomy
LRR	Locoregional recurrence rate
R	Recommendation
MSKCC	Memorial Sloan Kettering Cancer Center
NCDB	National cancer data base
SEER	Surveillance epidemiology, and end results

Case Discussion

Presentation

In January 2008, a 24-year-old woman saw her gynecologic nurse practitioner, who found an isthmic thyroid nodule. The patient was asymptomatic. She had no personal or family history of thyroid disease and had not been exposed in earlier life to head or neck irradiation. Her serum TSH was 2.1 mIU/L. A neck ultrasound (US) revealed a normal-sized thyroid gland and at the level of the isthmus just to the right of midline, a 9 mm isoechoic, solid nodule, correlating with the palpable finding. This nodule was avascular on color Doppler imaging and had no suspicious sonographic features. She was referred to an endocrinologist (the author), who felt that a guided biopsy was not indicated, but recommended a recheck neck US examination in 6 months.

Diagnosis

In August 2008, a repeat US showed the nodule to be slightly larger, now measuring 1.1×1.5×0.8 cm. An US-guided biopsy was performed; smears were positive for malignancy, and the cytologic features were consistent with papillary thyroid carcinoma (PTC). Chest X-ray was negative; vocal cord check showed normal motion bilaterally.

Surgical Management

After obtaining the diagnostic biopsy, the author discussed the expected outcome of patients presenting with a so-called "occult" PTC, as defined by Woolner et al. as a PTC with maximal tumor dimension of "1.5 cm or less" [1, 2]. The author recommended surgery, rather than observation, and advised a timely consultation with an experienced endocrine surgeon [3]. She noted that the neck US did not show any suspicious cervical adenopathy, but recommended for the patient a "near or total thyroidectomy with central compartment lymphadenectomy" [4–7]. She discussed the potential risks of the operation [8] and the need for lifelong thyroid hormone supplementation.

In August 2008, the patient underwent a "total thyroidectomy with central compartment lymphadenectomy." All removed specimens were submitted to immediate examination of frozen sections and the results conveyed intraoperatively to the surgeon in the operating room [9]. The final histologic report showed the primary tumor to be a histologic Broders [10–12] grade 1 (of 4) classical PTC, measuring 1.3 × 1.0 × 0.8 cm, and situated in the isthmus. The tumor focally extended into the peri-thyroidal soft tissue [13, 14], but the surgical margins were free of involvement. The contralateral lobe contained only benign thyroid tissue. Microscopic examination of the central compartment level VI dissection specimen revealed metastatic PTC in multiple (3 of 3) central compartment level VI nodes. Contemporary pTNM staging, according to the AJCC/UICC sixth edition [15], was stage I (pT3 N1A MO). The case would be classified as "low risk for cause-specific mortality" (CSM) because of an AGES score of 0.26 and a MACIS score of 3.47 but also by the AMES prognostic classification system [11, 16, 17].

Assessment During First Postoperative Year

The patient, despite the presence of microscopic extrathyroidal extension and central compartment neck nodal metastases (NNM), was classified on postoperative day 1 as having a PTC at minimal risk of CSM. With a MACIS score <6, as per our institutional practice since 1994 [18–21], she was advised to leave the hospital on thyroxine-suppressive therapy (TST) and return in 6–8 weeks for a neck ultrasound and a recheck of serum TSH and serum thyroglobulin (Tg). She was not advised to have radioiodine remnant ablation (RRA) nor was she given a recommendation for a postoperative whole body scan (WBS) with radioactive ^{123}I.

When she returned in October 2008, her serum TSH was 0.1 mIU/L, her Tg antibody screen was negative, and her serum Tg was 0.2 ng/ml. A neck US showed no evidence of thyroid bed nodules or suspicious neck adenopathy. The patient was advised to continue with her TST, return for review at one postoperative year with repeat studies, including a neck US as well as serum TSH and Tg measurements. She was told that her prognosis should be excellent [10–12] and that there was probably only a 5–10 % chance [4, 6, 18, 20] in future years of finding any further residual microscopic cervical lymphadenopathy. She was also advised that, if such cervical nodal metastatic disease was to be discovered, she would likely be treated with US-guided percutaneous ethanol ablation at the Mayo Clinic [22–24]. At 14 postoperative months, she returned for follow-up. Her neck US was again negative for locoregional recurrence; TSH was 0.08 mIU/L and serum Tg was again 0.2 ng/mL.

Surveillance from One Through Six Postoperative Years

For the next 5 years (2010–2014), the patient was followed annually. Serum TSH levels on TST during 2010 through 2013 varied between 0.1 and 0.3 mIU/L; Tg levels were on two visits, 0.1, and on three visits, 0.2 ng/mL. On the last review visit in November 2014 (at 74 postoperative months), the serum TSH was in the lower part of the normal range at 0.4 mIU/L, the serum Tg was stable at 0.2 ng/mL (<0.1 undetectable), and the neck US was negative for recurrence.

Literature Review

Postoperative Outcome in Woolner's "Occult" PTC

At the 1959 American Goiter Association meeting, Dr. LB Woolner drew attention to the increasing prevalence of small, possibly biologically unimportant, papillary carcinomas. Most, he found, were 3 mm–1 cm in diameter, but he considered that "an arbitrary upper limit of size of 1.5 cm in greatest dimension" was appropriate to describe this increasingly recognized group. In 1960, he defined OPTC [1] as a "papillary carcinoma 1.5 cm or less in diameter with or without lymph node metastases." In his earliest study of 140 such patients treated during 1920–1965, he reported that none developed distant metastases (DM) or died from OPTC [1]. In a later study published in 1980, he followed 137 cases for a mean of 25 years and was only able to define one possible death from OPTC, but he did note that the "exact cause of death remained in question" [2]. His 1980 study concluded that "radical surgery or medical extirpation of all thyroid tissue is unnecessary in the treatment of this (non-lethal and curable) disease" [2].

In a 1986 study of 859 PTC patients treated during 1946 through 1970, McConahey and colleagues identified 396 OPTC (46 %), and they noted that the risk of CSM increased progressively as the size of the tumors increased [10]. The CSM rate per 1000 cases was 0.8 for OPTC, 3.8 for tumors 1.6–3.9 cm diameter, and 12.6 for those 4 cm or larger ($p<0.0001$). In this study, four fatal cases of OPTC were identified. All four were middle aged or older men (47–70 years of age at diagnosis); one patient had a grade 2 tumor and two had distant metastases at the time of initial presentation.

In 2002, our group reported the postoperative course of 1205 OPTC patients consecutively treated during 1940–2000, over a median follow-up period of 14 years [25]. Bilateral lobar resection (BLR) was the preferred surgical procedure in 89 %. Neck nodes were resected in 52 % of cases; RRA was given within six postoperative months in 27 %. Of 1190 patients having potentially curative surgery (no distant metastases and complete primary tumor resection), five developed postoperative distant metastases and five died of OPTC (20-year CSM rate of only 0.4 %). Overall, 20-year rates for local and regional recurrences were 2 % and 7 %, respectively, and were higher after lobectomy than BLR ($p<0.001$). After BLR, the risks of local recurrence or distant spread were not decreased by RRA. When regional nodal recurrence (RNR) was studied after BLR in 367 node-positive patients, the 20-year rate of 15 % after RRA and BLR was insignificantly different ($p=0.23$) from the 13 % seen after only BLR. For the 693 node-negative patients treated by BLR alone, the 20-year RNR rate of 1 % was not improved by RRA. From these results, we concluded that routine RRA, after BLR with complete tumor excision, was no longer justifiable in the management of patients presenting with small (<16-mm diameter) PTC.

By 2008, management policies for treating OPTC ranged from observation without surgical therapy, to total thyroidectomy with selective use of RRA, to some Italian investigators suggesting "always performing a total thyroidectomy followed by radioiodine therapy in all papillary carcinomas independent of their size" [26]. In that year, we presented to the Endocrine Society a study [27] of the postoperative outcome in a series of 1421 consecutively treated OPTC patients managed at our institution during the six decades of the "nuclear era" (1945–2004). Follow-up ranged to 54 years and averaged 17 years (>24,300 patient-years of observation). Total or near-total thyroidectomy was performed in 75 %; only 11 % had unilateral lobectomy. RRA was performed in only 2, 4, and 7 % during the first three decades studied. RRA rates for 1975–1984 and 1985–1994 rose to 39 and 41 %, perhaps influenced by the recently published results of Beierwaltes and Mazzaferri [18]. During 1995–2004, the rate then fell to 24 %, perhaps related to the implications of the recently published MACIS prognostic scoring system, now being regularly used at Mayo to select the minority of PTC patients with scores of 6+, more likely to benefit from RRA.

In this study, 20- and 40-year tumor recurrence rates were only 7 and 10 %. Higher rates were seen with primary tumors which were multicentric, with patients who were node-positive at diagnosis, or who underwent unilateral lobectomy. [27]. The influence (or lack of it) of RRA on RNR was studied separately in 611 unifocal node-negative, 255 unifocal node-positive, 200 multifocal node-negative, and 164 multifocal node-positive OPTC patients treated with BLR with curative intent. RRA did not improve RNR rates in any of the four subsets studied. It was concluded that RRA should rarely be employed for OPTC and at our institution generally only given for patients with a postoperative MACIS score of six or greater [18–20].

Accordingly, when the patient came to be treated in August 2008, she was being managed by a multidisciplinary team, who were very familiar with the studies performed at Mayo on OPTC for almost 50 years, during 1959 through 2008. In the years since she was first treated, our database has been further developed, and we now have outcome data available on all 3595 PTC patients treated at Mayo Rochester during the seven decades from 1940 to 2009. Since the upcoming 2015 ATA Guidelines [32] are likely to provoke further controversy with regards to the role of UL in OPTC, I decided, for the purposes of this invited chapter, to analyze our latest results on OPTC outcome in our 1940-2009 cohort, results which to date have neither been presented nor published.

Since the mortality rates of patients with OPTC are essentially zero, it is more appropriate to assess possible differences in locoregional recurrence rates in patients treated with more or less aggressive surgery. In examining the differences in outcome after either UL or BLR (combination of BST, NTT, and TT) within the OPTC cohort of 1940–2009, we chose to confine our examination to those undergoing surgery with curative intent (i.e., no distant spread at diagnosis and complete initial tumor resection without postoperative gross residual disease). Looking at the 1757 patients as defined above, the 20-year locoregional (neck) recurrence rates (LRR) were 16 % after UL and 8 % after BLR ($p=0.06$). Since initial NNM are a significant predisposition to future recurrence in neck nodes [10, 12, 18], we looked separately at both the 1157 node-negative and the 600 node-positive cases. In the node-negative cases, the 20-year LRR were 7 % after UL and 2.5 % after BLR ($p=0.02$). For the node-positive cases, the comparable rates were, as expected, much higher, and the 20-year LRR of 40 % after UL significantly exceeded the 17 % rate seen after BLR ($p=0.0009$). Such, as yet unreported data, appear to confirm the "superiority" of a bilateral procedure in OPTC, a conclusion that is consistent with our earlier studies [11, 12, 18, 20]. However, they differ from the recent recommendations of Nixon and his colleagues from Memorial Sloan Kettering Cancer Center (MSKCC), who now have "an informed discussion" with (T1T2N0) patients about the options of thyroid lobectomy versus total thyroidectomy. If the thyroid mass is a single nodule less than 4 cm with no contralateral nodules in the opposite lobe, and no evidence of extrathyroidal extension, patients (at MSKCC) are given the option of thyroid lobectomy [28, 29].

What Would the ATA Guidelines Advise for the Patient Discussed?

In all three ATA Guidelines [30–32], the primary goal of initial management has been "to remove the primary tumor, disease that has extended beyond the thyroid capsule, and involved cervical lymph nodes." In 2009, Recommendation 26 stated that "for patients with thyroid cancer >1 cm, the initial surgical procedure should be a near-total or total thyroidectomy unless there are contraindications to the surgery," while Recommendation 27 (b), developed in collaboration with four endocrine and four head and neck surgeons, stated that "prophylactic central compartment neck dissection may be performed in patients with PTC with clinically uninvolved central neck lymph nodes, especially for advanced primary tumors (T3 or T4); Recommendation rating C." In the 2009 document, a novel three-level stratification for risk of recurrence was described, and by this classification, our patient, on the basis of her microscopic invasion (pT3) and cervical lymph node metastases (pN1A), would be considered as an "intermediate-risk" patient.

Recommendation 32 (b) stated that "RAI ablation is recommended for selected patients with 1–4 cm thyroid cancers confined to the thyroid, who have documented lymph node metastases or other higher risk features." Table 5 of the Guidelines [31] demonstrated that, for T3 tumors, RRA provided no decreased risk of CSM and there was "inadequate data" to define whether recurrence risk would decrease. Similarly, for N1 patients <45 years old, there was no expected benefit in terms of CSM and only "conflicting data" on recurrence. Therefore, in both these settings, RRA should be "selectively used" and the ATA taskforce could not "recommend either for or against RAI ablation" in these two groups [31].

Therefore, the initial management, employed in our discussed patient, conforms to the recommendations of the 2009 Guidelines and is consistent with the lessons learned at Mayo from five decades of studying outcome in OPTC.

How Therefore Should a Thyroidologist Advise Such a Patient in 2015?

In 2010, I was asked to write an editorial [5] to accompany a recent paper on the surgical management of patients with stage I (cT1N0M0) PTC, similar in fact to our discussed case. In that editorial, which was entitled "East versus West, whose policy is best?," I compared and contrasted the surgical policies currently pursued in Kobe City, Japan; Villejuif, France; and Rochester, Minnesota. In 2015, I would now add to this geographic survey, New York City, where the surgical policy at SKMCC, as reported by Nixon [28, 29], would be initial lobectomy and, thereafter, observation of clinically negative level VI nodes "rather than prophylactic central neck dissection" [29]. In my 2010 editorial, I concluded that "the shift in attitude worldwide towards more initial surgery and less postoperative radioiodine is gaining momentum [31, 33, 34]. In that respect, we in the West should be beholden to our colleagues in the East, such as Ito and Noguchi, who have long championed such an approach [5]."

I am not sure that in my own institution, the surgical pendulum has perhaps swung too far to the aggressive side [4, 6], although by our surgeon's standards, the present policy of "a moderate surgical approach of bilateral thyroid resection, with usual central neck nodal clearance, and lateral internal jugular lymphadenopathy for node-positive disease can be performed safely, and with about a 5 % recurrence rate." Clearly, we would be in agreement with the recently published findings from Sosa's group [35, 36] who found by analyzing patients from the NCDB dataset and the SEER database that total thyroidectomy, when compared to unilateral lobectomy, is not associated with improved overall survival, either in patients <45 years old with AJCC stage PTC and tumors 1.1–4 cm diameter or in patients of any age with tumors 1–4 cm diameter. My personal concern relates more to the regional recurrence rates that we may see in future years when we attempt to analyze the impact of near-routine prophylactic central node sampling in our cN0 patients. Moreover, such a "moderate" surgical policy, as advocated by Mayo's Professor Grant, in less experienced hands, could translate to an unacceptable rate of significant morbidity, without an improved recurrence rate [4, 6, 37].

On the other hand, I remain optimistic that our present management policies are reducing the likelihood in future postoperative years of discovering perplexing serum Tg levels and, in turn, US-identifiable NNM. I am personally delighted that we at Mayo are certainly using RRA in a much more selective fashion. As a consequence, I would say that, if I saw this patient in my clinic, but this time in 2015, I think I would likely treat her in the same fashion as I did before. I can certainly live with a stable serum Tg of 0.2 ng/mL on TST, and I truly believe that the likelihood of this patient ever seeing PTC again is now very close to zero.

Clinical Pearls/Pitfalls

- Occult papillary thyroid carcinoma (OPTC) is in the twenty-first century the world's most frequently recognized endocrine malignancy.
- Less than 0.5 % spread to distant sites or result in cancer-related death.
- About a third are node-positive at presentation, and almost 90 % of postoperative recurrences are in regional neck nodes.
- Controversy surrounds the ideal extent of primary thyroid surgical resection and the role of prophylactic central compartment level VI nodal dissection.
- Radioiodine remnant ablation should no longer be used in treating OPTC as it does not prevent recurrence at either locoregional or distant sites.
- Postoperative surveillance involves measurement of serum thyroglobulin on TST and careful neck ultrasound examinations.
- OPTC patients can be reassured that they will enjoy a normal life expectancy and 90 % will never have a recurrence.
- In OPTC, recurrent NNM can conveniently and cost-effectively be treated as outpatients with ultrasound-guided percutaneous ethanol ablation.

References

1. Woolner LB, Lemmon ML, Beahrs OH, Black BM, Keating Jr FR. Occult papillary carcinoma of the thyroid gland: a study of 140 cases observed in a 30-year period. J Clin Endocrinol. 1960;20:89–105.
2. Hubert Jr JP, Kiernan PD, Beahrs OH, McConahey WM, Woolner LB. Occult papillary carcinoma of the thyroid. Arch Surg. 1980;115:394–8.
3. Thompson NW, Nishiyama RH, Harness JK. Thyroid carcinoma: current controversies. Curr Probl Surg. 1978;15:1–67.
4. Grant CS, Stulak J, Thompson GB, Richards ML, Reading CC, Hay ID. Risks and adequacy of an optimized surgical approach to the primary surgical management of papillary thyroid carcinoma treated during 1999–2006. World J Surg. 2010;34:1239–46.
5. Hay ID. Managing patients with a preoperative diagnosis of AJCC/UICC stage I (T1N0M0) papillary thyroid carcinoma: East versus West, whose policy is best? World J Surg. 2010;34:1291–3.
6. Grant CS. Papillary thyroid cancer: strategies for optimal individualized surgical management. Clin Ther. 2014;36:1117–26.

7. Nixon IJ, Shaha AR. Management of regional nodes in thyroid cancer. Oral Oncol. 2013;49: 671–5.
8. Giordano D, Valcavi R, Thompson GB, Pedroni C, Renna L, Gradoni P, Brabieri V. Complications of central neck dissection in patients with papillary thyroid carcinoma: results of a study on 1087 patients and review of the literature. Thyroid. 2012;22:911–7.
9. Paphasavit A, Thompson GB, Hay ID, Grant CS, van Heereden JA, Ilstrup DM, Schleck C, Goellner JR. Follicular and Hurthle cell thyroid neoplasms: is frozen-section evaluation worthwhile? Arch Surg. 1997;132:674–9.
10. McConahey WM, Hay ID, Woolner LB, van Heerden JA, Taylor WF. Papillary thyroid cancer treated at the Mayo Clinic, 1946 through 1970: initial manifestations, pathologic findings, therapy, and outcome. Mayo Clin Proc. 1986;61:978–96.
11. Hay ID, Grant CS, Taylor WF, McConahey WM. Ipsilateral lobectomy versus bilateral lobar resection in papillary thyroid carcinoma; a retrospective analysis of surgical outcome using a novel prognostic scoring system. Surgery. 1987;102:1088–95.
12. Hay ID. Papillary thyroid carcinoma. Endocrinol Metab Clin North Am. 1990;19:545–76.
13. Rivera M, Ricarte-Filho J, Tuttle RM, Ganly I, Shaha A, Knauf J, Fagin J, Ghossein R. Molecular, morphologic, and outcome analysis of thyroid carcinomas according to degree of extrathyroid extension. Thyroid. 2010;20:1085–93.
14. Ito Y, Miyauchi A, Kihara M, Kobayashi K, Miya A. Prognostic values of clinical lymph node metastases and macroscopic extension in papillary thyroid carcinoma. Endocrinol J. 2014;61:745–60.
15. Ito Y, Tomoda C, Uruno T, Takamura Y, Miya A, Kobayashi K, Matsuzuka F, Kuma K, Miyauchi A. Prognostic significance of extrathyroid extension of papillary thyroid carcinoma: massive but not minimal extension affects the relapse-free survival. World J Surg. 2006;30:780–6.
16. Hay ID, Bergstralh EJ, Goellner JR, Ebersold JR, Grant CS. Predicting outcome in papillary thyroid carcinoma: development of a reliable prognostic scoring system in a cohort of 1779 patients surgically treated at one institution during 1940 through 1989. Surgery. 1987;114:1050–8.
17. Cady B, Rossi R. An expanded view of risk-group definition in differentiated thyroid carcinoma. Surgery. 1988;104:947–53.
18. Hay ID. Managing patients with papillary thyroid carcinoma: insights gained from the Mayo Clinic's experience of treating 2,512 consecutive patients during 1940 through 2000. Trans Am Clin Assoc. 2002;113:241–60.
19. Hay ID. Selective use of radioactive iodine in the postoperative management of patients with papillary and follicular thyroid carcinoma. J Surg Oncol. 2006;94:692–700.
20. Hay ID. Management of patients with low-risk papillary thyroid carcinoma. Endocr Pract. 2007;13:521–33.
21. Randolph GW, Thompson GB, Branovan DI, Tuttle RM. Treatment of thyroid cancer 2007 – a basic review. Int J Radiat Oncol Biol Phys. 2007;69 Suppl 2:892–7.
22. Lewis BD, Hay ID, Charboneau JW, McIver B, Reading CC, Goellner JR. Percutaneous ethanol injection for treatment of cervical node metastases in patients with papillary thyroid carcinoma. AJR Am J Roentgenol. 2002;178:699–704.
23. Heilo A, Sigstad E, Fagerlid KH, Haskjold OI, Groholt KK, Berner A, Bjoro T, Jorgensen LH. Efficacy of ultrasound-guided percutaneous ethanol injection treatment in patients with a limited number of metastatic cervical lymph nodes from papillary thyroid carcinoma. J Clin Endocrinol Metab. 2011;96:2750–5.
24. Hay ID, Lee RA, Davidge-Pitts C, Reading CC, Charboneau JW. Long-term outcome of ultrasound-guided percutaneous ethanol ablation of selected "recurrent" neck nodal metastases in 25 patients with TNM stages III or IVA papillary thyroid carcinoma previously treated by surgery and ^{131}I therapy. Surgery. 2013;154:1448–55.
25. Hay ID, Mullan BP, McIver B, Maurer M, Powell CC, Oberg AL, Wiseman GA, Goellner JR, Gorman CA. Radioiodine remnant ablation does not decrease recurrence rates in patients with small papillary thyroid carcinomas. J Nucl Med. 2002;43 Suppl 5:12P.
26. Cappelli C, Castellano M, Braga M, Gandossi E, Pirola I, De Martino E. Aggressiveness and outcome of papillary thyroid carcinoma versus microcarcinoma: a mono-institutional experience. J Surg Oncol. 2007;95:555–60.

27. Hay ID, Hutchinson ME, Reinalda MS, Grant CS, McIver B, Thompson GB. Woolner's "occult" papillary thyroid cancer revisited: 1421 cases treated at one institution during a 60-year period. Proceedings 90th Annual Meeting, Endocrine Society, San Francisco, CA; June 2008.
28. Nixon IJ, Ganly I, Patel SG, Palmer FL, Whitcher MM, Tuttle RM, Shaha A, Shah JP. Thyroid lobectomy for treatment of well differentiated intrathyroid malignancy. Surgery. 2012; 151:571–9.
29. Nixon IJ, Ganly I, Patel SG, Morris LG, Palmer FL, Thomas D, Tuttle RM, Shah JP, Shaha AR. Observation of clinically negative central compartment lymph nodes in papillary thyroid carcinoma. Surgery. 2013;154:1166–73.
30. Cooper DS, Doherty GM, Haugen BR, Kloos RT, Lee SL, Mandel SJ, Mazzaferri EL, Sherman SI, Tuttle RM, The American Thyroid Association Guidelines Taskforce. Management guidelines for patients with thyroid nodules and differentiated thyroid cancer. Thyroid. 2006;16:109–42.
31. Cooper DS, Doherty GM, Haugen BR, Kloos RT, Lee SL, Mandel SL, Mazzaferri EL, McIver B, Pacini F, Schlumberger M, Sherman SI, Steward DL, Tuttle RM. Revised American Thyroid Association management guidelines for patients with thyroid nodules and differentiated thyroid cancer. Thyroid. 2009;11:1–48.
32. Haugen BR, Alexander EK, Bible KC, Doherty GM, Mandel SJ, Nikiforov YE, Pacini F, Randolph GW, Sawka AM, Schlumberger M, Schuff K, Sherman SI, Sosa JA, Steward DL, Tuttle RM, Wartofsky L. American Thyroid Association Management Guidelines for Adult Patients with Thyroid Nodules and Differentiated Thyroid Cancer. Thyroid. 2015 (in press).
33. Hay ID, McDougall IR, Sisson JC. Perspective: the case against radioiodine remnant ablation in patients with differentiated thyroid carcinoma. J Nucl Med. 2008;49:1395–7.
34. Mazzaferri EL. A vision for the surgical management of papillary thyroid carcinoma: extensive lymph node compartmental dissections and selective use of radioiodine. J Clin Endocrinol Metab. 2009;94:1086–8.
35. Adam MA, Pura J, Gu L, Dinan MA, Tyler DS, Reed SD, Scheri R, Roman SA, Sosa JA. Extent of surgery for papillary thyroid cancer is not associated with survival: an analysis of 61,775 patients. Ann Surg. 2014;260:601–7.
36. Abdelgadir AM, Pura J, Goffredo P, Dinan M, Hyslop T, Reed SD, Scheri RP, Roman SA, Sosa JA. Impact of extent of surgery on survival for papillary thyroid cancer patients younger than 45 years. J Clin Endocrinol Metab. 2015;100:115–21.
37. Grant CS. Recurrence of papillary thyroid cancer after optimized surgery. Gland Surg. 2015;4:52–62.

Chapter 9
Papillary Thyroid Cancer with Central Neck Lymph Node Metastases

Alyse S. Goldberg, Lorne E. Rotstein, and Anna M. Sawka

Abbreviations

TSH	Thyroid-stimulating hormone concentration
micro-PTC	Micropapillary thyroid cancer
RAI	Radioactive iodine

Case Presentation

A previously healthy 30-year-old female was seen by her family physician for a general medical exam. As part of this evaluation, she underwent measurement of thyroid-stimulating hormone (TSH) concentration and a neck ultrasound. It was not clear why the ultrasound was ordered, as the patient was not aware of any abnormality in her thyroid exam. The patient had no compressive symptoms (i.e., no hoarseness, dysphagia, nor dyspnea). There was no family history of thyroid cancer, nor thyroid disorders. The patient had no significant history of head and neck radiation exposure.

Diagnosis/Assessment

For the case presented, the baseline TSH level was normal (2.49 mIU/L) and a neck ultrasound showed a left-sided solid, 1.0 cm hypoechoic thyroid nodule with smooth margins and no microcalcifications, and there were no other thyroid nodules and no enlarged/suspicious lymph nodes. Ultrasound-guided fine-needle aspiration

A.S. Goldberg, MD • L.E. Rotstein, MD • A.M. Sawka, MD, PhD (✉)
Toronto General Hospital, 200 Elizabeth Street, 12 Eaton North, Room 212,
Toronto, ON, Canada, M5G 2C4
e-mail: Alyse.goldberg@utoronto.ca; Lorne.Rotstein@uhn.ca; Annie.Sawka@uhn.ca

D.S. Cooper, C. Durante (eds.), *Thyroid Cancer*,
DOI 10.1007/978-3-319-22401-5_9

biopsy of the thyroid nodule was positive for papillary thyroid cancer. She underwent total thyroidectomy, and the intraoperative detection of an enlarged a paratracheal lymph node prompted therapeutic left pretracheal and left paratracheal nodal dissection as part of the same procedure. The final surgical pathology showed multifocal micropapillary thyroid cancer (micro-PTC, follicular variant), with two foci, measuring in maximal diameter, 0.9 cm (in the left lobe) and 0.2 cm (in the right lobe), respectively. There was no extrathyroidal extension of the primary tumor, with no lymphatic, vascular, nor capsular invasion. The resection margins were clear. There was evidence of chronic lymphocytic thyroiditis. Upon examination of the eight resected central neck lymph nodes, two of them were positive for PTC, measuring 8 mm and 3 mm, respectively, in maximal diameter, with no evidence of any extranodal extension.

The clinicopathologic stage of disease in this case was interpreted as follows:

T1aN1aMx (Stage I) per the AJCC/TNM VII system [1, 2]
Low risk (for thyroid cancer-related mortality) by the MACIS system (score 3.37) [3]
American Thyroid Association (ATA) intermediate risk of recurrence [4]

Postoperatively, the patient started taking levothyroxine and recovered uneventfully, with normal calcium and parathyroid hormone levels and no problems with her voice. Approximately 11 weeks following surgery, while on levothyroxine therapy (TSH 7.24 mIU/L with a normal free thyroxine concentration), the thyroglobulin was measured to be <0.9 ng/dl, but thyroglobulin antibodies were present at a level of 97 IU/L (thyroglobulin antibody reference range <39 IU/L and the assay detection limit 20 IU/L). Given the presence of thyroglobulin antibodies, the thyroglobulin measurement was considered unreliable, due to potential assay interference [5]. A postoperative ultrasound of the neck 12 weeks after surgery was negative. Her levothyroxine dose was increased, with the intention of suppressing the TSH concentration (<0.1 mIU/L). The patient's endocrinologist recommended radioactive iodine (RAI) adjuvant treatment, given the presence of nodal metastases associated with increased risk of disease recurrence; another reason why RAI was recommended was to facilitate disease follow-up. However, the patient indicated that she did not want to take RAI, unless there was proof that it could reduce the risk of dying from thyroid cancer or distant metastatic recurrence, specifically in her situation. She strongly disliked the idea of taking any form of "radiation," unless it was clear that it could prevent death or distant metastases (which were her primary concerns). She was then referred an endocrinologist at a tertiary care center for further counseling.

Literature Review

Classification of Lymph Node Disease

Randolph et al. of the ATA Surgical Affairs Committee have reviewed the literature on prognostic significance of nodal metastases of papillary thyroid carcinoma and have proposed a categorization system for nodal disease [6]. Pathologic N1 (pN1) is any metastatic papillary thyroid cancer detected on the pathologic specimen of any resected lymph nodes [6]. Clinically apparent nodal disease, referred to as clinical N1, (cN1) is defined as metastatic lymph nodes identified on either physical examination, diagnostic imaging studies, or intraoperative inspection by the surgeon, and the absence of such features is clinical N0 (cN0) [6]. The presence of one or more metastatic lymph nodes that are visible on preoperative physical examination, ultrasound, or during surgery (the latter according to surgical and pathologic reports) has been independently associated with increased risk of recurrence of disease in a multivariable analysis, including data from 545 patients [7]. However, in the central neck, the accuracy of intraoperative surgical inspection is only about 60 % [8], with larger affected nodes being more readily clinically detected [9]. Moreover, the significance of subclinical, low-volume nodal disease in the central neck is not clear.

Regardless of how cN1 disease is detected, resection of such affected nodes and relevant nodal compartments is termed "therapeutic neck dissection" [6]. In contrast, "prophylactic neck dissection" is defined as nodal dissection in the absence of any evidence of cN1 disease prior the procedure [6]. Randolph et al. divided nodal disease into two categories: lower-risk N1 disease and higher-risk N1 disease [6]. Lower-risk N1 disease has been defined by the presence of the following criteria: (a) clinical N0; (b) low-volume nodal disease, specifically micrometastatic nodes (i.e., largest node <0.2 cm in diameter) or small nodal metastases (0.2 to <1.0 cm in diameter); and (c) ≤5 small lymph node metastases (i.e., each measuring <1.0 cm in diameter) [6]. Higher-risk N1 disease has been defined by the presence of the following criteria: (a) clinically detectable lymph node metastases (cN1), (b) metastatic lymph node(s) >3 cm, and (c) >5 metastatic lymph nodes [6]. Randolph et al. have also reported that gross extranodal extension, increasing number of metastatic lymph nodes with microscopic extranodal extension, or the combination of microscopic extranodal extension and metastatic lymph nodes >1 cm is also predictive of a higher risk of disease recurrence [6]. However, the predictive performance of the ATA metastatic lymph node classification system from Randolph et al. [6] has not yet been independently validated. It is important to note that according to the TNM/AJCC VII system, pathologic N1 disease is categorized as follows: N1a (metastases to the pretracheal, paratracheal, and/or prelaryngeal or Delphian lymph nodes, which are in the central neck) and N1b (metastases to unilateral, bilateral, or contralateral cervical or superior mediastinal nodes) (i.e., including the lateral neck or mediastinum) [1, 2]. The location of nodal disease has been reported to be associated with the size of involved nodes in papillary thyroid cancer, particularly for bulky enlarged nodes. For example, Chow et al. reported that 13 % of N1a and 56 % of N1b papillary thyroid cancer patients had involved nodes >2 cm in diameter ($p<0.001$) [10]. Ito et al. suggested that for papillary thyroid cancer patients whose nodal disease is detected on preoperative imaging, the cause-specific survival of patients with N1b level nodal involvement is not significantly different from that of those with N1a nodal involvement [11]. However, in this study [11], the disease-free survival was adversely affected in papillary thyroid cancer patients with N1b level nodal involvement who had pathologic evidence of aggressive nodal disease, including the lymph nodes measuring >3 cm in diameter, extranodal extension, or ≥5 or more involved nodes [11]. Furthermore, the presence of two or more such adverse features in N1b disease was associated with reduced cause-specific survival [11]. Age also appears to be an important prognostic variable in N1 disease. For example, Verberg et al. reported that in differentiated thyroid cancer, patients aged ≥45 years who have lateral neck lymph node metastases have a reduced long-term life expectancy, but life expectancy is not significantly impacted in younger patients with similar disease features [12]. Furthermore, Hughes et al. have reported that in differentiated thyroid cancer patients with N1 disease, the recurrence rate was 8 % in those <45 years of age, as compared with 31 % in those ≥45 years of age [13]. In this study, all disease recurrences were successfully treated in the N1 patients aged <45 years, but only about a third of those aged ≥45 years of age [13]. In conclusion, the size and number, location of metastatic lymph nodes, the presence of extranodal extension, and patient age are relevant considerations in risk stratification of N1 disease.

Epidemiology of N1 Disease in Patients with Micro-PTC

Lymph node metastases are evident at the time of diagnosis in approximately 12–64 % of cases of micro-PTC [14–26]. If nodal metastases are present in this situation, the ipsilateral paratracheal compartments, followed by the pretracheal compartments, are the levels most frequently affected [20]. Lateral neck nodal metastases may be present in about 3–7 % of individuals with micro-PTC [15, 20, 24, 27, 28]. The presence of primary tumor extrathyroidal extension [14, 19, 29] and tumor multifocality [19, 29, 30] are risk factors for the presence of lymph node metastases with micro-PTC. In summary, N1 disease is not uncommon in patients with micro-PTC, and if it is present, it is most frequent in the central neck.

Prognosis of N1 Disease in Patients with Micro-PTC

The overall risk of disease recurrence of persistence in patients with papillary thyroid microcarcinoma and positive lymph nodes (without distant metastases at presentation) has been reported to range between 3.0 and 22 % [15–17, 19]. The risk of dying of thyroid cancer and developing distant metastatic recurrence in this context are important considerations. In a recent retrospective review of micro-PTCs, Mercante et al. reported that in a subgroup of 27 patients with T1aN1a disease, none of the patients died of disease nor developed distant metastases (follow-up about 8 years) [19]. Similarly, Kim et al. found that in a subgroup of 168 individuals with micro-PTC with no evidence of macroscopic extrathyroidal extension nor distant metastases at initial presentation, no patient died of thyroid cancer nor developed distant metastatic disease (mean follow-up about 5 years) [15]. In a retrospective review of micro-PTC cases from a hospital in Hong Kong, Chow et al. [22] reported that in a subgroup of 48 patients with micro-PTC and various degrees of severity of lymph node disease without distant metastases, 2 % died due to thyroid cancer (1/50) and 4.0 % (two patients) developed distant metastatic recurrence (mean follow-up about 8 years) [22]. In a retrospective chart review of patients with differentiated thyroid carcinoma ≤1 cm in diameter treated in the years 1962–1995 in France, Baudin et al. reported that in node-positive micro-PTC patients without distant metastases at primary presentation, none of the patients died from thyroid cancer (0/113), and only 1 % developed distant metastatic recurrence (1/113) (mean follow-up of about 7 years) [21]. Also, in a retrospective review of micro-PTC cases at the Mayo Clinic, Hay et al. studied that the outcomes of a subgroup of 273 patients had positive lymph nodes at diagnosis [17]. Hay et al. indicated that no female with initial disease confined to the neck ultimately died of disease or developed distant metastases, but one male with extensive bulky lateral neck disease at presentation developed bone metastases and died of the disease, approximately 30 years after presentation (mean study follow-up 17 years) [17]. In summary, in papillary thyroid microcarcinoma patients with limited nodal involvement, no evidence of other adverse disease features, and no distant metastatic disease at the time of presentation, the risk of dying of thyroid cancer is likely about 0–2 % and the risk of developing distant metastatic recurrence is likely about 0–4 %.

In patients with papillary thyroid microcarcinoma and lymph node metastases (T1aN1), the risk of local-regional recurrence of disease in the neck or lymph nodes is another relevant consideration. The risk of local-regional recurrence in T1aN1 micro-PTC has been reported to range from 3 to 16 % [15, 17, 21]. Furthermore, the incidence rate of local-regional recurrence has been subdivided according to the level of nodal involvement at the time of initial diagnosis as follows, in two of the more recent studies: N1a (central neck)—0 to 3 % and N1b (lateral neck or mediastinum)—2 to 11 % (excluding individuals with extrathyroidal extension of the primary tumor at initial diagnosis) [15, 19]. Based on these limited data, it appears that nodal recurrence of disease is relatively uncommon in patients with micro-PTC whose initial nodal disease is confined to the central neck, in the absence of other adverse disease characteristics.

Does RAI Adjuvant Treatment Reduce the Risk of Disease Recurrence in T1aN1 Disease?

There are limited data from observational studies examining whether radioactive adjuvant treatment reduces the risk of recurrence after total thyroidectomy in patients with node-positive micro-PTC. Hay et al. reported that of 253 node-positive patients with micro-PTC, RAI adjuvant treatment did not significantly reduce local recurrence in the neck (p=0.81) nor distant metastatic recurrence (p=0.68) [17]. Ross et al. of the National Thyroid Cancer Treatment Cooperative Study Group also reported that in a subgroup analysis of 135 node-positive patients with micro-PTC who were followed prospectively, RAI treatment did not significantly improve recurrence-free survival in node-positive patients (17 % without RAI, 11 % with RAI, $p > 0.05$) [16]. Kim et al. reported that in a subgroup of 168 micro-PTC patients who either had nodal disease, microscopic extrathyroidal extension of the primary tumor, or multifocality, RAI treatment did not significantly improve recurrence-free survival ($p = 0.52$) [15]. Chow et al. reported that in 50 micro-PTC patients with N1 disease, the administration of RAI did not significantly impact the risk of lymph node recurrence (nodal relapse rate 12.2 % (5/41) in the RAI-treated patients and 22.2 % (2/9) in those who did not receive RAI, $p = 0.6$) [22]. Creach et al. published a retrospective study of micro-PTC patients, which included a subgroup analysis of 153 individuals with N1 disease [26]. In this study, the 5-year recurrence-free survival rate was significantly higher in node-positive micro-PTC patients treated with RAI (93.2 %) compared to those not treated with RAI (42.9 %) ($p < 0.0001$) [26]. An important limitation of the latter study is that not all of the patients had total thyroidectomy, so it is not clear if the surgical extent was the same in both groups [26]. Thus, there is conflicting evidence on whether RAI adjuvant treatment reduces the risk of disease recurrence in node-positive patients with micro-PTC. The relatively small population size, limited follow-up, retrospective nature, and potential bias in selection of patients for RAI, in many of the aforementioned studies, are limitations that need to be considered in interpreting the results, which appear to be conflicting. Furthermore, none of these studies risk-stratified node-positive patients according to the number, size, or levels of involved nodes or the presence of extranodal extension. Given the low event rates, none of these studies would have been likely to be sufficiently statistically powered to detect differences in incidence rates of distant metastatic recurrence nor thyroid cancer-related mortality between RAI treatment and control groups. These studies also did not examine the potential benefit of RAI adjuvant treatment in disease staging (e.g., pre- or posttherapy RAI scans) or facilitating disease follow-up. So et al. recently reported that in patients with micro-PTC who had positive central neck nodal disease in the absence of preoperative evidence on the examination or ultrasound of abnormal nodes, the intensity of sodium iodine symporter (NIS) expression in affected nodes was highly variable [31] and may potentially lead to variability of RAI treatment efficacy among different individuals and populations. However, there are currently no data examining long-term RAI treatment outcomes according to NIS expression in metastatic nodes of patients with micro-PTC. Randomized controlled trials are clearly needed to better define the role of RAI adjuvant treatment in node-positive micro-PTC patients. Ideally, treatment effect according to potential molecular or other biomarkers should be explored in such trials.

Management Considerations and Outcome

Our patient presented with micro-PTC, with no preoperative evidence of nodal metastases, but with intraoperative palpation of a suspicious paratracheal lymph node prompting ipsilateral para- and pretracheal lymph node dissection, yielding two small metastatic lymph nodes (maximal diameter 8 mm) out of eight nodes that were removed. The finding of the largest node being palpable intraoperatively in this case would technically upstage the disease to the "higher-risk" nodal disease category as defined by Randolph et al. [6], but the relatively small size and number of involved nodes and negative pre- and postoperative imaging would be more suggestive of a lower-risk nodal disease. The inherent limitations of accuracy of intraoperative detection of nodal disease in the central neck [7, 8] and the lack of data on independent prognostic significance of this finding are important considerations. The risk stratification of this case was largely based on the number, size, and levels of involved lymph nodes, in the context of the patient's young age, the absence of an adverse histologic subtype, the lack of extrathyroidal extension or vascular invasion of the primary tumor, and negative postoperative ultrasound imaging of the neck. Diagnostic I-123 scanning was not available at the treating institution, and I-131 pretherapy scans were generally not employed in the treating institution. However, there are some data, in centers experienced in the use of pretherapy I-123 or I-131 diagnostic scans, that such imaging may be helpful in evaluating disease status and other relevant variables, in patients being considered for RAI remnant ablation or treatment [32, 33]. The addition of single photon emission computed tomography–computed tomography (SPECT-CT) to iodine radioisotope planar imaging may provide additional information, clarifying the structural correlates of areas of increased uptake [34]. If an interfering thyroglobulin antibody were not present, measurement of a stimulated thyroglobulin could have also been helpful in postoperative risk stratification and related deliberation on RAI treatment, as previously respectively reported by Walfish et al. [35] and Rosario et al. [36]. The potential strengths and limitations of various postsurgical diagnostic test options for patients being considered for RAI remnant ablation or therapy are weighed in the new ATA guidelines on the management of thyroid nodules and differentiated thyroid cancer in adults [37].

The patient was counseled on disease prognosis, risks, benefits, and evidence uncertainties relating to RAI treatment in the context of her disease stage. Follow-up implications, including the limitation of biochemical follow-up in the presence of thyroglobulin antibodies, were also explained. The patient ultimately declined RAI treatment, reiterating her general opposition to "radiation" and indicating that the available evidence was not sufficiently convincing, in terms of reducing the risk of dying of thyroid cancer or developing distant metastatic disease, in her situation. She was less concerned about the potential for local-regional recurrence and understood the possibility of needing additional surgery, in the event of a recurrence. The patient agreed to close surveillance by ultrasound imaging of the neck and measurement of thyroglobulin and thyroglobulin antibody levels, with the intention of accepting additional treatment in the event of disease recurrence. She also accepted thyroid hormone suppressive treatment, with the intention of suppressing TSH to levels <0.1 mIU/L.

The thyroglobulin antibody positivity at the time of diagnosis was consistent with the pathologic evidence of Hashimoto's thyroiditis. The baseline thyroglobulin antibody titer (97 IU/L) decreased by 67 % within 10 months following surgery and continued to slowly decrease to undetectable levels over the next 4 years, with continued concurrent undetectable serum thyroglobulin measurements. The patient was maintained on thyroid hormone suppressive therapy, keeping the TSH <0.1 mIU/L with normal free thyroxine levels. The continuing presence of thyroglobulin antibody has been reported to be associated with the presence of residual disease [38, 39]. However, a decrease in thyroglobulin antibody titers of ≥50 % in the first postoperative year after total thyroidectomy is associated with a risk of disease recurrence or persistence of 0–2 % [38, 39]. Furthermore, Tsushima et al. reported that in a multivariable model adjusted for other relevant prognostic factors, a thyroglobulin antibody reduction of <50 % from baseline or rise in this measurement over 1–2 years following thyroidectomy was independently associated with significantly increased risk of recurrence in lymph nodes [40]. Spencer and Fatemi have proposed a classification system for thyroglobulin antibody trends during long-term follow-up of papillary thyroid cancer, including the following categories: (a) falling thyroglobulin antibody trend (>50 % reduction from initial value, associated with <3 % risk of recurrence), (b) stable but significantly elevated thyroglobulin antibody (<50 % change from initial value, approximately 20 % risk of disease recurrence), and (c) rising thyroglobulin antibody trend (progressive, sustained rise in thyroglobulin antibody of >50 % from initial value, approximately 40 % risk of disease recurrence) [41]. Our patient continues to be followed, but as of 5 years after her surgery, she has had no evidence of structural disease on ultrasound imaging, and her thyroglobulin antibodies are continuing to slowly drop, currently bordering the detection limit of the assay; there has been no change in her undetectable thyroglobulin levels. In follow-up visits, she asserts that she is satisfied and she made the right choice for her, relating to not taking RAI, and she is highly compliant with close surveillance and TSH suppressive therapy.

Clinical Pearls/Pitfalls

- The risk of recurrence of patients with papillary thyroid carcinoma who have nodal metastases is dependent on factors such as the size, number, and presence or absence of extranodal extension of involved nodes and patient age, in addition to consideration of other disease features.
- Lymph node metastases are not uncommon in patients with micro-PTC.
- The risk of disease recurrence or persistence in node-positive patients with papillary thyroid microcarcinoma is variable; however, some of the lowest recurrence rates in this group appear to be in patients with relatively low-volume nodal disease confined to the central neck, in the absence of other adverse prognostic features or clinically detectable disease preoperatively.
- There is conflicting evidence as to whether adjuvant RAI treatment significantly impacts the risk of disease recurrence in node-positive micro-PTC patients, particularly for lower-risk nodal disease; however, RAI use may facilitate follow-up.

- Thyroglobulin antibodies interfere with thyroglobulin interpretation, but monitoring changes in antithyroglobulin antibody titers, in conjunction with structural imaging, may be helpful in disease surveillance.
- Patient preferences are important to consider in RAI decision-making, especially when there is conflicting or unclear evidence of long-term outcome benefit.

References

1. Edge SB, Byrd DR, Carducci MA, Compton CC, editors. AJCC cancer staging manual. 7th ed. New York: Springer; 2009.
2. Sobin LH, et al. TNM classification of malignant tumours. 7th ed. Chichester: Wiley; 2009.
3. Hay ID, Bergstralh EJ, Goellner JR, Ebersold JR, Grant CS. Predicting outcome in papillary thyroid carcinoma: development of a reliable prognostic scoring system in a cohort of 1779 patients surgically treated at one institution during 1940 through 1989. Surgery. 1993; 114:1050–7.
4. Cooper DS, Doherty GM, Haugen BR, Kloos RT, Lee SL, American Thyroid Association (ATA) Guidelines Taskforce on Thyroid Nodules and Differentiated Thyroid Cancer, et al. Revised American thyroid association management guidelines for patients with thyroid nodules and differentiated thyroid cancer. Thyroid. 2009;19:1167–214.
5. Spencer CA, Takeuchi M, Kazarosyan M, Wang CC, Guttler RB, Singer PA, et al. Serum thyroglobulin autoantibodies: prevalence, influence on serum thyroglobulin measurement, and prognostic significance in patients with differentiated thyroid carcinoma. J Clin Endocrinol Metab. 1998;83:1121–7.
6. Randolph GW, Duh QY, Heller KS, LiVolsi VA, Mandel SJ, Steward DL, American Thyroid Association Surgical Affairs Committee's Taskforce on Thyroid Cancer Nodal Surgery, et al. The prognostic significance of nodal metastases from papillary thyroid carcinoma can be stratified based on the size and number of metastatic lymph nodes, as well as the presence of extranodal extension. Thyroid. 2012;22:1144–52.
7. Bardet S, Malville E, Rame JP, Babin E, Samama G, De Raucourt D, et al. Macroscopic lymph-node involvement and neck dissection predict lymph-node recurrence in papillary thyroid carcinoma. Eur J Endocrinol. 2008;158(4):551–60.
8. Ji YB, Lee DW, Song CM, Kim KR, Park CW, Tae K. Accuracy of intraoperative determination of central node metastasis by the surgeon in papillary thyroid carcinoma. Otolaryngol Head Neck Surg. 2014;150(4):542–7.
9. Scherl S, Mehra S, Clain J, Dos Reis LL, Persky M, Turk A, et al. The effect of surgeon experience on the detection of metastatic lymph nodes in the central compartment and the pathologic features of clinically unapparent metastatic lymph nodes: what are we missing when we don't perform a prophylactic dissection of central compartment lymph nodes in papillary thyroid cancer? Thyroid. 2014;24(8):1282–8.
10. Chow SM, Yau S, Kwan CK, Poon PC, Law SC. Local and regional control in patients with papillary thyroid carcinoma: specific indications of external radiotherapy and radioactive iodine according to T and N categories in AJCC 6th edition. Endocr Relat Cancer. 2006; 13:1159–72.
11. Ito Y, Fukushima M, Tomoda C, Inoue H, Kihara M, Higashiyama T, et al. Prognosis of patients with papillary thyroid carcinoma having clinically apparent metastasis to the lateral compartment. Endocr J. 2009;56(6):759–66.
12. Verburg FA, Mäder U, Tanase K, Thies ED, Diessl S, Buck AK, et al. Life expectancy is reduced in differentiated thyroid cancer patients ≥45 years old with extensive local tumor invasion, lateral lymph node, or distant metastases at diagnosis and normal in all other DTC patients. J Clin Endocrinol Metab. 2013;98:172–80.

13. Hughes CJ, Shaha AR, Shah JP, Loree TR. Impact of lymph node metastasis in differentiated carcinoma of the thyroid: a matched-pair analysis. Head Neck. 1996;18:127–32.
14. Varshney R, Pakdaman MN, Sands N, Hier MP, Rochon L, Black MJ, et al. Lymph node metastasis in thyroid papillary microcarcinoma: a study of 170 patients. J Laryngol Otol. 2014;128(10):922–5.
15. Kim HJ, Kim NK, Choi JH, Kim SW, Jin SM, Suh S, et al. Radioactive iodine ablation does not prevent recurrences in patients with papillary thyroid microcarcinoma. Clin Endocrinol (Oxf). 2013;78:614–20.
16. Ross DS, Litofsky D, Ain KB, Bigos T, Brierley JD, Cooper DS, et al. Recurrence after treatment of micropapillary thyroid cancer. Thyroid. 2009;19:1043–8.
17. Hay ID, Hutchinson ME, Gonzalez-Losada T, McIver B, Reinalda ME, Grant CS, et al. Papillary thyroid microcarcinoma: a study of 900 cases observed in a 60-year period. Surgery. 2008;144:980–8.
18. Wada N, Duh QY, Sugino K, Iwasaki H, Kameyama K, Mimura T, et al. Lymph node metastasis from 259 papillary thyroid microcarcinomas: frequency, pattern of occurrence and recurrence, and optimal strategy for neck dissection. Ann Surg. 2003;237:399–407.
19. Mercante G, Frasoldati A, Pedroni C, Formisano D, Renna L, Piana S, et al. Prognostic factors affecting neck lymph node recurrence and distant metastasis in papillary microcarcinoma of the thyroid: results of a study in 445 patients. Thyroid. 2009;19:707–16.
20. Roh JL, Kim JM, Park CI. Central cervical nodal metastasis from papillary thyroid microcarcinoma: pattern and factors predictive of nodal metastasis. Ann Surg Oncol. 2008; 15(9):2482–6.
21. Baudin E, Travagli JP, Ropers J, Mancusi F, Bruno-Bossio G, Caillou B, et al. Microcarcinoma of the thyroid gland: the Gustave-Roussy Institute experience. Cancer. 1998;83(3):553–9.
22. Chow SM, Law SC, Chan JK, Au SK, Yau S, Lau WH. Papillary microcarcinoma of the thyroid-prognostic significance of lymph node metastasis and multifocality. Cancer. 2003; 98(1):31–40.
23. Roti E, degli Uberti EC, Bondanelli M, Braverman LE. Thyroid papillary microcarcinoma: a descriptive and meta-analysis study. Eur J Endocrinol. 2008;159(6):659–73.
24. Pelizzo MR, Boschin IM, Toniato A, Piotto A, Bernante P, Pagetta C, et al. Papillary thyroid microcarcinoma (PTMC): prognostic factors, management and outcome in 403 patients. Eur J Surg Oncol. 2006;32(10):1144–8.
25. Yu XM, Wan Y, Sippel RS, Chen H. Should all papillary thyroid microcarcinomas be aggressively treated? An analysis of 18,445 cases. Ann Surg. 2011;254(4):653–60.
26. Creach KM, Siegel BA, Nussenbaum B, Grigsby PW. Radioactive iodine therapy decreases recurrence in thyroid papillary microcarcinoma. ISRN Endocrinol. 2012;2012:816386.
27. Kwak JY, Kim EK, Kim MJ, Son EJ, Chung WY, Park CS, et al. Papillary microcarcinoma of the thyroid: predicting factors of lateral neck node metastasis. Ann Surg Oncol. 2009;16:1348–55.
28. Kim YS. Patterns and predictive factors of lateral lymph node metastasis in papillary thyroid microcarcinoma. Otolaryngol Head Neck Surg. 2012;147:15–9.
29. Zhang L, Wei WJ, Ji QH, Zhu YX, Wang ZY, Wang Y, et al. Risk factors for neck nodal metastasis in papillary thyroid microcarcinoma: a study of 1066 patients. J Clin Endocrinol Metab. 2012;97:1250–7.
30. Vasileiadis I, Karakostas E, Charitoudis G, Stavrianaki A, Kapetanakis S, Kouraklis G, et al. Papillary thyroid microcarcinoma: clinicopathological characteristics and implications for treatment in 276 patients. Eur J Clin Invest. 2012;42:657–64.
31. So YK, Son YI, Baek CH, Jeong HS, Chung MK, Ko YH. Expression of sodium-iodide symporter and TSH receptor in subclinical metastatic lymph nodes of papillary thyroid microcarcinoma. Ann Surg Oncol. 2012;19(3):990–5.
32. Van Nostrand D, Aiken M, Atkins F, Moreau S, Garcia C, Acio E, et al. The utility of radioiodine scans prior to iodine 131 ablation in patients with well-differentiated thyroid cancer. Thyroid. 2009;19:849–55.
33. Chen MK, Yasrebi M, Samii J, Staib LH, Doddamane I, Cheng DW. The utility of I-123 pretherapy scan in 1-131 radioiodine therapy for thyroid cancer. Thyroid. 2012;22:304–9.

34. Wong K, Sisson JC, Koral KF, Frey KA, Avram AM. Staging of differentiated thyroid carcinoma using diagnostic 131I SPECT/CT. Am J Roentgenol. 2010;195:730–6.
35. Vaisman A, Orlov S, Yip J, Hu C, Lim T, Dowar M, et al. Application of post-surgical stimulated thyroglobulin for radioiodine remnant ablation selection in low-risk papillary thyroid carcinoma. Head Neck. 2010;32(6):689–98.
36. Rosario PW, Mineiro Filho AF, Prates BS, Silva LC, Calsolari MR. Postoperative stimulated thyroglobulin of less than 1 ng/mL as a criterion to spare low-risk patients with papillary thyroid cancer from radioactive iodine ablation. Thyroid. 2012;22:1140–3.
37. Haugen BR, Alexander EK, Bible KC, Doherty GM, Mandel SJ, Nikiforov YE, American Thyroid Association Guidelines Task Force on Differentiated Thyroid Cancer, et al. American thyroid association management guidelines for adults with thyroid nodules and differentiated thyroid cancer. Thyroid. 2014 (To be submitted).
38. Yamada O, Miyauchi A, Ito Y, Nakayama A, Yabuta T, Masuoka H, et al. Changes in serum thyroglobulin antibody levels as a dynamic prognostic factor for early-phase recurrence of thyroglobulin antibody-positive papillary thyroid carcinoma after total thyroidectomy. Endocr J. 2014;61(10):961–5.
39. Kim WG, Yoon JH, Kim WB, Kim TY, Kim EY, Kim JM, et al. Change of serum antithyroglobulin antibody levels is useful for prediction of clinical recurrence in thyroglobulin-negative patients with differentiated thyroid carcinoma. J Clin Endocrinol Metab. 2008;93:4683–9.
40. Tsushima Y, Miyauchi A, Ito Y, Kudo T, Masuoka H, Yabuta T, et al. Prognostic significance of changes in serum thyroglobulin antibody levels of pre- and post-total thyroidectomy in thyroglobulin antibody-positive papillary thyroid carcinoma patients. Endocr J. 2013; 60:871–6.
41. Spencer C, Fatemi S. Thyroglobulin antibody (TgAb) methods – Strengths, pitfalls and clinical utility for monitoring TgAb-positive patients with differentiated thyroid cancer. Best Pract Res Clin Endocrinol Metab. 2013;27:701–12.

Chapter 10
A Patient with a Large Minimally Invasive Follicular Thyroid Cancer

Tracy S. Wang, Paolo Goffredo, and Julie Ann Sosa

Case Presentation

A 40-year-old man was found to have a thyroid nodule discovered on physical examination. He was clinically and biochemically euthyroid and had no symptoms of compression; specifically, he denied dysphagia, dyspnea, and voice changes. Thyroid ultrasound was performed, demonstrating a right thyroid nodule measuring $1.5 \times 1.3 \times 3.0$ cm and a normal left thyroid lobe. There was no evidence of cervical lymphadenopathy on ultrasound. Fine needle aspiration (FNA) biopsy was performed of the right thyroid nodule, and the cytology demonstrated "atypical follicular cells of undetermined significance (Bethesda category III)."

Given the cytological findings, a right thyroid lobectomy was performed. The final pathology demonstrated "a $1.5 \times 1.3 \times 3.0$ cm partially encapsulated follicular carcinoma, with >3 foci of transcapsular invasion, consistent with a minimally invasive follicular carcinoma" (Fig. 10.1). There was no evidence of vascular invasion. The patient did not undergo additional surgery and did not require thyroid hormone replacement.

T.S. Wang, MD, MPH (✉)
Section of Endocrine Surgery, Division of Surgical Oncology, Department of Surgery
Medical College of Wisconsin, 9200 W. Wisconsin Avenue, Milwaukee, WI 53226, USA
e-mail: tswang@mcw.edu

P. Goffredo, MD
Duke Clinical Research Institute, Duke University, 2400 Pratt St, Durham, NC 27705, USA
e-mail: paolo.goffredo@duke.edu

J.A. Sosa, MD, MA
Section of Endocrine Surgery, Dept of Surgery, Endocrine Neoplasia Diseases Group,
Duke Cancer Institute and Duke Clinical Research Institute, Duke University, DUMC #2945,
Durham, NC 27710, USA
e-mail: julie.sosa@duke.edu

D.S. Cooper, C. Durante (eds.), *Thyroid Cancer*,
DOI 10.1007/978-3-319-22401-5_10

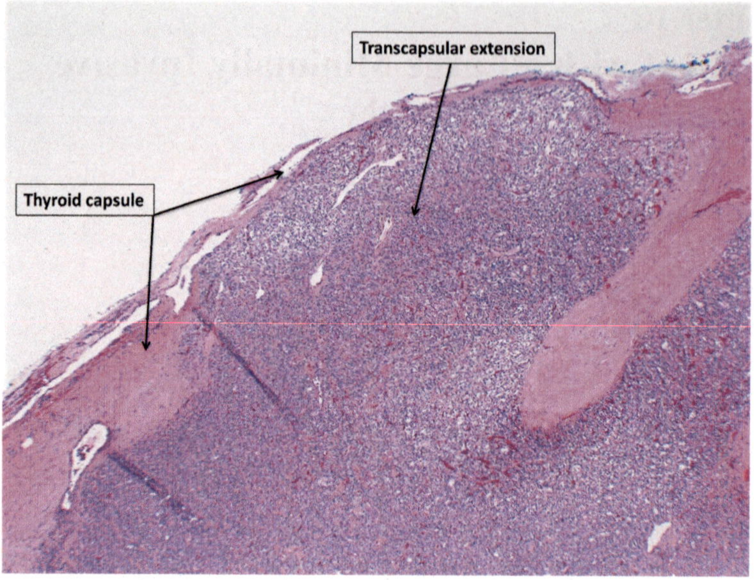

Fig. 10.1 Follicular thyroid cancer demonstrating capsular invasion of tumor

Literature Review

Definition

Follicular thyroid cancer (FTC) is a differentiated thyroid cancer, representing approximately 5.5 % of all thyroid malignancies [1]. Histologically, FTC is characterized by the absence of nuclear features of papillary thyroid carcinoma and the presence of capsular or vascular invasion; therefore, histologic rather than cytologic evaluation of tumors is mandatory to discern between malignant lesions and benign adenomas [2, 3]. The World Health Organization (WHO) histologic classification of thyroid tumors suggests a subclassification of FTC based on the degree of invasiveness, into minimally invasive follicular cancer (MIFC) and widely invasive follicular thyroid cancer (WIFC). According to the WHO, MIFC is an encapsulated follicular tumor of low malignant potential; unequivocal invasion of the blood vessels within or immediately outside of the tumor capsule and/or invasion that penetrates the full thickness of the capsule is required for diagnosis. WIFC is characterized by widespread infiltration of blood vessels and/or surrounding parenchyma and tissues, often lacking complete encapsulation [4]. FTC also may present as an oncocytic variant, Hürthle cell FTC, which is recognized by the WHO and characterized by the presence of >75 % of metaplastic cells, along with an abnormal accumulation of altered mitochondria [3, 5].

However, the criteria for diagnosis of MIFC are still controversial, even among experienced pathologists [6–12]. Although the WHO definition of a MIFC is a follicular tumor with complete capsular invasion, some consider even a focal extension into the capsule to be diagnostic for malignancy [10, 13, 14]. This diagnosis is made more difficult by the potential for disruption of the nodule at the time of FNA, by an intraoperative disruption of the capsule during thyroidectomy, or pathologic artifacts; all of these factors may be difficult to distinguish from neoplastic capsular invasion. Hence, the integrity of the tumor capsule is fundamental to allow proper diagnosis [15].

Similarly, the definition of vascular invasion is not consistent in the literature; some investigators diagnose MIFC only when fewer than four blood vessels are involved [16, 17]. In contrast, an update to the College of American Pathologists' thyroid cancer protocol published in 2009 reports that some authors believe that the presence of any vascular infiltration negates a diagnosis of MIFC due to the more aggressive behavior that these tumors demonstrate [8, 18]. In spite of controversies, there is consensus that histological examination of a minimum of ten tissue blocks is necessary for confirmation of FTC in encapsulated neoplasia.

Molecular Analysis

Over the past decade, research has focused on identifying potential genetic mutations in thyroid cancer that could be translated into clinical practice to complement preoperative FNA testing [19–21]. More than 70 % of differentiated thyroid cancers are found to carry identified genetic mutations, including *BRAF* and *RAS* point mutations and *RET*/*PTC* and *PAX8*/*PPARγ* gene fusions. These alterations can be detected in thyroid FNA and surgical specimens and molecular markers of diagnostic and prognostic significance. In fact, the 2009 revised American Thyroid Association (ATA) guidelines suggest that molecular markers such as *BRAF*, *RAS*, *RET*/*PTC*, and *PAX8*/*PPARγ* can be considered in the management of patients with indeterminate FNA cytology reports [22]. Specifically, *PAX8*/*PPARγ* rearrangement, which is a fusion of the PAX8 gene and the peroxisome proliferator-activated receptor (*PPARγ*) gene, is present in 30–40 % of conventional FTC and less often in oncocytic variants of FTC [20]. FTC patients with the mutation often present at a younger age have smaller tumors, and the tumors often have vascular invasion. While the presence of the mutation is not diagnostic of malignancy, it should prompt a more thorough search for potential capsular and vascular invasion. FTC also is associated with Cowden syndrome, which is within the spectrum of the phosphatase and tensin (PTEN)—hamartoma tumor syndrome caused by a germline mutation of the PTEN tumor suppressor gene. Up to 10 % of patients will develop thyroid cancer, most commonly FTC [23].

Recent studies have focused on other molecular analyses to identify potential markers of MIFC. Hunt et al. assessed a panel of ten tumor suppressor genes (*L-MYC*, *CMM*, *hOGG1*, *VHL*, *APC*, *MCC*, *MTS1*/*p16*, *pTEN*, *p53*, and *NF2*) to study loss of heterozygosity mutations, with the hypothesis that genotyping follicular-derived thyroid neoplasms may predict histologic aggressiveness [24].

Despite a limited sample size (8 follicular adenomas, 5 MIFC, and 5 WIFC), the authors found that the frequency of allelic loss (FAL) did correlate with histologic aggressiveness; follicular adenomas had a FAL of only 9 %, compared with a FAL of 30 % for MIFC and 53 % for WIFC. Lubitz et al. performed a microarray analysis of 13 follicular adenomas, seven MIFC, and seven WIFC to generate a list of differentially expressed genes and found that while many MIFCs were genetically similar, MIFC had 223 differently expressed genes, compared with follicular adenomas, and 365 differently expressed genes compared with WIFC [25]. This suggests that gene profiling may be useful in the molecular pathogenesis of MIFC and in predicting malignancy potential. Lastly, in a study of 34 patients with MIFC, including 12 with distant metastases and 13 patients with WIFC, comprehensive expression profiling was performed utilizing real-time PCR and PCR arrays to identify novel prognostic factors for metastatic MIFC using microRNA [26]. The authors found that several microRNA clusters correlated with metastatic MIFC, and that these expression levels were similar to those of patients with WIFC, suggesting a close similarity between metastatic MIFC and WIFC.

Prognosis

The subclassification between MIFC and WIFC carries a relevant prognostic meaning, given the excellent long-term prognosis and low rates of recurrent disease associated with MIFC [6, 10, 27, 28]. One of the earliest studies on the outcomes of patients with FTC was a review of 72 patients at the Mayo Clinic; 20 patients had capsular invasion only, and 45 patients had vascular invasion, with or without capsular invasion. After a median follow-up of 11 years, 10-year cause-specific mortality was 0 % for patients with capsular invasion and 28 % for patients with vascular invasion ($p=0.019$); the 10-year rates of development of distant metastases were 0 % and 19 %, respectively ($p=0.052$). This suggests that patients with FTC and only capsular invasion (the equivalent of the current definition of MIFC) represent a subgroup of patients that have excellent outcomes and therefore can be managed more conservatively [11).

A recent retrospective study from the Surveillance, Epidemiology, and End Results (SEER) database analyzed the largest published series of MIFC; a total of 1,200 patients with MIFC and 4,208 with WIFC were identified between 2000 and 2009. MIFC tumors were less likely than WIFC tumors to involve lymph nodes (0.9 vs. 3.6 %; $p<0.001$) and metastasize (0.5 vs. 8.9 %; $p<0001$). At last follow-up, a significantly greater proportion of patients with MIFC were alive (96.8 vs. 86.5 % WIFC; $p<0.001$). Of particular interest was that only two MIFC patients died of disease-specific causes (disease-specific survival rate, 99.8 %), compared to a disease-specific survival rate of 94.8 % in patients with WIFC ($p<0.001$). The overall survival rate of patients with MIFC was found to be comparable to that of the general US population (Fig. 10.2) [29]. In contrast, in a single institutional series of 251 Japanese patients diagnosed with MIFC from 1989 to 2006, Sugino et al. found

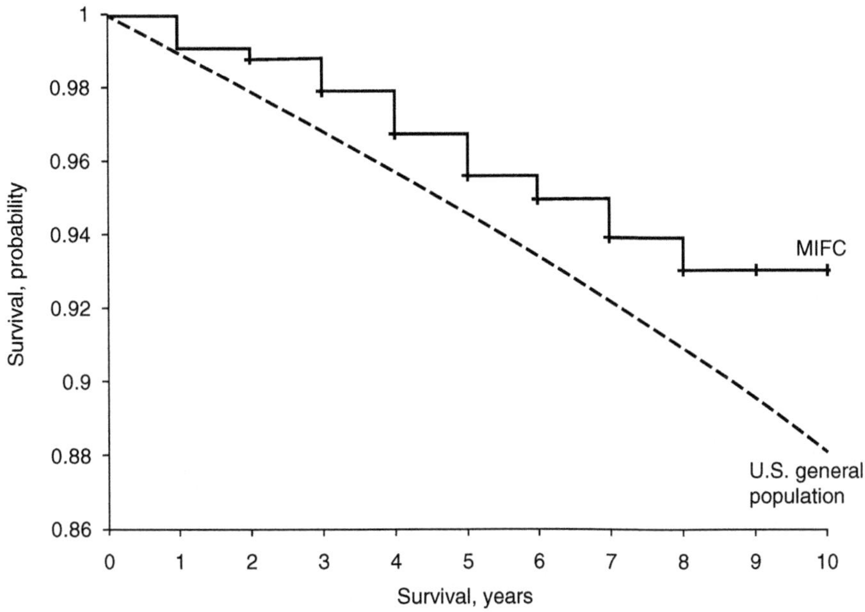

Fig. 10.2 Overall survival of MIFC versus U.S. general population [29]

a compromised cause-specific survival of 95.2, 89.5, and 84.5 % at 10, 15, and 20 years, respectively [30]. Distant metastases were identified in 54 (22 %) patients, including 22 patients with metastases identified at the time of initial surgery. On univariate analysis, tumor size ≥4 cm and patient age ≥45 years were associated with distant metastases. An explanation for such a divergence in survival between this study and the SEER study could be secondary to the higher rate of metastatic MIFC of the Sugino study: 21.5 % compared to 0.6 % of patients in the SEER database. The reason for the different rates of metastases between these two studies is not clear but may be due to differences in the cohort of analyzed patients; the Japanese manuscript included MIFCs with a larger mean tumor size than the US population-based analysis (4.4 cm vs. 3.4 cm, respectively) as well as pediatric patients, while the SEER study was limited to adults only.

Several other factors have been reported to affect prognosis of patients with MIFC. Patient age ≥45 years at the time of diagnosis is an established predictor of compromised survival for patients with differentiated thyroid cancers; the American Joint Committee on Cancer (AJCC) staging system utilizes two different staging systems for patients with differentiated thyroid cancer [31–33]. Patients <45 years are considered to have stage I disease, irrespective of the extent of locoregional metastases, unless distant metastases are present, in which patients are considered to have stage II disease. In contrast, patients ≥45 years are divided into stage I–IV disease, and those with locoregional lymph node metastases are classified as having stage III (N1a) or stage IV (N1b) disease. Ito et al. recently analyzed a cohort of 292 patients who underwent initial surgery between 1983 and 2007 and showed that MIFC in patients ≥45 years had compromised disease-free survival and cause-specific survival compared to similar patients who were younger [34]. Interestingly, the disease-free survival of patients <20 years of age tended to be reduced compared to patients aged 20–44 years; nevertheless, none of the patients <20 years died of their disease. Whereas previous studies have failed to demonstrate that vascular invasion was a negative prognostic factor, in 2013 two sets of investigators, Kim et al. and Ito et al., showed that extensive involvement of blood vessels was associated with increased disease-specific mortality in series of 165 and 292 MIFCs, respectively [11, 13, 27, 35]. This finding might be a helpful contribution to the debate regarding the definition of pathologic criteria for MIFC. Moreover, tumor size >4.0 cm has been reported to be associated with compromised outcomes in these patients [30, 36]. This is not surprising, considering that the 4.0 cm cutoff is taken into account both in the AJCC staging system and in the ATA guidelines for the management of thyroid nodules and differentiated thyroid cancer [22, 33].

The prognosis of the Hürthle cell variant of FTC has been controversial and ranges from a low malignant potential tumor to a more aggressive one. In a review of all thyroid cancer cases captured in the National Cancer Data Base, Hundahl et al. demonstrated that patients with the Hürthle cell variant of FTC had similar 5-year survival rates to patients with FTC, but at 10 years, patients with the Hürthle cell variant had a lower overall survival rate (76 vs. 85 %), suggesting that the prognosis for this variant may be compromised [37]. In contrast, in a SEER study of 172 patients with the Hürthle cell variant and 783 patients with non-Hürthle cell FTC, the histological distinction was less important than patient's age and gender and tumor stage with regard to association with the 10-year survival rate [38].

Treatment

The appropriate management of MIFC has not reached universal consensus. Based on the low rate of metastases and disease-specific mortality, there are proponents of thyroid lobectomy (with or without isthmusectomy) as an adequate treatment for MIFC [6, 10, 13, 15, 29, 39–41]. In one recent study, 124 patients with FTC were divided into three groups: MIFC, MIFC with vascular invasion, and WIFC. Overall, the disease-free survival rate was 85 % at a median follow-up of 40 months, but disease-free survival differed significantly among the groups, with rates ranging from 97 % for the MIFC group to 81 % for the MIFC withvascular invasion group to 46 % for the WIFC group. Only patients <45 years with MIFC (no vascular invasion) had 100 % disease-free survival, suggesting that in these patients, thyroid lobectomy alone may be sufficient, and that total thyroidectomy [with or without radioactive iodine ablation (RAI)] should be performed in all other patients with FTC [39].

In contrast, others have emphasized that MIFC can metastasize and is associated with compromised patient survival; therefore, total thyroidectomy followed by RAI has been advocated by some [30, 42–44]. In the Japanese series by Sugino et al., routine completion total thyroidectomy and RAI appeared not to be necessary for MIFC, particularly for small tumors and in young patients. However, a subsequent study from these researchers published in 2014 focused on the outcomes of MIFC patients who had a completion thyroidectomy; there, the authors reviewed 324 patients who underwent thyroid lobectomy for MIFC. Of these, 101 patients underwent completion thyroidectomy within 6 months of initial surgery, and 81 patients had radioiodine ablation. The remaining patients did not undergo further treatment. Overall cause-specific survival rates were 97.5, 94.8, and 92.8 % at 10, 15, and 20 years, and distant metastasis-free survival rates were 85.5, 75.2, and 73.5 % over the same time periods. After adjusting for possible confounders, the multivariate model appeared to show higher rates of distant metastases-free survival in patients who underwent completion thyroidectomy [44].

A consensus report on MIFC by the European Society of Endocrine Surgeons (ESES) recommended (recommendation rating: C) that thyroid lobectomy be performed for neoplasms with exclusive capsular invasion at diagnosis, without vascular invasion, without any lymph node or distant metastases, tumors <4.0 cm, and in patients <45 years [45]. Candidates for total thyroidectomy are patients ≥45 years, tumor size ≥4.0 cm, vascular invasion, and presence of lymph node or distant metastases. Lymphadenectomy was considered only when clinical evidence of lymph node metastasis was present. Lastly, ESES suggested using RAI when criteria for total thyroidectomy are met and if recurrence is observed in follow-up.

The current ATA guidelines do not make specific recommendations regarding extent of surgery for patients with MIFC [22]. The guidelines published by the National Comprehensive Cancer Network (NCCN) define MIFC as "a well-defined tumor with microscopic capsular and/or a few foci of vascular invasion" and suggest that thyroid lobectomy alone may be sufficient for patients with MIFC. In the NCCN recommendations, RAI is only recommended for patients with WIFC [46].

Clinical Pearls/Pitfalls

- MIFC is a follicular tumor with capsular invasion but minimal, if any, vascular invasion and is typically associated with excellent prognosis. Extent of surgery is controversial, with some guidelines suggesting that thyroid lobectomy alone may be sufficient and others implying that total thyroidectomy might be necessary for a higher-risk subset of MIFC patients (i.e., patients ≥45 years, tumor size ≥4.0 cm, vascular invasion, and presence of lymph node or distant metastases).
- WIFC is a follicular tumor with extensive capsular and vascular invasion. It carries a compromised prognosis. Total thyroidectomy, with consideration of RAI, should be performed.
- The optimal extent of surgery for patients with MIFC would be informed by additional research on this relatively uncommon histologic entity. Long-term follow-up will be necessary in such a cohort of patients in order to be able to detect meaningful differences, given the overall bright prognosis.

References

1. SEER Cancer Statistics Review 1975–2011. Cancer of the Thyroid (Invasive). http://seer.cancer.gov/csr/1975_2011/browse_csr.php?sectionSEL=26&pageSEL=sect_26_table.22.html. National Cancer Institute. Surveillance, Epidemiology, and End Results (SEER) Program; 2014 (cited 1 Aug 2014).
2. Franssila KO, Ackerman LV, Brown CL, Hedinger CE. Follicular carcinoma. Semin Diagn Pathol. 1985;2(2):101–22.
3. DeLellis RALR, Heitz PU, Eng C. WHO classification of tumours, pathology and genetics of tumours of endocrine organs. 1st ed. Lyon: World Health Organization/IARC Press; 2004.
4. Hedinger CEWE, Sobin LH. Histological typing of thyroid tumours. International histological classification of tumours, vol. 11. Berlin: Springer; 1988.
5. Goffredo P, Roman SA, Sosa JA. Hurthle cell carcinoma: a population-level analysis of 3311 patients. Cancer. 2013;119(3):504–11.
6. Huang CC, Hsueh C, Liu FH, Chao TC, Lin JD. Diagnostic and therapeutic strategies for minimally and widely invasive follicular thyroid carcinomas. Surg Oncol. 2011;20(1):1–6.
7. D'Avanzo A, Treseler P, Ituarte PH, Wong M, Streja L, Greenspan FS, et al. Follicular thyroid carcinoma: histology and prognosis. Cancer. 2004;100(6):1123–9.
8. Ghossein R. Update to the College of American Pathologists reporting on thyroid carcinomas. Head Neck Pathol. 2009;3(1):86–93.
9. Carcangiu ML. Minimally invasive follicular carcinoma. Endocr Pathol. 1997;8(3):231–4.
10. Heffess CS, Thompson LD. Minimally invasive follicular thyroid carcinoma. Endocr Pathol. 2001;12(4):417–22.
11. van Heerden JA, Hay ID, Goellner JR, Salomao D, Ebersold JR, Bergstralh EJ, et al. Follicular thyroid carcinoma with capsular invasion alone: a nonthreatening malignancy. Surgery. 1992;112(6):1130–6. discussion 6–8.
12. Baloch ZW, LiVolsi VA. Follicular-patterned afflictions of the thyroid gland: reappraisal of the most discussed entity in endocrine pathology. Endocr Pathol. 2014;25(1):12–20.
13. Thompson LD, Wieneke JA, Paal E, Frommelt RA, Adair CF, Heffess CS. A clinicopathologic study of minimally invasive follicular carcinoma of the thyroid gland with a review of the English literature. Cancer. 2001;91(3):505–24.
14. Rosai JCM, DeLellis RA. Tumours of the thyroid gland. Atlas of tumor pathology 3rd series, fascicle 5. Washington: Armed Forces Institute of Pathology; 1992. p. 49–63.
15. Hermann M, Tonninger K, Kober F, Furtlehner EM, Schultheis A, Neuhold N. [Minimally invasive follicular thyroid carcinoma: Not always total thyroidectomy]. Chirurg. 2010; 81(7):627–30. 632–5.
16. Rosai J. Handling of thyroid follicular patterned lesions. Endocr Pathol. 2005;16(4):279–83.
17. Lang BH, Lo CY, Chan WF, Lam KY, Wan KY. Staging systems for follicular thyroid carcinoma: application to 171 consecutive patients treated in a tertiary referral centre. Endocr Relat Cancer. 2007;14(1):29–42.
18. Baloch ZW, Livolsi VA. Follicular-patterned lesions of the thyroid: the bane of the pathologist. Am J Clin Pathol. 2002;117(1):143–50.
19. Raman P, Koenig RJ. Pax-8-PPAR-gamma fusion protein in thyroid carcinoma. Nat Rev Endocrinol. 2014;10:616–23.
20. Bhaijee F, Nikiforov YE. Molecular analysis of thyroid tumors. Endocr Pathol. 2011;22(3):126–33.
21. Nikiforov YE, Steward DL, Robinson-Smith TM, Haugen BR, Klopper JP, Zhu Z, et al. Molecular testing for mutations in improving the fine-needle aspiration diagnosis of thyroid nodules. J Clin Endocrinol Metab. 2009;94(6):2092–8.
22. Cooper DS, Doherty GM, Haugen BR, Kloos RT, Lee SL, Mandel SJ, et al. Revised American Thyroid Association management guidelines for patients with thyroid nodules and differentiated thyroid cancer. Thyroid. 2009;19(11):1167–214.

23. Laury AR, Bongiovanni M, Tille JC, Kozakewich H, Nose V. Thyroid pathology in PTEN-hamartoma tumor syndrome: characteristic findings of a distinct entity. Thyroid. 2011; 21(2):135–44.
24. Hunt JL, Livolsi VA, Baloch ZW, Swalsky PA, Bakker A, Sasatomi E, et al. A novel microdissection and genotyping of follicular-derived thyroid tumors to predict aggressiveness. Hum Pathol. 2003;34(4):375–80.
25. Lubitz CC, Gallagher LA, Finley DJ, Zhu B, Fahey 3rd TJ. Molecular analysis of minimally invasive follicular carcinomas by gene profiling. Surgery. 2005;138(6):1042–8. discussion 8–9.
26. Jikuzono T, Kawamoto M, Yoshitake H, Kikuchi K, Akasu H, Ishikawa H, et al. The miR-221/222 cluster, miR-10b and miR-92a are highly upregulated in metastatic minimally invasive follicular thyroid carcinoma. Int J Oncol. 2013;42(6):1858–68.
27. Ito Y, Hirokawa M, Masuoka H, Yabuta T, Kihara M, Higashiyama T, et al. Prognostic factors of minimally invasive follicular thyroid carcinoma: extensive vascular invasion significantly affects patient prognosis. Endocr J. 2013;60(5):637–42.
28. Ito Y, Hirokawa M, Masuoka H, Yabuta T, Fukushima M, Kihara M, et al. Distant metastasis at diagnosis and large tumor size are significant prognostic factors of widely invasive follicular thyroid carcinoma. Endocr J. 2013;60(6):829–33.
29. Goffredo P, Cheung K, Roman SA, Sosa JA. Can minimally invasive follicular thyroid cancer be approached as a benign lesion?: a population-level analysis of survival among 1,200 patients. Ann Surg Oncol. 2013;20(3):767–72.
30. Sugino K, Kameyama K, Ito K, Nagahama M, Kitagawa W, Shibuya H, et al. Outcomes and prognostic factors of 251 patients with minimally invasive follicular thyroid carcinoma. Thyroid. 2012;22(8):798–804.
31. Cho SW, Choi HS, Yeom GJ, Lim JA, Moon JH, Park YJ, et al. Long-term prognosis of differentiated thyroid cancer with lung metastasis in Korea and its prognostic factors. Thyroid. 2014;24(2):277–86.
32. Tran Cao HS, Johnston LE, Chang DC, Bouvet M. A critical analysis of the American Joint Committee on Cancer (AJCC) staging system for differentiated thyroid carcinoma in young patients on the basis of the surveillance, epidemiology, and end results (SEER) registry. Surgery. 2012;152(2):145–51.
33. Staging information for thyroid cancer http://cancer.gov/cancertopics/pdq/treatment/thyroid/HealthProfessional/page3: National Cancer Institute; 2014 (cited 1 Jun 2014).
34. Ito Y, Miyauchi A, Tomoda C, Hirokawa M, Kobayashi K, Miya A. Prognostic significance of patient age in minimally and widely invasive follicular thyroid carcinoma: investigation of three age groups. Endocr J. 2014;61(3):265–71.
35. Kim HJ, Sung JY, Oh YL, Kim JH, Son YI, Min YK, et al. Association of vascular invasion with increased mortality in patients with minimally invasive follicular thyroid carcinoma but not widely invasive follicular thyroid carcinoma. Head Neck 2014;36(12):1695–700.
36. Goldstein NS, Czako P, Neill JS. Metastatic minimally invasive (encapsulated) follicular and Hurthle cell thyroid carcinoma: a study of 34 patients. Mod Pathol. 2000;13(2):123–30.
37. Hundahl SA, Fleming ID, Fremgen AM, Menck HR. A national cancer data base report on 53,856 cases of thyroid carcinoma treated in the U.S., 1985–1995 (see comments). Cancer. 1998;83(12):2638–48.
38. Haigh PI, Urbach DR. The treatment and prognosis of Hurthle cell follicular thyroid carcinoma compared with its non-Hurthle cell counterpart. Surgery. 2005;138(6):1152–7. discussion 7–8.
39. O'Neill CJ, Vaughan L, Learoyd DL, Sidhu SB, Delbridge LW, Sywak MS. Management of follicular thyroid carcinoma should be individualised based on degree of capsular and vascular invasion. Eur J Surg Oncol. 2011;37(2):181–5.
40. Collini P, Sampietro G, Rosai J, Pilotti S. Minimally invasive (encapsulated) follicular carcinoma of the thyroid gland is the low-risk counterpart of widely invasive follicular carcinoma but not of insular carcinoma. Virchows Arch. 2003;442(1):71–6.

41. Shaha AR. Invited commentary: minimally invasive follicular thyroid carcinoma. Surgery. 2001;130(1):119–20.
42. Ban EJ, Andrabi A, Grodski S, Yeung M, McLean C, Serpell J. Follicular thyroid cancer: minimally invasive tumours can give rise to metastases. ANZ J Surg. 2012;82(3):136–9.
43. Delbridge L, Parkyn R, Philips J, Barraclough B, Robinson B. Minimally invasive follicular thyroid carcinoma: completion thyroidectomy or not? ANZ J Surg. 2002;72(11):844–5.
44. Sugino K, Kameyama K, Nagahama M, Kitagawa W, Shibuya H, Ohkuwa K, et al. Does completion thyroidectomy improve the outcome of patients with minimally invasive follicular carcinoma of the thyroid? Ann Surg Oncol. 2014;21(9):2981–6.
45. Dionigi G, Kraimps JL, Schmid KW, Hermann M, Sheu-Grabellus SY, De Wailly P, et al. Minimally invasive follicular thyroid cancer (MIFTC)—a consensus report of the European Society of Endocrine Surgeons (ESES). Langenbeck's Arch Surg. 2014;399(2):165–84.
46. NCCN guidelines: thyroid carcinoma. https://www.nccn.org/store/login/login.aspx?ReturnURL=http://www.nccn.org/professionals/physician_gls/PDF/thyroid.pdf. National Comprehensive Cancer Network 2012 (cited 1 Aug 2014).

Chapter 11
A Young Patient with Intrathyroidal Papillary Thyroid Cancer and Family History of Differentiated Thyroid Cancer

Cosimo Durante, Fabiana Trulli, and Sebastiano Filetti

Case Presentation

A general practitioner referred an asymptomatic 39-year-old man to our center for thyroid ultrasonography. The patient had no evidence of thyroid disease, and his past medical history was unremarkable. However, his mother and his uncle had both been diagnosed with papillary thyroid cancer (PTC). Both had been treated with thyroidectomy followed by radioactive iodine (RAI) remnant ablation (RRA), and the uncle also had had multiple RAI therapies for RAI-avid lung metastases. At the time of the patient's referral, they had been disease-free for 5 and 1.5 years, respectively. There was no documentable history of radiation exposure.

The patient's physical examination was negative, but thyroid and neck ultrasonography revealed multiple hypoechoic lesions in both lobes of the thyroid. The largest nodule, which was located in the left lobe, measured 10 mm and exhibited intranodular punctate hyperechogenicity and signs of central and perilesional vascularity. There was no clinical or sonographic evidence of lymph node involvement. The patient was euthyroid (serum TSH: 1.4 mIU/L). The dominant nodule was subjected to fine-needle aspiration biopsy (FNAB), and the cytology findings were consistent with PTC (Bethesda class VI) [1]. A total thyroidectomy was performed. The pathology showed multifocal, bilateral, classic variant PTC (lesion diameters: left lobe, 9 and 2 mm; isthmus, 4 mm; right lobe, 5 mm). There was no evidence of extrathyroidal extension or vascular invasion (pT1am, Nx—AJCC/TNM VII Edition Stage 1) [2]. Based on the 2009 American Thyroid Association (ATA) Initial Risk Stratification System [3], the patient's disease was considered at low risk for

C. Durante, MD (✉) • S. Filetti, MD
Department of Internal Medicine and Medical Specialties, University of Rome "Sapienza", Viale del Policlinico 155, 00161 Rome, Italy
e-mail: cosimo.durante@uniroma1.it

F. Trulli, MD
Gustave Roussy and University Paris Sud, 114 rue Edouard Vaillant, 94800 Villejuif, France

D.S. Cooper, C. Durante (eds.), *Thyroid Cancer*,
DOI 10.1007/978-3-319-22401-5_11

recurrence. Because the case met the current criteria for familial nonmedullary thyroid cancer (FNMTC), however, the possibilities that the patient might actually be at higher risk than he seemed to be, and that other members of his family might be genetically predisposed to thyroid cancer, had to be considered.

Literature Review

Approximately 3–10 % of all NMTCs appear to be familial [4, 5]. Excluding those tumors linked to familial adenomatous polyposis, Gardner's syndrome, Cowden disease, Werner's syndrome, or Carney's complex, most of these cases have not been linked to specific genetic causes [4]. Therefore, the diagnosis is generally made when NMTC has been found in two or more first-degree relatives. When cases are defined in this manner, the probability that affected family members actually have sporadic tumors has been estimated at about 30–40 %, but when three of more members of a kindred are affected, the probability of hereditary disease climbs to over 96 % [6].

Management of patients with FNMTC should be based for the most part on the ATA risk class of the individual patient, although a positive family history is a potential risk modifier. In terms of surgery, for example, the 2015 ATA guidelines list familial disease as one of the *possible* indications for choosing thyroidectomy over lobectomy (others being age>45 years, the presence of nodules in the contralateral lobe, or a personal history of radiation therapy to the head and neck) [5]. The issue of RRA in this context is even more of a gray area. Our patient had multiple foci of PTC, each with a maximum diameter of less than 1 cm, and his risk for recurrence was thus classified as low. There is an appreciable difference between the risks of recurrence associated with unifocal and multifocal papillary microcarcinomas (1–2 % vs. 4–6 %, respectively), especially when the sum of the diameters of the tumor foci exceeds 1 cm (as it did in our patient) [7]. Nonetheless, the risk remains low in both cases, and there is no evidence that RRA improves the disease-specific or disease-free survival in either case—unless there are other high-risk features [5].

Does the fact that the multifocal disease is familial rather than sporadic constitute an additional high-risk feature that could tip the scales in favor of RRA? Conflicting data have been published on the clinical behavior of FNMTCs. Some studies suggest that they are indeed more aggressive than their sporadic counterparts, as reflected by higher rates of extrathyroidal invasion, lymph node metastases, and postoperative recurrence and significantly lower rates of disease-free survival [8]. Others studies, however, have found that the prognosis for FNMTC (even in kindreds with three or more affected members) is not significantly different from that of similarly treated sporadic NMTCs, even though the familial cases were associated with higher rates of multifocal involvement in index cases and a possibly greater tendency to spread outside the thyroid [9–11]. The discrepancies between these findings have been attributed to the possible/probable polygenetic etiology of FNMTC suggested by the wide variation in penetrance documented in many large pedigrees [4]. It has also been suggested that closer surveillance of the relatives of patients who have FNMTCs leads to earlier diagnosis and treatment of familial forms of the disease, thereby improving the prognosis and attenuating evidence of their increased aggressiveness relative to sporadic NMTCs [4].

The actual value of screening thyroid ultrasonography for unaffected family members is also uncertain. Formal cost-benefit studies have yet to be undertaken, but the results will in any case reflect features of the local health-care system. In general, screening of apparently healthy family members believed to be at increased risk for cancer is recommended when the following criteria are satisfied. First, the familial form of the cancer should be more aggressive than the sporadic form; otherwise, the early diagnosis offered by the screening program would probably not represent any clinically important benefit. As noted above, there is no conclusive evidence that familial NMTCs are more aggressive than their nonfamilial counterparts. Second, the screening test itself should be simple and safe to perform, clinically validated, and accurate (high sensitivity and specificity for detecting early-stage disease). Thyroid ultrasonography with FNAb confirmation meets all of these criteria [5]. Third, for disease that is identified early through screening, there must be some treatment or intervention capable of improving the outcome (in terms of recurrence and/or mortality rates) over that associated with later detection. There are no data from RCTs on interventions of this sort for relatives of patients with FNMTC. The 2015 ATA guidelines acknowledge that ultrasound-based screening may lead to earlier diagnosis of thyroid cancer in these cases, but the panel refrains from recommending for or against this practice since evidence is lacking that it would diminish morbidity or mortality [5].

Back to the Patient

In kindreds with only two members having DTCs, the possibility that the cancers may actually be sporadic is substantial. Our patient, however, was the third member of his family to develop PTC, so the likelihood of true familial disease was much higher. We discussed the fact that his own cancer had all the earmarks of being low risk for recurrence, and we reviewed the pros and cons of RRA. In the end, the patient opted for ablation, noting that both his mother and uncle had received the same treatment and "they seem to be doing pretty well." He was also strongly in favor of sonographic screening for his siblings and his children. Following the diagnosis of her brother's thyroid cancer, he said, his mother had had a thyroid scan (it was not clear who had ordered the test) and that "as a result of that precaution," she had experienced far less morbidity than her brother.

The patient underwent RRA (administered activity: 30 mCi), and at the 1-year follow-up visit, the cervical ultrasound examination revealed no macroscopic evidence of residual thyroid tissue and no findings suggestive of lymph node involvement. The recombinant human TSH-stimulated thyroglobulin level was 0.8 ng/mL (normal: <1), and the thyroglobulin antibody assay was negative. His sister (age 41) and his two brothers (51 and 48 years old) have all undergone screening sonography in our center. The sister's examination revealed a 12-mm nodule in the right lobe, with suspicious sonographic and cytologic features (Bethesda class V) [1]. She is scheduled for surgery in the near future and promises to become the fourth member of the family with thyroid cancer. The patient's two children, currently 2 and 3 years old, will be screened after puberty.

Clinical Pearls

- At present, there is no convincing evidence that the treatment strategies indicated by the initial ATA Risk Classification of NMTC should be substantially modified solely because the disease seems to be familial rather than sporadic.
- Likewise, there is no evidence that sonographic screening of unaffected family members in these kindreds will have any significant impact on morbidity or mortality.
- Treatment planning with patients who have been diagnosed with familial neoplastic disease can be "complicated" by psychological factors that are absent in cases of sporadic cancer, e.g., the patient's recall of loved ones who have had the disease and anxiety over the prospect of other cases in the family.

References

1. Cibas ES, Ali SZ. The Bethesda system for reporting thyroid cytopathology. Am J Clin Pathol. 2009;132(5):658–65.
2. Edge SB, Byrd DR, Carducci MA, Compton CC, editors. AJCC cancer staging manual. 7th ed. New York: Springer; 2009.
3. Cooper DS, Doherty GM, Haugen BR, Kloos RT, Lee SL, Mandel SJ, Mazzaferri EL, McIver B, Pacini F, Schlumberger M, Sherman SI, Steward DL, Tuttle RM. Revised American Thyroid Association management guidelines for patients with thyroid nodules and differentiated thyroid cancer. American Thyroid Association (ATA) Guidelines Taskforce on Thyroid Nodules and Differentiated Thyroid Cancer. Thyroid. 2009;19(11):1167–214.
4. Mazeh H, Sippel RS. Familial nonmedullary thyroid carcinoma. Thyroid. 2013;23(9): 1049–56.
5. Haugen BR, Alexander EK, Bible KC, Doherty GM, Mandel SJ, Nikiforov YE, Pacini F, Randolph GW, Sawka AM, Schlumberger M, Schuff K, Sherman SI, Sosa JA, Steward DL, Tuttle RM, Wartofsky L. American Thyroid Association management guidelines for patients with thyroid nodules and differentiated thyroid cancer. Thyroid. 2015 (in press).
6. Charkes ND. On the prevalence of familial nonmedullary thyroid cancer in multiply affected kindreds. Thyroid. 2006;16(2):181–6.
7. Roti E, degli Uberti EC, Bondanelli M, Braverman LE. Thyroid papillary microcarcinoma: a descriptive and meta-analysis study. Eur J Endocrinol. 2008;159(6):659–73.
8. Uchino S, Noguchi S, Kawamoto H, Yamashita H, Watanabe S, Yamashita H, Shuto S. Familial nonmedullary thyroid carcinoma characterized by multifocality and a high recurrence rate in a large study population. World J Surg. 2002;26(8):897–902.

9. Maxwell EL, Hall FT, Freeman JL. Familial non-medullary thyroid cancer: a matched-case control study. Laryngoscope. 2004;114(12):2182–6.
10. Robenshtok E, Tzvetov G, Grozinsky-Glasberg S, Shraga-Slutzky I, Weinstein R, Lazar L, Serov S, Singer J, Hirsch D, Shimon I, Benbassat C. Clinical characteristics and outcome of familial nonmedullary thyroid cancer: a retrospective controlled study. Thyroid. 2011;21(1):43–8.
11. Pinto AE, Silva GL, Henrique R, Menezes FD, Teixeira MR, Leite V, Cavaco BM. Familial vs sporadic papillary thyroid carcinoma: a matched-case comparative study showing similar clinical/prognostic behaviour. Eur J Endocrinol. 2013;170(2):321–7.

Chapter 12
A Child with Papillary Thyroid Cancer and Locally Advanced Disease but No Distant Metastasis

Sarah J. Bottomley and Steven G. Waguespack

Introduction

Papillary thyroid carcinoma (PTC) is the most common type of thyroid cancer in the pediatric population, representing 90 % or more of cases in patients ≤18 years of age. Children with PTC are more likely to present with regional lymph node involvement and extra-thyroidal extension. Despite often having advanced cervical disease at presentation, pediatric patients have very favorable outcomes with long-term survival decades after diagnosis being the norm. The management of lymph node metastases is primarily surgical, and the role of radioactive iodine (RAI) in the treatment of cervical disease in children is evolving.

Case Presentation

A 17-year-old female was found by her primary care provider to have a palpable right thyroid mass. She had no personal risk factors for thyroid cancer and was clinically and biochemically euthyroid. Neck ultrasound revealed a dominant solid nodule in the right lobe measuring 3.5 × 2.1 × 2.4 cm; cervical lymph nodes were not interrogated. The patient was seen by a local general surgeon, who performed a

S.J. Bottomley, MSN, RN, CPNP (✉)
The Children's Cancer Hospital, MD Anderson Cancer Center,
University of Texas, 1515 Holcombe Blvd, Unit 87, Houston, TX 77080, USA
e-mail: sjbottom@mdanderson.org

S.G. Waguespack, MD, FAAP, FACE
Department of Endocrine Neoplasia and Hormonal Disorders, MD Anderson Cancer Center,
University of Texas, Unit 1461, PO Box 301402, Houston, TX 77230, USA
e-mail: swagues@mdanderson.org

D.S. Cooper, C. Durante (eds.), *Thyroid Cancer*,
DOI 10.1007/978-3-319-22401-5_12

right thyroid lobectomy without a preoperative fine-needle aspiration biopsy (FNAB). Pathology revealed a T2N0Mx PTC, classical subtype, with focal angioinvasion and positive surgical margins. There was one small lymph node adjacent to the gland that was disease-free. Three days later, the patient underwent a completion thyroidectomy with a central neck dissection (CND). The left lobe of the thyroid was without evidence of disease, and in the central compartment, 16/26 lymph nodes (overall sizes ranging from 0.2 to 1.5 cm; no extranodal extension) were positive for PTC.

The patient presented to a tertiary cancer center for further evaluation. Neck US revealed a suspicious, 1.3 cm right level IV lymph node (Fig. 12.1a) that was positive for PTC on FNAB. Because the patient was already hypothyroid, a ^{123}I thyroid scan and a stimulated thyroglobulin (Tg) level (TSH 86 mIU/L) were obtained after the patient followed a strict low iodine diet for a week. There was uptake identified in the thyroid bed, but no lateral cervical uptake was seen (Fig. 12.1b). The stimulated Tg was 2.0 ng/ml but with a mildly positive Tg antibody (46 IU/ml; normal ≤40). Given these results, a right lateral neck dissection was undertaken, and pathology revealed 8/26 lymph nodes positive for PTC (overall sizes ranging

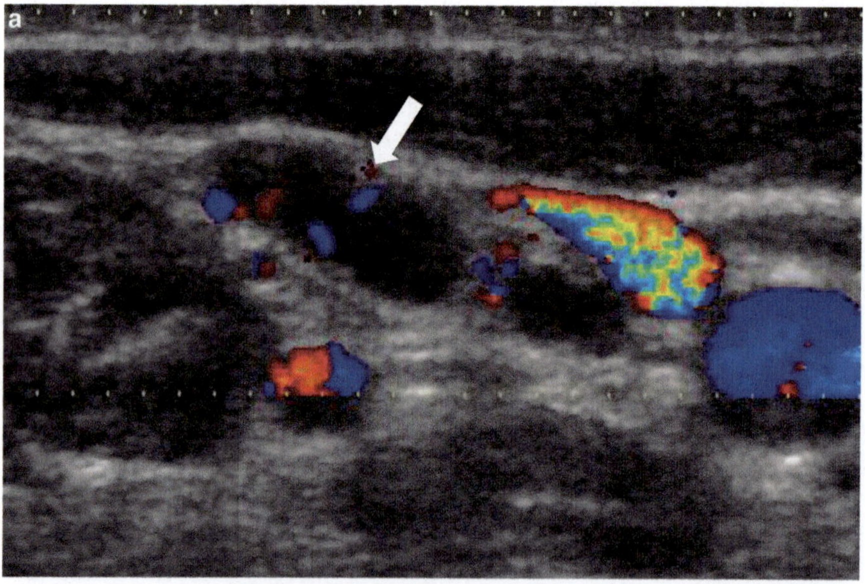

Fig. 12.1 A 17-year-old female with a locally metastatic PTC presented for further evaluation at a tertiary cancer center after having already had two surgeries. Cervical ultrasonography revealed a suspicious, 1.3 cm right level IV lymph node (**a**, *arrow*), which was proven to be PTC after fine-needle aspiration biopsy. Despite the presence of residual lymph node disease, there was no indication of iodine-avid lateral neck metastases on a diagnostic ^{123}I thyroid scan (**b**). Preoperative contrast-enhanced CT also identified a suspicious lymph node in the right tracheoesophageal groove (**c**, *arrow*), which was resected and proven to be PTC. Subsequent to her third surgery, the patient had no evidence of residual PTC, and she remains disease-free greater than 4 years after her last surgery.

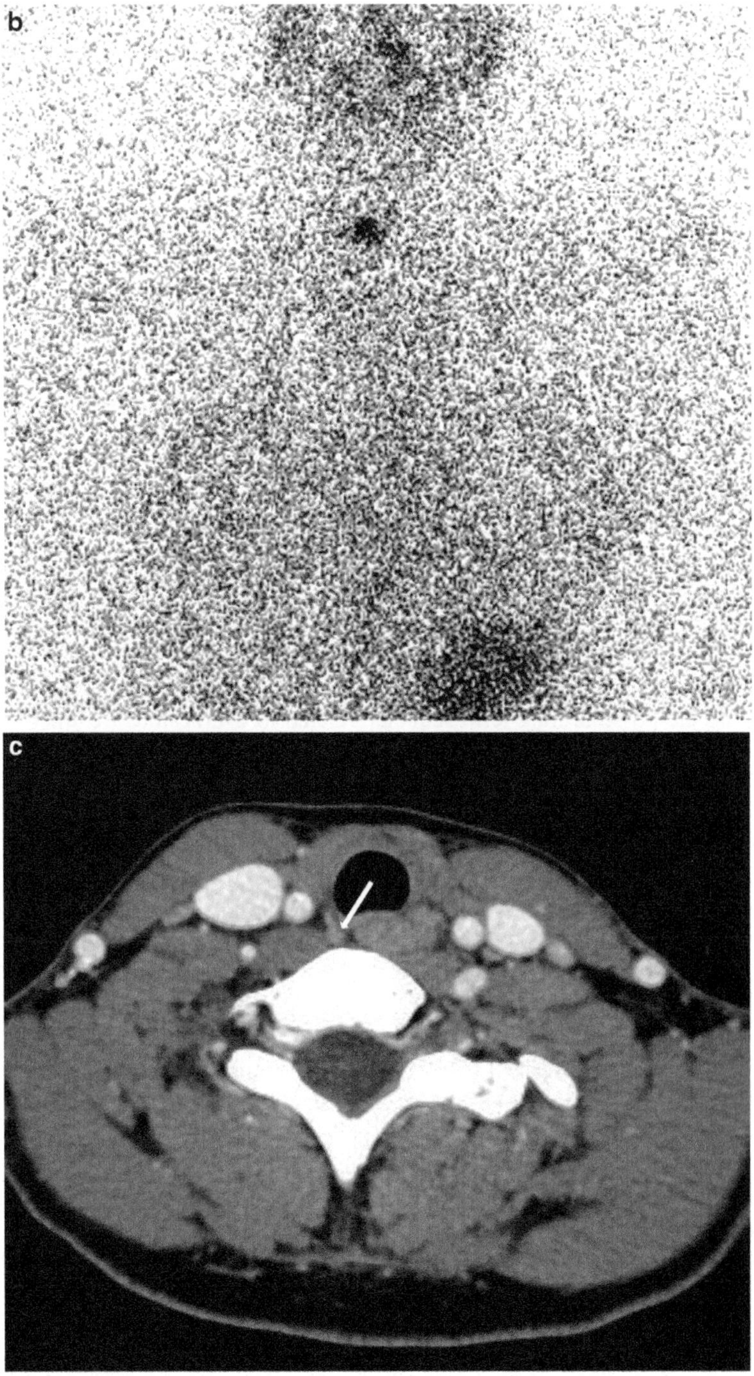

Fig. 12.1 (continued)

from 0.1 to 1.6 cm; no extranodal extension); the tumor was negative for the *BRAF* V600E mutation. In addition to the right neck dissection, the right central compartment was reexplored because a preoperative contrast-enhanced CT suggested an abnormal lymph node in the right tracheoesophageal groove (Fig. 12.1c); on pathology, a single right paratracheal lymph node (0.5 cm; no extranodal extension) was positive for PTC.

Assessment and Literature Review

Thyroid cancer is rare in the pediatric population, but the incidence appears to be increasing, especially in adolescents. PTC is the most common type, accounting for 90 % or more of childhood thyroid cancers, followed by follicular and, rarely, medullary thyroid carcinoma. PTC is frequently multifocal and bilateral, and in children, regional lymph node metastases occur in >80 % of cases at diagnosis [1–7]. Patients with a significant volume of cervical disease are at the highest risk of hematogenous metastases to the lungs [3, 4], which occur in up to 25 % of pediatric cases in some series [5, 8–10]. Despite more extensive disease at clinical presentation, pediatric PTC is biologically distinct from PTC diagnosed in older adults, and children with PTC have an extremely low disease-specific mortality (2 % or less decades after diagnosis) [9, 11]. This excellent prognosis, coupled with unique concerns regarding the possible long-term sequelae related to overzealous treatment during childhood, makes the management of pediatric PTC challenging. It is only recently that formal guidelines for the management of pediatric PTC have been developed by the American Thyroid Association (ATA) [12].

Children with PTC typically present with a palpable thyroid nodule and/or overt cervical lymphadenopathy [1, 2], which is not uncommonly treated with an antibiotic before the diagnosis of PTC is recognized. The initial workup of suspected PTC should include a comprehensive cervical and soft tissue neck US by an experienced ultrasonographer, given the high rate of lymph node metastases. US-guided FNAB in children is a sensitive and specific tool for the diagnosis and management of PTC, and it is recommended in all children to confirm the diagnosis and properly stage the extent of cervical disease. FNAB of suspicious lymph nodes is also essential for planning the appropriate initial surgical approach, which is the mainstay of therapy in pediatric PTC.

Contemporary guidelines recommend that children with PTC be cared for at centers where there is multidisciplinary expertise in the management of pediatric thyroid cancer [12], and it is always preferred that surgery be performed by a high-volume thyroid surgeon, defined in previous studies as a surgeon who performs 30 or more cervical endocrine procedures annually [12, 13]. Most pediatric patients with PTC will require a total thyroidectomy (TT) with or without a compartment-oriented neck dissection. The type of surgery planned is based on the results of preoperative comprehensive neck ultrasonography and FNAB. Additionally, cross-sectional imaging, using either a contrast-enhanced CT of the neck or MRI, is recommended for those with fixed thyroid masses, vocal cord paralysis, or bulky lymphadenopathy [12, 14]. Although the use of iodinated CT contrast may delay postoperative evaluation and treatment with RAI, it is considered the best diagnostic study in which to inform the surgeon about the extent of cervical disease and its anatomic relationship with critical aerodigestive structures.

Current data suggest that the single most important factor for improving long-term disease-free survival is the extent of the initial surgery, with more comprehensive surgery decreasing or eliminating the need for additional surgery and decreasing the risk of recurrence [4, 7, 9–11, 15, 16]. However, previous studies are confounded by the routine use of RAI, and so further studies are required. Current ATA guidelines recommend a CND in children who have gross extrathyroidal invasion and/or locoregional metastasis identified either pre- or intraoperatively [12]. Lateral neck dissection is recommended in those with FNAB-proven lateral neck disease.

The role of prophylactic CND in pediatric PTC without imaging evidence of lymph node metastases is very controversial. Due to the very high prevalence of cervical metastasis in children, prophylactic CND may be selectively considered based upon tumor size and focality. For patients with unifocal PTC, especially tumors >1 cm [17], an ipsilateral CND, with pursuit of contralateral CND only if intraoperative findings suggest central compartment disease, may help to balance the risks and benefits. In all cases, the plan for CND should be driven by the experience of the surgeon. Preservation of parathyroid and voice function is paramount, even if all central neck disease is not removed.

The inaugural ATA guidelines introduced a new risk categorization (ATA pediatric low, intermediate, and high risk) that helps to identify patients at risk of persistent cervical disease and to determine which patients should undergo more intensive postoperative staging [12]. Children with incidental, microscopic central lymph node disease are considered low risk, with recommendations to monitor thyroglobulin (Tg) levels and neck US after the initial surgery. Children with more significant central or lateral neck disease are considered ATA pediatric intermediate (clinical N1a or microscopic N1b disease) or high risk (clinical N1b disease), and postoperative staging with a diagnostic RAI scan and a TSH-stimulated Tg is recommended to identify persistent locoregional or distantly metastatic disease [12, 14]. Children who are found or suspected to have iodine-avid nodal disease may benefit from ^{131}I therapy if the disease is not amenable to further surgery, as determined by consultation with a thyroid cancer surgeon. Children who have no scintigraphic or Tg evidence of residual cervical disease or distant metastases may not benefit from routine adjuvant ^{131}I therapy [12, 14], but further research is needed. Nevertheless, decisions regarding ^{131}I therapy in pediatric PTC should weigh the long-term risks of RAI (primarily second malignancies [11]) against the potential benefits of therapy.

All children with PTC are replaced with exogenous thyroid hormone, and the goal of TSH depends on initial clinical and pathologic staging [12, 14]. In most children with lymph node metastases, the TSH is initially maintained around 0.1 mIU/L, and TSH suppression can eventually be reduced in children who have no evidence of disease after a 1–3-year period of follow-up. Similar to adults and even when ^{131}I therapy is not used, Tg levels can be used as a marker of residual or recurrent disease, assuming there are no interfering Tg autoantibodies. However, the degree of Tg elevation that correlates to disease is not well studied in children, and current Tg cutoffs employed in the care of adults with PTC may not be applicable to young children. In any event, the trend of the Tg level over time is more informative than an isolated measurement. Finally, cervical US is a highly sensitive clinical tool to identify residual/recurrent PTC, and it is recommended at 6–12-month intervals early in the follow-up period and then with a frequency based upon the patient's ATA pediatric risk level and clinical concern for disease [12].

Back to the Case

Postoperatively, the patient was categorized as ATA pediatric intermediate risk due to extensive N1a and minimal N1b lymph node disease. Therefore, postoperative restaging was undertaken with a hypothyroid ^{123}I thyroid scan (2.2 mCi) and a stimulated Tg, which revealed 0.1 % uptake in the right thyroid bed and a value of <0.9 ng/ml with an undetectable Tg antibody, respectively. ^{131}I therapy was not recommended due to the reassuring clinical data, the unclear benefit of RAI in this young patient, as well as the knowledge that previous residual right neck disease did not clearly concentrate iodine on a ^{123}I diagnostic scan. Expectant monitoring and mild TSH suppression were recommended, and over 4 years after her third surgery, she remained without evidence of disease based upon neck US and non-stimulated Tg and Tg antibody levels, both of which remained undetectable.

Clinical Pearls

- In the child presenting with a thyroid nodule, FNAB is safe and effective in making a diagnosis of PTC, which in turn allows for the most appropriate surgery (usually total thyroidectomy ± lymph node dissection) to be performed at the outset.
- Lymph node metastases are very common in children with PTC and are best treated by surgical resection.
- Preoperative staging with a comprehensive cervical US and FNAB of suspicious lymph nodes is essential; in addition, contrast-enhanced CT (preferred) or MRI may help to identify additional sites of disease and clarify anatomic relationships, both of which can enhance surgical planning and oncologic outcome.
- Comprehensive surgery, including a compartment-oriented lymph node resection dictated by imaging findings and clinical presentation, should be performed by a high-volume thyroid surgeon.
- ^{131}I therapy may not be necessary in all children with lymph node metastases, especially if there is no clinical evidence for residual cervical disease at the time of postoperative staging.

- Not all lymph node disease is iodine avid, and the role of RAI in eradicating cervical disease in children remains poorly studied; for persistent macroscopic LN disease, repeat surgery by a high-volume thyroid surgeon is preferred over RAI in most cases.
- The follow-up of children with PTC incorporates routine cervical ultrasonography and the measurement of Tg levels; the goal of TSH suppression depends on the extent of initial disease and current disease status.

References

1. Zimmerman D, Hay ID, Gough IR, Goellner JR, Ryan JJ, Grant CS, McConahey WM. Papillary thyroid carcinoma in children and adults: long-term follow-up of 1039 patients conservatively treated at one institution during three decades. Surgery. 1988;104:1157–66.
2. Frankenthaler RA, Sellin RV, Cangir A, Goepfert H. Lymph node metastasis from papillary-follicular thyroid carcinoma in young patients. Am J Surg. 1990;160:341–3.
3. Wada N, Sugino K, Mimura T, Nagahama M, Kitagawa W, Shibuya H, Ohkuwa K, Nakayama H, Hirakawa S, Yukawa N, Rino Y, Masuda M, Ito K. Treatment strategy of papillary thyroid carcinoma in children and adolescents: clinical significance of the initial nodal manifestation. Ann Surg Oncol. 2009;16:3442–9.
4. Machens A, Lorenz K, Nguyen Thanh P, Brauckhoff M, Dralle H. Papillary thyroid cancer in children and adolescents does not differ in growth pattern and metastatic behavior. J Pediatr. 2010;157:648–52.
5. Newman KD, Black T, Heller G, Azizkhan RG, Holcomb 3rd GW, Sklar C, Vlamis V, Haase GM, La Quaglia MP. Differentiated thyroid cancer: determinants of disease progression in patients <21 years of age at diagnosis: a report from the Surgical Discipline Committee of the Children's Cancer Group. Ann Surg. 1998;227:533–41.
6. Popovtzer A, Shpitzer T, Bahar G, Feinmesser R, Segal K. Thyroid cancer in children: management and outcome experience of a referral center. Otolaryngol Head Neck Surg. 2006;135:581–4.
7. Savio R, Gosnell J, Palazzo FF, Sywak M, Agarwal G, Cowell C, Shun A, Robinson B, Delbridge LW. The role of a more extensive surgical approach in the initial multimodality management of papillary thyroid cancer in children. J Pediatr Surg. 2005;40:1696–700.
8. Bal CS, Kumar A, Chandra P, Dwivedi SN, Mukhopadhyaya S. Is chest x-ray or high-resolution computed tomography scan of the chest sufficient investigation to detect pulmonary metastasis in pediatric differentiated thyroid cancer? Thyroid. 2004;14:217–25.
9. Demidchik YE, Demidchik EP, Reiners C, Biko J, Mine M, Saenko VA, Yamashita S. Comprehensive clinical assessment of 740 cases of surgically treated thyroid cancer in children of Belarus. Ann Surg. 2006;243:525–32.
10. Handkiewicz-Junak D, Wloch J, Roskosz J, Krajewska J, Kropinska A, Pomorski L, Kukulska A, Prokurat A, Wygoda Z, Jarzab B. Total thyroidectomy and adjuvant radioiodine treatment independently decrease locoregional recurrence risk in childhood and adolescent differentiated thyroid cancer. J Nucl Med. 2007;48:879–88.
11. Hay ID, Gonzalez-Losada T, Reinalda MS, Honetschlager JA, Richards ML, Thompson GB. Long-term outcome in 215 children and adolescents with papillary thyroid cancer treated during 1940 through 2008. World J Surg. 2010;34:1192–202.
12. Francis GL, Waguespack SG, Bauer AJ, Angelos P, Benvenga S, Cerutti JM, Dinauer CA, Hamilton J, Hay ID, Luster M, Parisi MT, Rachmiel M, Thompson GB, Yamashita S. Management guidelines for children with thyroid nodules and differentiated thyroid cancer: The American Thyroid Association guidelines task force on pediatric thyroid cancer. Thyroid. 2015;25(7):716–59.

13. Tuggle CT, Roman SA, Wang TS, Boudourakis L, Thomas DC, Udelsman R, Ann Sosa J. Pediatric endocrine surgery: who is operating on our children? Surgery. 2008;144:869–77. discussion 877.
14. Waguespack SG, Francis G. Initial management and follow-up of differentiated thyroid cancer in children. J Natl Compr Canc Netw. 2010;8:1289–300.
15. Jarzab B, Handkiewicz Junak D, Wloch J, Kalemba B, Roskosz J, Kukulska A, Puch Z. Multivariate analysis of prognostic factors for differentiated thyroid carcinoma in children. Eur J Nucl Med. 2000;27:833–41.
16. Sywak M, Cornford L, Roach P, Stalberg P, Sidhu S, Delbridge L. Routine ipsilateral level VI lymphadenectomy reduces postoperative thyroglobulin levels in papillary thyroid cancer. Surgery. 2006;140:1000–5. discussion 1005–7.
17. Lee KE, Chung IY, Kang E, Koo do H, Kim KH, Kim SW, Youn YK, Oh SK. Ipsilateral and contralateral central lymph node metastasis in papillary thyroid cancer: patterns and predictive factors of nodal metastasis. Head Neck. 2013;35:672–6.

Part III
Low Risk Differentiated Thyroid Cancer: *Postoperative Follow-Up*

Chapter 13
A Patient with Papillary Thyroid Cancer and Biochemical Evidence of Disease at the One-Year Follow-Up Visit

Cosimo Durante and Sebastiano Filetti

Case Presentation

A 54-year-old man with type 2 diabetes and hypertension underwent Doppler ultrasound assessment of the carotid arteries as part of a primary cardiovascular prevention program. He was referred to our staff because the examination disclosed an asymptomatic nodule in the right lobe of the thyroid. Ultrasonography (US) of the thyroid and neck performed by our staff revealed a hypoechoic nodule measuring 24 mm with signs of central and perilesional vascularization. No suspicious lymph nodes were seen. The patient was euthyroid with a serum TSH level of 1.6 mIU/L. The nodule was subjected to fine-needle aspiration biopsy (FNAb), and the cytological findings were suggestive of papillary thyroid cancer (PTC) (Bethesda class V).

The patient underwent total thyroidectomy. Pathology examination of the surgical specimen revealed a follicular-variant PTC measuring 22 mm with no evidence of extrathyroidal extension or vascular invasion [pT2, Nx (stage 2) according to the AJCC/TNM VII Edition] [1]. The risk of recurrence was classified as low according to the 2009 American Thyroid Association (ATA) staging system [2]. After discussion of these findings and the pros and cons of radioactive iodine remnant ablation (RRA), the patient chose to forego ablation and to be followed with simple surveillance. The cervical ultrasound examination performed during the first 1-year follow-up visit revealed no gross evidence of residual tumor and no suspicious lymph node findings. However, the serum thyroglobulin (Tg) level was 3.5 ng/mL (normal after total thyroidectomy <0.2 ng/mL) with a TSH level of 1.1 mIU/L and no evidence of thyroglobulin antibodies.

C. Durante, MD (✉) • S. Filetti, MD
Department of Internal Medicine and Medical Specialties, University of Rome "Sapienza", Viale del Policlinico 155, 00161 Rome, Italy
e-mail: cosimo.durante@uniroma1.it

D.S. Cooper, C. Durante (eds.), *Thyroid Cancer*,
DOI 10.1007/978-3-319-22401-5_13

Literature Review

What Is the Role of Serum Tg Measurement in Patients Who Have not Undergone Radioiodine Remnant Ablation?

The role played by serum Tg assays in the postoperative management of patients with PTC continues to evolve. Because Tg is produced solely by cells of thyroid follicular origin, its presence in the serum of a patient with PTC who has undergone thyroidectomy followed by RRA is a highly specific marker of residual or recurrent tumor tissue [2, 3]. But, in the growing number of cases in which RRA is omitted (i.e., those characterized by a low to intermediate ATA risk for recurrence), the specificity of assay positivity is lost, since there is no reliable cutoff for distinguishing Tg production by recurrent tumor tissue from that synthesized by nests of normal thyrocytes left behind after surgery. The specificity has been further diminished by the introduction of increasingly sensitive immunometric Tg assays [4]. A few years ago, levels <1 ng/mL were considered "undetectable," but most assays being used today have functional sensitivity limits of 0.2 ng/mL, and second-generation assays can detect serum concentrations as low as 0.1 ng/mL. The clinical significance of this low-level production is uncertain, and large prospective studies are needed to define the cutoff between benign and malignant Tg production.

While the clinical significance of a single positive serum Tg assay is obviously uncertain in a non-radioiodine-ablated patient, *serial* measurements can still provide valuable information on the likelihood of persistent/recurrent disease [5, 6]. Benign production by the normal thyroid remnant is characterized by progressive, spontaneous decline over time, and studies of ATA low-risk nonablated populations indicate that in well over half (60 %) of all cases, unstimulated Tg levels will drop below 0.2 ng/mL during the first year after surgery. By 5 years, this subgroup will comprise close to 80 % of the population [5]. Once these levels have been achieved, nonablated patients are on equal footing with their ablated counterparts in terms of the diagnostic value of serum Tg assays for detecting persistent/recurrent disease. In 20 % of the low-risk patients studied, however, Tg production declined steadily and subsequently plateaued at low but still detectable levels, but this pattern was also associated with the absence of structural disease at the end of follow-up (median 5 years). The single case of recurrence observed in the entire study population ($n=290$) was heralded by a progressive rise in previously stable Tg levels [5]. Indeed, increasing Tg production (in particular, a Tg doubling time of <1 year) has repeatedly emerged as a strong predictor of the presence of locoregional and/or distant recurrence, even if RRA has been omitted [7].

Technically speaking, it is important to recall that serum thyroglobulin assays should always be calibrated against the international CRM457 standard, and serial measurements for a given patient should ideally be performed by the same laboratory with the same assay. Thyroglobulin autoantibodies should also be quantitatively assessed with each measurement of serum Tg [2]. These autoantibodies are present in approximately 20 % of all patients with differentiated thyroid cancers, and they can cause false negatives or falsely low levels in immunometric assays for Tg [2]. There is no method that can reliably eliminate this interference. Radioimmunoassays are advocated by some as a less susceptible alternative, but they have limitations of their own (low availability and sensitivity and potential for falsely elevated Tg values), and their role in patient management is uncertain [2]. Temporal trends in serum anti-Tg antibody titers (again, measured with the same assay) have been used to distinguish residual normal thyroid tissue from recurrent tumor although they are less precise than serum Tg trends [8–11].

What Is the Role of Neck US or Other Imaging Techniques?

While the results of serum Tg assays in nonablated PTC patients become more informative as follow-up progresses, neck US provides valuable information right from the start, and it plays an indispensable role in the initial months/years of follow-up, when Tg assay results are difficult to interpret. Disease spread or recurrence almost always begins in the cervical lymph nodes, where it can be readily detected by ultrasound imaging, especially after thyroidectomy. Sonographic criteria for identifying nodal metastases in the neck are well established [12], and in experienced hands neck ultrasound consistently proves to be much more sensitive for detecting this type of involvement than diagnostic I^{131}WBS [13, 14]. Its negative predictive power is excellent, even in the first preoperative scan (3–12 months after surgery), approaching 100 % in patients with an ATA low risk of recurrence [15]. Its specificity can be improved if suspicious nodes are subjected to fine-needle aspiration biopsy (FNAb) for cytologic confirmation (or assessment of Tg levels in the needle washout) [14]. The examination also furnishes important information for surgeons on the location of involved nodes.

In the absence of positive neck findings on the ultrasound, distant metastases are rare. However, if Tg levels are increasing or the patient has suspicious signs/symptoms, the presence of extracervical lesions should in any case be excluded with second-line imaging studies. These include both cross-sectional modalities (computed tomography or magnetic resonance imaging) and nuclear medicine procedures (WBS and 2-[18 F]fluoro-2-deoxyglucose–positron emission tomography [18FDG–PET]) [2, 3]. 18FDG–PET findings are also potentially helpful for treatment planning since FDG-avid lesions are almost invariably refractory to high-dose radioiodine therapy, and they are associated with very high rates of disease-specific mortality [16].

What Are the Criteria for the Absence of Persistent Tumor?

According to the 2015 ATA guidelines [17], patients who have undergone RRA can be considered disease-free when three conditions have been met: (1) the absence of clinical evidence of disease, (2) negative imaging studies (i.e., no extrathyroidal uptake on the initial postoperative WBS and/or outside the thyroid bed on the initial posttreatment WBS, if performed, or, if uptake outside the thyroid bed had been present, no imaging evidence of tumor on a recent diagnostic or post-therapy WBS) and/or neck US, and (3) serum Tg levels that are <0.2 ng/mL during TSH suppression and <1 ng/mL after stimulation in the absence of interfering antibodies. The final criterion cannot be applied in cases in which RRA has been omitted: the persistence of low-level Tg production that exceeds these limits but remains stable over time may be indicative of "minimal residual disease," but it may also stem from the normal thyroid remnant. It is important to recall that PTCs are slow-growing tumors and the likelihood of distant metastases in the absence of cervical lymph node involvement is extremely low. Therefore, if there is no sonographic evidence of neck disease, most cases of this type can still be safely managed with watchful waiting based on yearly US and periodic Tg assays. The risk declines substantially after the first 5 years of follow-up since 77 % of all recurrences are observed during this interval [18].

Back to the Patient

The possibility of a positive Tg assay at the 1-year visit had already been discussed with the patient when the decision had been made to omit RRA. When the results were back, the significance of the findings was reviewed and management options were discussed. Given the low risk of recurrence and the negative sonographic findings, the proposal was made to proceed with follow-up as originally planned with yearly neck US and serum Tg assays, and the patient agreed. The imaging findings continued to be unequivocally negative, and the serum Tg levels were already lower by the second-year visit. They declined steadily thereafter and dropped below 0.2 ng/mL at the 4-year visit (Fig. 13.1). Five years have passed since the thyroidectomy, and the patient remains symptom-free with no evidence of disease.

Clinical Pearls

- Neck ultrasound is the mainstay of follow-up for PTC patients who have not undergone post-thyroidectomy RRA, especially during the first 5 years when serum Tg levels may be relatively uninformative.
- In over half of all PTC patients who have not undergone RRA, benign Tg production is already undetectable (i.e., <0.2 ng/mL) at the 1-year follow-up visit, and the percentage approaches 80 % by year 5. For this subset of patients, the specificity of a positive serum Tg assay for predicting persistent/recurrent disease is the same as it is in ablated patients.
- Roughly one out of five nonablated patients will have persistent, stable low-level production (≥0.2 ng/mL). In the absence of clinical or imaging evidence of disease, watchful waiting may be the most appropriate course in these cases.

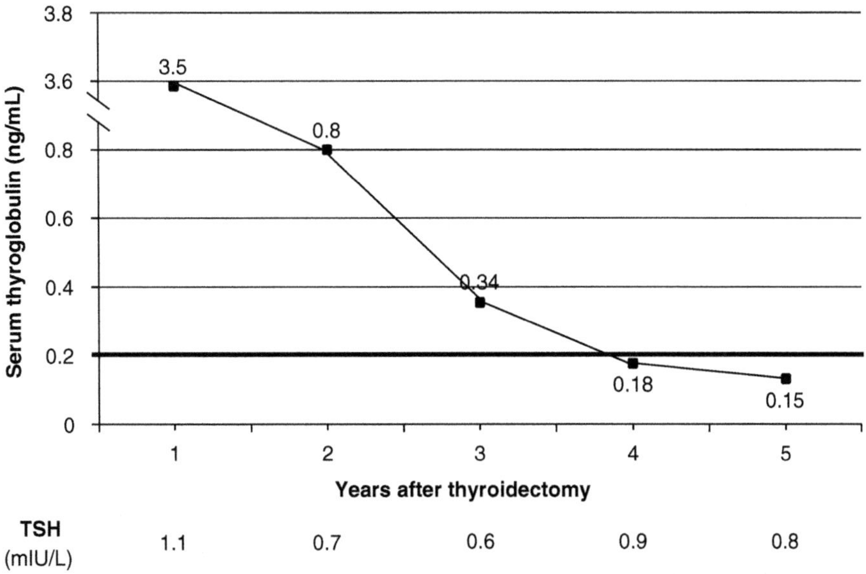

Fig. 13.1 Trend of serial basal Tg determination during the first 5 years after thyroidectomy. The graph line displays the Tg levels obtained with a highly sensitive immunometric assay (functional sensitivity, 0.2 ng/mL) at each annual visit. The corresponding TSH values are reported in the graph

References

1. Edge SB, Byrd DR, Carducci MA, Compton CC, editors. AJCC cancer staging manual. 7th ed. New York: Springer; 2009.
2. Cooper DS, Doherty GM, Haugen BR, Kloos RT, Lee SL, Mandel SJ, Mazzaferri EL, McIver B, Pacini F, Schlumberger M, Sherman SI, Steward DL, Tuttle RM, American Thyroid Association (ATA) Guidelines Taskforce on Thyroid Nodules and Differentiated Thyroid Cancer. Revised American Thyroid Association management guidelines for patients with thyroid nodules and differentiated thyroid cancer. Thyroid. 2009;19(11):1167–214.
3. Pacini F, Schlumberger M, Dralle H, Elisei R, Smit JW, Wiersinga W, European Thyroid Cancer Taskforce. European consensus for the management of patients with differentiated thyroid carcinoma of the follicular epithelium. Eur J Endocrinol. 2006;154(6):787–803.
4. Schlumberger M, Hitzel A, Toubert ME, Corone C, Troalen F, Schlageter MH, Claustrat F, Koscielny S, Taieb D, Toubeau M, Bonichon F, Borson-Chazot F, Leenhardt L, Schvartz C, Dejax C, Brenot-Rossi I, Torlontano M, Tenenbaum F, Bardet S, Bussière F, Girard JJ, Morel O, Schneegans O, Schlienger JL, Prost A, So D, Archambeaud F, Ricard M, Benhamou E. Comparison of seven serum thyroglobulin assays in the follow-up of papillary and follicular thyroid cancer patients. J Clin Endocrinol Metab. 2007;92(7):2487–95.
5. Durante C, Montesano T, Attard M, Torlontano M, Monzani F, Costante G, Meringolo D, Ferdeghini M, Tumino S, Lamartina L, Paciaroni A, Massa M, Giacomelli L, Ronga G, Filetti S, PTC Study Group. Long-term surveillance of papillary thyroid cancer patients who do not undergo postoperative radioiodine remnant ablation: is there a role for serum thyroglobulin measurement? J Clin Endocrinol Metab. 2012;97(8):2748–53.

6. Angell TE, Spencer CA, Rubino BD, Nicoloff JT, LoPresti JS. In search of an unstimulated thyroglobulin baseline value in low-risk papillary thyroid carcinoma patients not receiving radioactive iodine ablation. Thyroid. 2014;24(7):1127–33.
7. Miyauchi A, Kudo T, Miya A, Kobayashi K, Ito Y, Takamura Y, Higashiyama T, Fukushima M, Kihara M, Inoue H, Tomoda C, Yabuta T, Masuoka H. Prognostic impact of serum thyroglobulin doubling-time under thyrotropin suppression in patients with papillary thyroid carcinoma who underwent total thyroidectomy. Thyroid. 2011;21(7):707–16.
8. Spencer CA, Takeuchi M, Kazarosyan M, Wang CC, Guttler RB, Singer PA, Fatemi S, LoPresti JS, Nicoloff JT. Serum thyroglobulin autoantibodies: prevalence, influence on serum thyroglobulin measurement, and prognostic significance in patients with differentiated thyroid carcinoma. J Clin Endocrinol Metab. 1998;83(4):1121–7.
9. Chiovato L, Latrofa F, Braverman LE, Pacini F, Capezzone M, Masserini L, Grasso L, Pinchera A. Disappearance of humoral thyroid autoimmunity after complete removal of thyroid antigens. Ann Intern Med. 2003;139:346–51.
10. Kim WG, Yoon JH, Kim WB, Kim TY, Kim EY, Kim JM, Ryu JS, Gong G, Hong SJ, Shong YK. Change of serum antithyroglobulin antibody levels is useful for prediction of clinical recurrence in thyroglobulin-negative patients with differentiated thyroid carcinoma. J Clin Endocrinol Metab. 2008;93(12):4683–9.
11. Durante C, Tognini S, Montesano T, Orlandi F, Torlontano M, Puxeddu E, Attard M, Costante G, Tumino S, Meringolo D, Bruno R, Trulli F, Toteda M, Redler A, Ronga G, Filetti S, Monzani F, PTC Study Group. Clinical aggressiveness and long-term outcome in patients with papillary thyroid cancer and circulating anti-thyroglobulin autoantibodies. Thyroid. 2014;24(7): 1139–45.
12. Leboulleux S, Girard E, Rose M, Travagli JP, Sabbah N, Caillou B, Hartl DM, Lassau N, Baudin E, Schlumberger M. Ultrasound criteria of malignancy for cervical lymph nodes in patients followed up for differentiated thyroid cancer. J Clin Endocrinol Metab. 2007; 92(9):3590–4.
13. Pacini F, Molinaro E, Castagna MG, Agate L, Elisei R, Ceccarelli C, Lippi F, Taddei D, Grasso L, Pinchera A. Recombinant human thyrotropin-stimulated serum thyroglobulin combined with neck ultrasonography has the highest sensitivity in monitoring differentiated thyroid carcinoma. J Clin Endocrinol Metab. 2003;88(8):3668–73.
14. Torlontano M, Attard M, Crocetti U, Tumino S, Bruno R, Costante G, D'Azzò G, Meringolo D, Ferretti E, Sacco R, Arturi F, Filetti S. Follow-up of low risk patients with papillary thyroid cancer: role of neck ultrasonography in detecting lymph node metastases. J Clin Endocrinol Metab. 2004;89(7):3402–7.
15. Durante C, Attard M, Torlontano M, Ronga G, Monzani F, Costante G, Ferdeghini M, Tumino S, Meringolo D, Bruno R, De Toma G, Crocetti U, Montesano T, Dardano A, Lamartina L, Maniglia A, Giacomelli L, Filetti S, Papillary Thyroid Cancer Study Group. Identification and optimal postsurgical follow-up of patients with very low-risk papillary thyroid microcarcinomas. J Clin Endocrinol Metab. 2010;95(11):4882–8.
16. Robbins RJ, Wan Q, Grewal RK, Reibke R, Gonen M, Strauss HW, Tuttle RM, Drucker W, Larson SM. Real-time prognosis for metastatic thyroid carcinoma based on 2-[18F]fluoro-2-deoxy-D-glucose-positron emission tomography scanning. J Clin Endocrinol Metab. 2006;91(2):498–505.
17. Haugen BR, Alexander EK, Bible KC, Doherty GM, Mandel SJ, Nikiforov YE, Pacini F, Randolph GW, Sawka AM, Schlumberger M, Schuff K, Sherman SI, Sosa JA, Steward DL, Tuttle RM, Wartofsky L. American Thyroid Association management guidelines for patients with thyroid nodules and differentiated thyroid cancer. Thyroid. 2015 (in press).
18. Durante C, Montesano T, Torlontano M, Attard M, Monzani F, Tumino S, Costante G, Meringolo D, Bruno R, Trulli F, Massa M, Maniglia A, D'Apollo R, Giacomelli L, Ronga G, Filetti S, PTC Study Group. Papillary thyroid cancer: time course of recurrences during postsurgery surveillance. J Clin Endocrinol Metab. 2013;98(2):636–42.

Chapter 14
Low but Detectable Suppressed Thyroglobulin Levels in the Follow-Up of Differentiated Thyroid Cancer

Fernanda Vaisman

Case Presentation

A 27-year-old woman was referred to the endocrine clinic for a 2.5 cm right thyroid nodule found on a "routine" thyroid ultrasound. Because of suspicious sonographic characteristics, she underwent a fine-needle aspiration biopsy that suggested papillary thyroid cancer (PTC). Preoperative neck ultrasound showed normal lymph nodes. A total thyroidectomy was performed, and the pathology showed a 2.7 cm classic PTC in the right lobe, with microscopic extrathyroidal extension and two perithyroidal lymph nodes with metastatic foci; the larger was 0.7 cm and showed extranodal extension. She underwent radioiodine ablation with 30 mCi ^{131}I and the post-therapy scan showed uptake only in the thyroid bed; the stimulated thyroglobulin (Tg) pre-ablation was 15 ng/ml. One year later she had a negative neck ultrasound and a suppressed serum Tg of 3.0 ng/ml (serum TSH 0.2 mUI/L) and negative antithyroglobulin antibodies. Computed tomography of the chest was also performed and it was normal as well.

Two years later she still has serum Tg levels in the range of 3.0 ng/ml and no evidence of structural disease on neck ultrasound.

Assessment and Literature Review

Over the past two decades, an increase in the incidence of PTC has been observed all over the world [1], the majority of which are small low- and intermediate-risk tumors, thus, with very low impact on mortality rates [2]. Thus, it is very important

F. Vaisman, MD, PhD (✉)
Instituto Nacional do Cancer do Rio de Janeiro (INCA) – Endocrinology,
Praça da Cruz Vermelha 23 – 8° andar Centro, CEP: 20230-130 Rio de Janeiro, Brazil
e-mail: fevaisman@globo.com

D.S. Cooper, C. Durante (eds.), *Thyroid Cancer*,
DOI 10.1007/978-3-319-22401-5_14

that the treatment and follow-up have to be individualized to avoid unnecessary therapy for those who have a very low risk of recurrence and to focus efforts and resources to treat those with a greater risk of recurrence and disease-specific death.

Risk Stratification

Tg is a specific marker of thyroid tissue and serum Tg measurement is a cornerstone in the long-term follow-up of PTC, being considered a highly sensitive and specific method to detect persistent and/or recurrent disease.

During the past decade, increased attention has been paid to the concept of risk stratification, in an effort to identify those patients who require aggressive treatment and those that can be managed more conservatively. To this end, many risk stratification systems- have been developed over the years, focusing mainly on the pathological features of the primary tumor, including size, histologic subtype and local invasion, extent of the surgical resection, presence of regional or distant metastases at diagnoses, and the age at the time the diagnosis of thyroid cancer is made [3–14]. However, for most of these schemes, it is the disease-specific mortality, rather than the risk of recurrence, that is the predicted outcome variable. In contrast, low- and intermediate-risk PTC patients have low to no mortality from their cancer, and it is the prediction of the recurrence rate (likely due to persistent disease) that is most appropriate to their long-term management.

Recently, Tuttle et al. showed [15] the importance of including the response to initial therapy by re-stratifying patients after initial treatment in an effort to predict the likelihood of recurrence. In this new approach, data regarding serum thyroglobulin levels were incorporated into the risk assessment.

In this system, patients can be classified as having an "excellent" response to initial therapy (if patients have negative ultrasound, suppressed and stimulated Tg <1 ng/ml 6–24 months after therapy), a response that is "favorable" or "acceptable" (if patients have a suppressed serum Tg <1 ng/nl but a stimulated Tg between 1 and 10 ng/ml and/or nonspecific changes in any cross-sectional images performed that cannot definitely rule out persistent disease), or an "incomplete" response, including a structurally incomplete (if any definite structural disease is found) or biochemically incomplete (if the suppressed Tg is >1 ng/ml and/or the stimulated Tg is >10 ng/ml with no structural disease found).

After the re-stratification, the risk of recurrence is often modified. For low- and intermediate-risk patients (using the ATA initial risk stratification system), if they present at 6–24 months with an excellent response to initial therapy, their risk of long-term recurrence drops dramatically from 12 % and 37 %, respectively, to around 2 %. On the other hand, if one has a structural incomplete response at the 6–24-month follow-up evaluation, the risk of recurrent disease can be increased up to 77 % [15, 16].

Recent data have also demonstrated that two clinically distinct cohorts can be identified within those patients classified as having an incomplete response to therapy

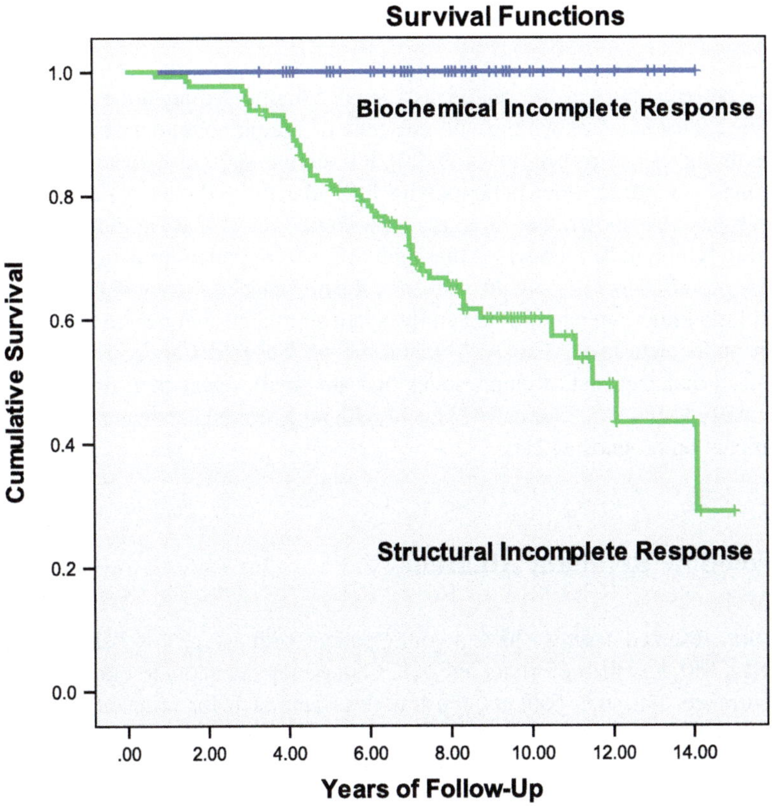

Fig. 14.1 Overall survival is significantly better in patients demonstrating a biochemical incomplete response to therapy than patients demonstrating a structural incomplete response to therapy (Kaplan–Meier analysis, $p<0.0001$) (Adapted from Ref. [16] with permission)

regarding overall survival. Patients with only biochemical evidence of disease have a significantly better clinical outcomes in terms of having a higher likelihood of being free of disease at final follow-up, a lower likelihood of having biochemical or structural disease progression, and a much lower likelihood of dying from thyroid cancer than patients exhibiting a structural incomplete response to therapy; no deaths were seen in the biochemical incomplete response group vs. 38 % in the structural incomplete response group during the 8 years of median follow-up [16]. Figure 14.1 shows the difference in overall survival between the two groups.

Furthermore, studies have shown that serum Tg levels can spontaneously decrease and become undetectable over years of time in both patients treated [17] or not treated with radioactive iodine after surgical treatment [18]. In the two cited studies [17, 18], with a median of 5–10 years of follow-up, serum Tg levels became undetectable in up to 72–79 % of the patients at the end of follow-up, especially in those who had low serum Tg levels at the beginning.

Lymph Node Involvement

The patient that was presented had small-volume lymph node involvement. Several studies have shown that the presence of lymph node metastases is associated with higher recurrence rates [19, 20], but its role in disease-specific survival is very small, except in older patients with follicular thyroid cancer [20]. However, research has also shown that there are pathologic factors that should be evaluated related to lymph node metastases that may differ from patient to patient: for example, size, number, locations in the neck, and the presence of extranodal extension are some of the important pathologic variables that should be analyzed in a patient with lymph node metastasis. The ATA Taskforce on Thyroid Cancer Nodal Surgery concluded that metastatic lymph nodes that are small, fewer than five in number, incidentally found (i.e., clinically N0, and with no extranodal extension have a very low impact on prognosis [21]).

Radioiodine Remnant Ablation

In the presented case, we have a young patient with a very low risk of mortality [T3, N1a, M0, less than 45 years old (AJCC stage 1)] and a low to intermediate risk of recurrence. For such patients, the low-dose approach for remnant ablation has been recently validated. In two randomized controlled trials, it was demonstrated that radioiodine ablation could be performed using 30 mCi with recombinant human TSH preparation [22, 23]. Some authors have also shown that these patients might even be followed without radioiodine ablation, especially if their postoperative stimulated Tg is less than 1 ng/ml [24] or even if the unstimulated Tg is <1 ng/ml [25].

In patients with stable or declining serum Tg values during follow-up, an empirical dose of radioiodine was shown to have no benefit [26]. This approach should be restricted to carefully selected patients with documented progression of serum Tg [26]. The selected group that might benefit from empirical treatment is high-risk patients with increasing serum Tg levels that had radioiodine-sensitive disease to begin with and in whom it was not possible to find the source of Tg production in cross-sectional imaging [13].

TSH Suppression

TSH suppression is usually defined as a serum TSH level below the lower limit of the reference range. It can be "full" (serum TSH <0.1 mU/L) or "partial" (serum TSH between 0.1 and 0.5 mU/L).

Most clinical practice guidelines [12] recommend that low-risk patients, especially those with an excellent response to initial therapy, do not need TSH suppression.

In contrast, TSH suppression, either full or partial, is thought to be beneficial in the incomplete response group (both biochemical and structural incomplete) but always taking into account the patient's clinical status. In young patients like the one presented here, this strategy seems to be appropriate.

Case Management

The patient under discussion is a young woman with an incomplete biochemical response to therapy (surgery and radioiodine therapy), with intermediate risk of recurrence tumor and a very low risk of death from thyroid cancer based on the current stratification systems mentioned above. After initial therapy she has an elevated but stable serum Tg, with no evidence of structural disease. Based on the data presented above, this patient should be followed only with surveillance at this point. As suppressed Tg is already elevated, it should be used to follow this patient's trend, and Tg stimulation is not necessary. Neck ultrasound should be ordered, at least annually, in the first five years and after that it would depend on the suppressed serum Tg trend.

Clinical Pearls/Pitfalls

- Risk assessment for recurrent PTC should include not only the initial pathological findings and patient age but also a more dynamic assessment that includes the response to initial therapy.
- An isolated elevated serum Tg should not be treated with empiric radioiodine therapy since, in the absence of identifiable structural disease, the overall survival is very high and structural recurrence seems to be low.
- A great number of low- to intermediate-risk patients will have a spontaneous decrease in serum Tg levels with no additional therapy.

References

1. Hundahl SA, Fleming ID, Fremgen AM, et al. A national cancer data base report on 53,856 cases of thyroid cancer treated in the US 1985–1995. Cancer. 1998;83:2638–848.
2. McLeod DS, Sawka AM, Cooper DS. Controversies in primary treatment of low-risk papillary thyroid cancer. Lancet. 2013;381(9871):1046–57.
3. Akslen LA. Prognostic importance of histologic grading in papillary thyroid carcinoma. Cancer. 1993;72:2680–5.
4. De Groot LJ, Kaplan EL, McCormick M, et al. Natural history, treatment, and course of papillary thyroid carcinoma. J Clin Endocrinol Metab. 1990;71:414–24.
5. Noguchi S, Murakami N, Kawamoto H. Classification of papillary cancer of thyroid based on prognosis. World J Surg. 1994;18:552–8.

6. Greene FL, Page DL, Fleming ID, et al., editors. AJCC cancer staging handbook: TNM classification of malignant tumors. 6th ed. New York: Springer; 2002.
7. Sugitani I, Kasai N, Fujimoto Y, et al. A novel classification system for patients with PTC: addition of the new variables of large (3 cm or greater) nodal metastases and reclassification during the follow-up period. Surgery. 2004;135:139–48.
8. Yildirim E. A model for predicting outcomes in patients with differentiated thyroid cancer and model performance in comparison with other classification systems. J Am Coll Surg. 2005;200:378–92.
9. Byar DP, Green SB, Dor P, et al. A prognostic index for thyroid carcinoma: a study of the EORTC thyroid cancer cooperative group. Eur J Cancer. 1979;15:1033–41.
10. Cady B, Rossi R. An expanded view of risk-group definition in differentiated thyroid carcinoma. Surgery. 1988;104:947–53.
11. Shaha AR, Ore TR, Shah JP. Intermediate-risk group for differentiated carcinoma of the thyroid. Surgery. 1994;116:1036–41.
12. Cooper DS, Doherty GM, Haugen BR, et al. Revised American thyroid association management guidelines for patients with thyroid nodules and differentiated thyroid cancer. Thyroid. 2009;19(11):1167–214.
13. Pacini F, Schlumberger M, Dralle H, et al. European consensus for the management of patients with differentiated thyroid carcinoma of the follicular epithelium. Eur J Endocrinol. 2006;154:787–803.
14. Rosario PW, Ward L, Carvalho GA, et al. Thyroid nodules and differentiated thyroid cancer: update on the Brazilian consensus. Arq Bras Endocrinol Metab. 2013;57:240–64.
15. Tuttle RM, Tala H, Shah J, et al. Estimating risk of recurrence in differentiated thyroid cancer after total thyroidectomy and radioactive iodine remnant ablation: using response to therapy variables to modify the initial risk estimates predicted by the new American Thyroid Association staging system. Thyroid. 2010;20:1341–9.
16. Vaisman F, Tala H, Grewal R, Tuttle RM. In differentiated thyroid cancer, an incomplete structural response to therapy is associated with significantly worse clinical outcomes than only an incomplete thyroglobulin response. Thyroid. 2011;21(12):1317–22.
17. Vaisman F, Momesso D, Bulzico DA, Pessoa CH, Dias F, Corbo R, Vaisman M, Tuttle RM. Spontaneous remission in thyroid cancer patients after biochemical incomplete response to initial therapy. Clin Endocrinol (Oxf). 2012;77(1):132–8.
18. Durante C, Montesano T, Attard M, Torlontano M, Monzani F, Costante G, Meringolo D, Ferdeghini M, Tumino S, Lamartina L, Paciaroni A, Massa M, Giacomelli L, Ronga G, Filetti S, PTC Study Group. Long-term surveillance of papillary thyroid cancer patients who do not undergo postoperative radioiodine remnant ablation: is there a role for serum thyroglobulin measurement? J Clin Endocrinol Metab. 2012;97(8):2748–53.
19. Schneider DF, Chen H, Sippel RS, et al. Impact of lymph node ratio on survival in papillary thyroid cancer. Ann Surg Oncol. 2013;20:1906–11.
20. Zaydfudim V, Feurer ID, Griffin MR, et al. The impact of lymph node involvement on survival in papillary and follicular thyroid cancer. Sugery. 2008;144:1070–8.
21. Randolph G, Duh QY, Heller KS, Livolsi VA, Mandel SJ, Steward D, Tufano RP, Tuttle RM, ATA Surgical Affairs Committee's Taskforce on Thyroid Cancer Nodal Surgery. The prognostic significance of nodal metastases from papillary thyroid carcinoma can be stratified based on the size and number of metastatic lymph nodes, as well as the presence of extranodal extension. Thyroid. 2012;22(11):1144–52.
22. Schlumberger M, Catargi B, Borget I, Deandreis D, Zerdoud S, Bridji B, Bardet S, Leenhardt L, Bastie D, Schvartz C, Vera P, Morel O, Benisvy D, Bournaud C, Bonichon F, Dejax C, Toubert ME, Leboulleux S, Ricard M, Benhamou E, Tumeurs de la Thyroïde Refractaires Network for the Essai Stimulation Ablation Equivalence Trial. Strategies of radioiodine ablation in patients with low-risk thyroid cancer. N Engl J Med. 2012;366(18):1663–73.
23. Mallick U, Harmer C, Yap B, Wadsley J, Clarke S, Moss L, Nicol A, Clark PM, Farnell K, McCready R, Smellie J, Franklyn JA, John R, Nutting CM, Newbold K, Lemon C, Gerrard G,

Abdel-Hamid A, Hardman J, Macias E, Roques T, Whitaker S, Vijayan R, Alvarez P, Beare S, Forsyth S, Kadalayil L, Hackshaw A. Ablation with low-dose radioiodine and thyrotropin alfa in thyroid cancer. N Engl J Med. 2012;366(18):1674–85.

24. Rosario PW, Mineiro Filho AF, Prates BS, Silva LC, Calsolari MR. Postoperative stimulated thyroglobulin of less than 1 ng/ml as a criterion to spare low-risk patients with papillary thyroid cancer from radioactive iodine ablation. Thyroid. 2012;22(11):1140–3.
25. Ibrahimpasic T, Nixon IJ, Palmer FL, Whitcher MM, Tuttle RM, Shaha A, Patel SG, Shah JP, Ganly I. Undetectable thyroglobulin after total thyroidectomy in patients with low- and intermediate-risk papillary thyroid cancer – is there a need for radioactive iodine therapy? Surgery. 2012;152(6):1096–105. doi:10.1016/j.surg.2012.08.034.
26. Rosario PW, Mourão GF, dos Santos JB, Calsolari MR. Is empirical radioactive iodine therapy still a valid approach to patients with thyroid cancer and elevated thyroglobulin? Thyroid. 2014;24(3):533–6.

Chapter 15
A Patient with Papillary Thyroid Carcinoma and Biochemical Evidence of Disease at Follow-Up Visits and Increasing Serum Tg Values at the Follow-Up Assessments

Yasuhiro Ito and Akira Miyauchi

Case Presentation

A 70-year-old Japanese woman was referred to Kuma Hospital for the evaluation of a thyroid mass detected through an ultrasound examination for the purpose of screening for carotid atherosclerosis in August 2001. She had undergone surgery for colon cancer 3 years earlier and had no other notable medical history. She had no family history of thyroid cancer. Ultrasound examination at Kuma Hospital revealed a solid tumor measuring 32×24 mm in the right lobe of her thyroid and lymph nodes suspicious for metastasis in both lateral compartments (level IV). She had no hoarseness or other compressive symptoms. Laryngotracheal fiberscopy showed that her bilateral vocal cords were functioning and that the tumor in the right lobe protruded into the tracheal mucosa (approx. one-third of the circumference of the trachea) and bled easily when the tip of the fiberscope touched it. No pulmonary metastases were detected on the preoperative chest CT scan.

In November 2001, we performed a total thyroidectomy with bilateral modified radical neck dissection. A window resection of the trachea (26×15 mm) was performed due to the tracheal invasion, and an airtight tracheocutaneostomy was created [1], which was closed using a local skin flap in March 2002. We were able to preserve the bilateral recurrent laryngeal nerves. The pathological diagnosis was

Y. Ito, MD, PhD
Clinical Trial Management Center, Kuma Hospital, Center for Excellence in Thyroid Care, Kobe 650-0011, Japan

Department of Surgery, Kuma Hospital, Center for Excellence in Thyroid Care, Kobe 650-0011, Japan

A. Miyauchi, MD, PhD (✉)
Department of Surgery, Kuma Hospital, Center for Excellence in Thyroid Care, Kobe 650-0011, Japan
e-mail: miyauchi@kuma-h.or.jp

D.S. Cooper, C. Durante (eds.), *Thyroid Cancer*,
DOI 10.1007/978-3-319-22401-5_15

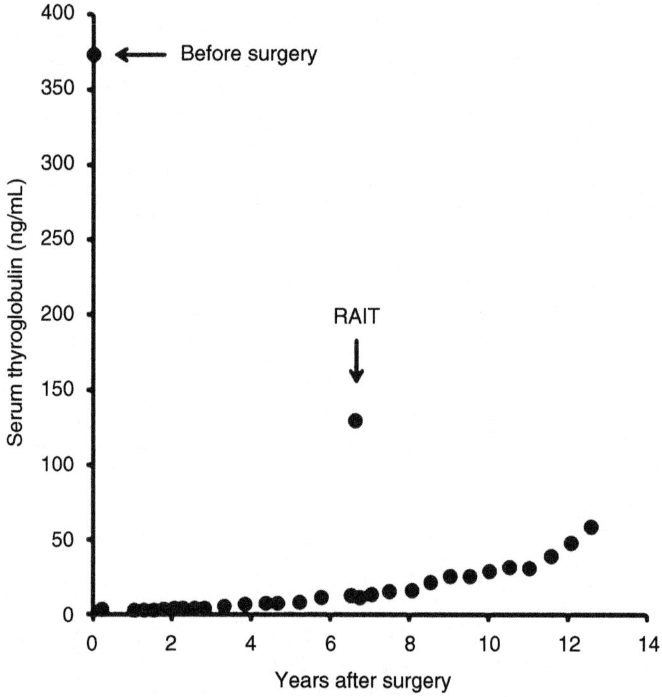

Fig. 15.1 Changes in serum non-stimulated thyroglobulin levels in the patient, a 70-year-old Japanese woman. *RAIT* radioactive iodine treatment

poorly differentiated thyroid carcinoma with a solid growth pattern with invasion into the tracheal mucosa. The cranial margin of the tracheal resection was positive on the final pathology report. The numbers of lymph node metastases were small at 1, 2, and 1 at right level VI, right level IV, and left level IV, respectively. All of the nodal metastases were smaller than 3 cm, and no extranodal extension was observed based on intraoperative and pathological findings. There were no metastases in levels II or III on either side.

Postoperative ablation using 100 mCi of radioactive iodine (RAI) was performed in April 2002, but only thyroid bed uptake was seen on the posttreatment scan. The stimulated Tg was 59.4 ng/ml. Since the margin of the tracheal resection was positive, external beam radiotherapy (50 Gy) was also performed from April to May 2002. The patient was followed with thyroid-stimulating hormone (TSH) suppression (<0.1 mU/L) because of the possible residual tumor at the tracheal resection site and detectable serum Tg levels.

The patient's non-stimulated Tg levels gradually increased from 2.8 to 11.4 ng/mL between June 2002 and August 2007 (Fig. 15.1). Her anti-Tg antibody test results were always negative. In November 2007, several lung metastases were detected on chest CT image; the sizes of the largest metastases were 9.3 × 6.7 mm and 8.4 × 4.3 mm on the left and right sides, respectively (Fig. 15.2). In June 2008,

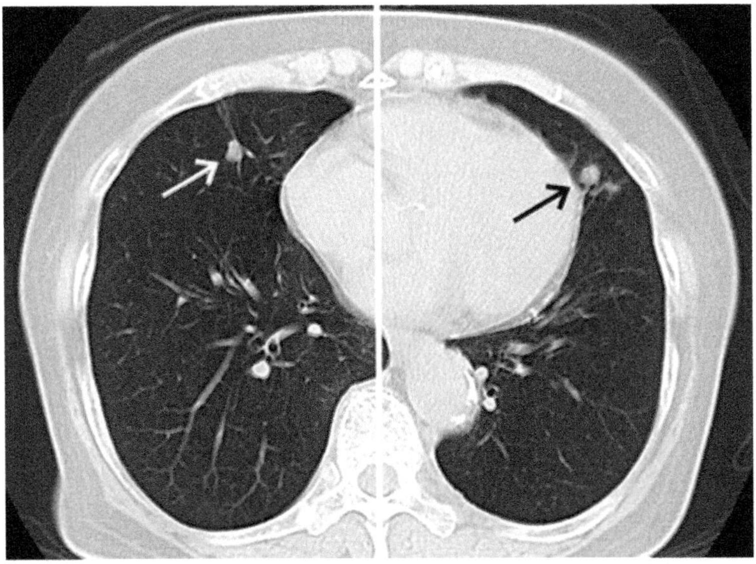

Fig. 15.2 November 2007 chest CT scan showing pulmonary metastases

RAI therapy (100 mCi) was performed, but no uptake was detected in the metastatic lesions. The patient was maintained on TSH suppressive therapy. Her serum Tg levels continued to gradually increase (Fig. 15.1).

In November 2012, an ultrasound examination detected suspicious lymph nodes measuring 11 mm and 9 mm in her right level II. However, fine-needle aspiration biopsy was not performed, since performing a reoperation for such small nodal metastases would be unlikely to improve her prognosis because of the presence of multiple lung metastases. Lung metastases had enlarged to 16.6×11.4 mm and 14.3×7.0 mm on the left and right sides, respectively, in December 2013 (Fig. 15.3), although the size of the suspicious nodes was unchanged.

As of June 2014, the patient was 83 years old with no symptoms of metastases, and her serum Tg level was 58.8 ng/mL (Fig. 15.1). Although she had been on prolonged TSH suppressive therapy, her bone density did not change between September 2005 and December 2012. Her TSH was suppressed to around 0.01 mIU/L.

The changes in the patient's serum non-stimulated Tg levels showed a gradual and exponential increase over time (Fig. 15.1). When we used a log scale for the vertical axis of the graph of the patient's Tg values, the change was basically linear and the slope of the regression line did not change between before and after the therapy (Fig. 15.4). We calculated the Tg-doubling time (DT) from the slope of the regression line, as we reported for the calcitonin DT in patients with medullary thyroid carcinoma [2]. A regression line, $\log y = \log a + bx$, was computed by non-linear least square regression (x, years after surgery; y, Tg level), and thyroglobulin-doubling time (Tg-DT) was given as $(\log 2)/b$. The calculated Tg-DT was 2.7 years.

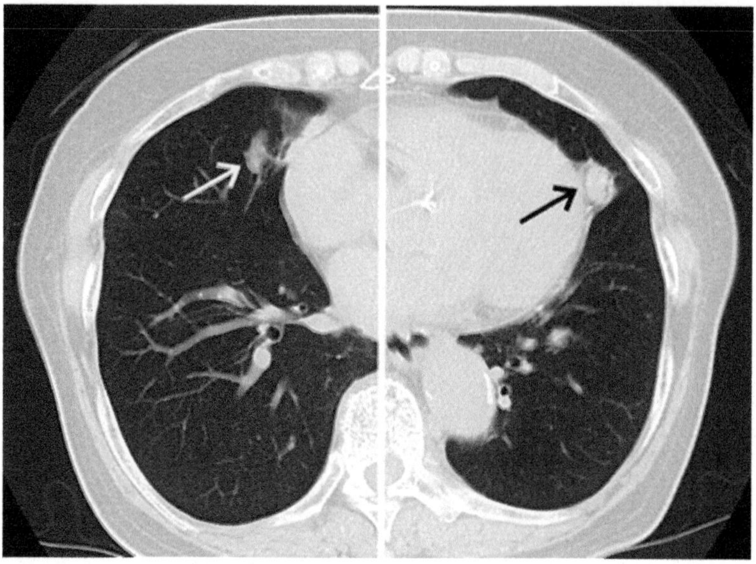

Fig. 15.3 December 2013 chest CT scan showing that the pulmonary metastases had slightly increased in size

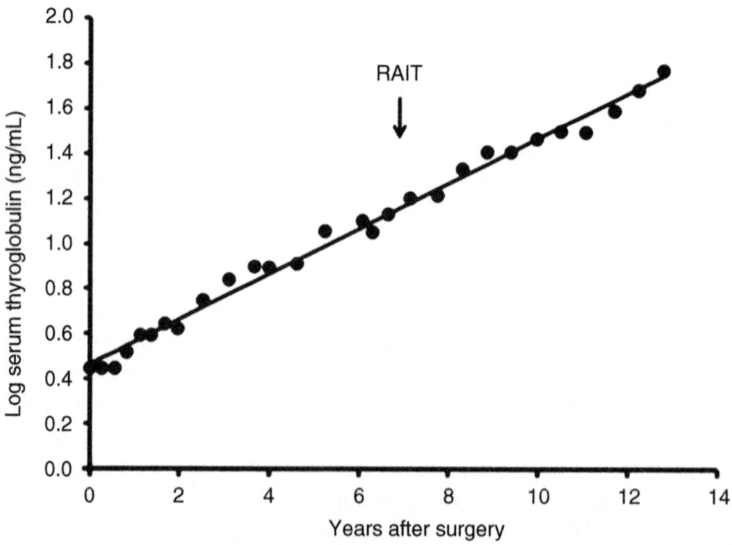

Fig. 15.4 Semilogarithmic graph showing the linear change in the patient's serum non-stimulated thyroglobulin levels. The *vertical axis* is shown in log scale for serum thyroglobulin levels. The *straight line* represents the regression line. The thyroglobulin-doubling time was calculated from the slope of the regression line. *RAIT* radioactive iodine treatment

We also calculated tumor volume DTs from the sizes of the pulmonary metastatic lesions on CT images in November 2007 and December 2013. The values were 2.6 and 2.8 years for the left and right metastatic lesions, respectively. These values were very similar to the Tg-DT.

Assessment and Literature Review

Therapies for Metastatic PTC

Papillary thyroid carcinoma (PTC) metastasizes not only to lymph nodes but also to distant sites such as the lung and bone, for which RAI therapy is the first-line treatment. However, no therapy was available for the patient's RAI-refractory metastases except for TSH suppression. Some molecular-targeted agents were recently reported to be effective for differentiated thyroid carcinomas (DTCs), including PTCs, with RAI-refractory metastases [3, 4]. However, in clinical practice, it remains unclear whether and when molecular-targeted agents should be administered, since not all RAI-refractory cancers are rapidly progressive and life threatening.

Representative Molecular-Target Agents for RAI-Refractory PTC

It was reported that sorafenib and lenvatinib significantly prolonged the progression-free survival (PFS) of DTC patients in randomized phase III studies [3, 4]. However, these agents displayed a high frequency of various adverse events, e.g., hand-foot syndrome (76 %), diarrhea (69 %), alopecia (67 %), rash (50 %), and hypertension (41 %), for sorafenib [3] and hypertension (68 %), diarrhea (60 %), fatigue/asthenia (59 %), decreased appetite (50 %), and nausea/vomiting (46 %) for lenvatinib [4]. The median PFS and hazard ratio (HR) with 95 % confidence intervals (CI) of the DECISION (sorafenib) and SELECT (lenvatinib) trials were 10.8 months (vs. 5.8 months for placebo), 0.59 (0.45–0.76) and 18.3 months (vs. 3.6 months for placebo), 0.21 (0.14–0.31), respectively [3, 4]. These agents are very costly, and since these trials were crossover studies, it was not proved that they prolong overall survival of patients. Clinicians must therefore carefully weigh the advantages and disadvantages of using these agents for individual patients.

Prognosis of DTC Patients with RAI-Refractory Metastases

Not all RAI-refractory metastases are progressive or immediately life threatening. In our prior series, the 5- and 10-year carcinoma-related death rates of 74 DTC patients with RAI-refractory metastases (metastases without RAI uptake from the time of the initial treatment) were 5 % and 30 %, respectively [5]. Therefore, these data suggest that not all patients with RAI-refractory thyroid cancer require treatment with molecular-targeted agents. Without appropriate selection, many of these patients would likely suffer various adverse events without clear improvement in quality of life or survival.

We also demonstrated by a multivariate analysis that older age (≥60 years) was an independent prognostic factor for cause-specific survival (CSS) [6], indicating that RAI-refractory metastases are more progressive in elderly patients. Therefore, molecular-targeted agents are more likely to be administered to elderly patients. We have to be careful in this clinical context, because elderly patients more often have comorbidities such as hypertension, liver and renal dysfunctions, and diabetes mellitus, and they have lower immune resistance than younger patients.

Thyroglobulin-Doubling Time

The change in serum Tg levels is the most important prognostic factor for thyroglobulin antibody (TgAb)-negative patients who have undergone a total thyroidectomy for PTC. We reported that a short Tg-DT (<1 year) after total thyroidectomy strongly predicted a poor disease-free survival (DFS) and CSS (Table 15.1) and that the Tg-DT shorter than 1 year was a very strong predictor of disease recurrence and carcinoma-related death: HR with 95 % CIs for locoregional recurrence, distant recurrence, and carcinoma-related death were 2.38 (1.20–4.71), 4.20 (1.73–10.21), and 47.06 (5.47–405.13), respectively (superior to other conventional prognostic factors in a multivariate analysis) [7]. We also found that the incidence of persistent disease was significantly higher in young (<40 years) and old (≥60 years) patients than in middle-aged patients (40–59 years), whereas short Tg-DT was more frequently observed in old patients than others [8].

These findings were consistent with the findings that younger and older patients were likely to show recurrence, but that older, but not younger, patients were likely to die of carcinoma, in studies by Mazzaferri and Jhiang [9] and our group [6].

Table 15.1 Relationship between cause-specific survival (CSS), distant (DRS) and locoregional recurrence-free survival rate (RFS), and Tg-DT/(first four data)[a,b]

	CSS		DRS		RFS	
	5 years (%)	10 years (%)	5 years (%)	10 years (%)	5 years (%)	10 years (%)
Tg-DT						
<1 year	90	60	72	31	63	38
1–3 years	95	95	90	63	84	58
≥3 years	100	100	92	64	71	54

[a]Tg-DT/(first four data): Thyroglobulin-doubling time was calculated using the first four available data
[b]Miyauchi et al. [7]

In addition, Tg-DT significantly reflects cell proliferative activity because of the inverse relationship between Tg-DT and the Ki 67 labeling index [10]. These findings indicate that Tg-DT might allow a quantified prediction of the prognosis for PTC patients. Therefore, it is suggested that Tg-DT is a useful support to predict disease progression and thus to determine the optimal time for initiating treatment such as tyrosine kinase inhibitors, although imaging confirmation of disease progression (tumor burden) is also necessary.

Management of the Case

Initial Management After Surgery

Older age, clinical lymph node metastases, and significant extrathyroid extension (corresponding to T4 in the UICC TNM classification; [11]) are representative conventional predictors of a poor prognosis for disease-free and CSS [12, 13]. We therefore speculated that our patient was likely to develop a recurrence, even though macroscopically curative surgery was performed. We therefore added RAI ablation and external beam radiotherapy because of the positive pathological margin, in order to prevent local recurrence [1]. She did not develop local recurrence, especially at the resection margin of the trachea. But, her serum Tg remained detectable and increased gradually over time. This indicated that she would likely develop a clinically apparent recurrence in the future; unfortunately this was the case.

Management After Detection of RAI-Refractory Recurrences

Eleven years after her surgery, our patient's PTC recurred at the lung, and the recurrent tumors were RAI-refractory. It is debatable whether and when molecular-targeted agents should be prescribed for her.

The metastatic foci in her lung did not accumulate RAI, and her Tg-DT also did not change following the RAI therapy. During the follow-up with TSH suppressive therapy, the pulmonary metastatic lesions gradually increased in size. Based on these findings, the patient can be considered as having radioiodine-refractory distant metastases. The question is, should we prescribe sorafenib or lenvatinib for her?

The tumor DTs calculated from the sizes of the metastatic foci on CT images were 2.6 and 2.8 years for the left and right sides, respectively. These were very close to the Tg-DT (2.7 years). A tumor with a DT of 2.7 years will grow to a volume 16 times the original volume after four doublings (10.8 years later in this case). When the present patient becomes 95 years old, the metastatic tumor of the left lung would become 42×29 mm in size. Furthermore, the site of lung target lesions was not risky, unlike adjacent lesion to the trachea and hilar area. Based on this calculation and metastatic sites, this patient is unlikely to die of lung metastases. We therefore did not think that molecular-targeted agents were indicated for her at present.

We showed that a Tg-DT <1 year accurately reflects carcinoma recurrence and carcinoma-related death, regardless of the patient's background and clinicopathological features [7]. Patients with a Tg-DT >2 years were very unlikely to die of PTC [7]. Molecular-targeted agents are costly and produce various adverse events, which may be even life threatening. In a clinical trial of sorafenib, therapy had to be discontinued in as many as 18.8 % of patients because of severe adverse events (median treatment period 10.6 months; [3]). Molecular-targeted agents should thus be administered to patients only when they are truly required. RAI-refractory thyroid cancer with rapid growth should be the indication for these agents. We propose a short Tg-DT (<1 year) as a convenient criterion of rapid tumor growth and a possible criterion for consideration of the use of these agents together with the findings of imaging studies.

In conclusion: our patient has RAI-refractory pulmonary metastases. We do not think that the currently available molecular-targeted agents are indicated at present, because of a moderately long tumor-DT or Tg-DT. Watchful follow-up under TSH suppression is recommended.

Clinical Pearls

- Molecular-targeted agents have been proven to be effective for DTC patients with RAI-refractory metastases, but these agents can cause severe adverse events, damaging the patients' quality of life.
- To evaluate when and whether molecular-targeted agents should be administered to patients, we propose a short Tg-DT (<1 year) as a convenient criterion of rapid tumor growth as a possible reason to consider the indication for these agents together with the findings of imaging studies.
- Molecular-targeted agents should be used only after carefully weighing their advantages and disadvantages.

References

1. Ito Y, Miyauchi A, Kihara M, Higashiyama T, Kobayashi K, Miya A. Airtight tracheocutaneostomy after window resection of the trachea for invasive papillary thyroid carcinoma: experience of 109 cases. World J Surg. 2014;38:660–6.
2. Miyauchi A, Onishi T, Morimoto S, Takai S, Matsuzuka F, Kuma K, Maeda M, Kumahara Y. Relation of doubling time of plasma calcitonin levels to prognosis and recurrence of medullary thyroid carcinoma. Ann Surg. 1984;199:461–6.
3. Brose M, Nutting C, Jarzab B, Elisei R, Sieno S, et al. Sorafenib in radioactive iodine-refractory, locally advanced or metastatic differentiated thyroid cancer: a randomized, double-blind phase 3 trial. Lancet. 2014;384:319–28.
4. Schlumberger M, Tahara M, Wirth LJ, Robinson B, Brose MS, Elisei R, et al. Lenvatinib versus placebo in radioiodine-refractory thyroid cancer. N Engl J Med. 2015; 372:621-30.

5. Ito Y, Miyauchi A, Ito M, Yabuta T, Masuoka H, Higashiyama T, et al. Prognosis and prognostic factors of differentiated thyroid carcinoma after the appearance of metastasis refractory to radioactive iodine therapy. Endocr J. 2014;61:821–4.
6. Ito Y, Miyauchi A, Kihara M, Higashiyama T, Kobayashi K, Miya A. Prognostic significance of young age in papillary thyroid carcinoma: analysis of 5733 patients with 150 months' median follow-up. Endocr J. 2014;61:491–7.
7. Miyauchi A, Kudo T, Miya A, Kobayashi K, Ito Y, Takamura Y, et al. Prognostic impact of serum thyroglobulin doubling-time under thyrotropin suppression in patients with papillary thyroid carcinoma who underwent total thyroidectomy. Thyroid. 2011;21:707–16.
8. Miyauchi A, Kudo T, Kihara M, Higashiyama T, Ito Y, Kobayashi K, et al. Relationship of biochemically persistent disease and thyroglobulin-doubling time to age at surgery in patients with papillary thyroid carcinoma. Endocr J. 2013;60:415–21.
9. Mazzaferri EL, Jhiang SM. Long-term impact of initial surgical and medical therapy on papillary and follicular thyroid cancer. Am J Med. 1994;97:418–28.
10. Miyauchi A, Kudo T, Hirokawa M, Ito Y, Kihara M, Higashiyama T, et al. Ki-67 labeling index is a predictor of postoperative persistent disease and cancer growth and a prognostic indicator in papillary thyroid carcinoma. Eur Thyroid J. 2013;2:57–64.
11. Sobin LH, Wittekind CH, editors. UICC: TNM classification of malignant tumors. 7th ed. New York: Wiley-Liss; 2009.
12. Ito M, Miyauchi A, Morita S, Kudo T, Nishihara E, Kihara M, Takamura Y, Ito Y, Kobayashi K, Miya A, Kubota S, Amino N. TSH-suppressive doses of levothyroxine are required to achieve preoperative native serum triiodothyronine levels in patients who have undergone total thyroidectomy. Eur J Endocrinol. 2012;167:373–8.
13. Ito Y, Kudo T, Kobayashi K, Miya A, Ichihara K, Miyauchi A. Prognostic factors for recurrence of papillary thyroid carcinoma in the lymph nodes, lung, and bone: analysis of 5768 patients with average 10-year follow-up. World J Surg. 2012;36:1274–8.

Chapter 16
A Young Patient with Recurrent Lymph Node Involvement: Imaging, Cytology, and Thyroglobulin Washout

Livia Lamartina, Sebastiano Filetti, and Cosimo Durante

Case Presentation

A 34-year-old woman was referred to our clinic with a small, firm mass in the left anterior neck, which had been discovered by her general practitioner during a physical examination. Neck ultrasound (US) demonstrated a hypoechoic thyroid nodule measuring approximately 20 mm. Fine-needle aspiration biopsy (FNAb) findings were consistent with papillary thyroid cancer (PTC) (Bethesda class VI) [1]. The patient underwent total thyroidectomy with central neck dissection prompted by intraoperative detection of suspicious lymph nodes. Pathology review disclosed an intracapsular PTC measuring 18 mm (largest diameter) in the left lobe of the gland and metastatic involvement of six of the ten central lymph nodes that had been removed (all six less than 3 mm in diameter). There was no evidence of extra-nodal extension (pT1b, pN1b [stage I] per the AJCC/TNM VII system) [2]. Radioiodine remnant ablation (RRA) with 30 mCi was performed after stimulation with recombinant human TSH (rhTSH). At the time of the ablation, the stimulated serum thyroglobulin (Tg) level was 10.6 ng/mL, and the thyroglobulin antibody (AbTg) levels were below assay sensitivity (<4.11 U/mL). The posttreatment whole body scan (WBS) showed radioiodine uptake only in the thyroid bed.

One year later, the stimulated serum Tg level had dropped to 3.2 ng/mL, and AbTg levels were still undetectable. Neck US revealed a round (12.5 × 11.2 × 11.6 mm) lymph node in the left lateral neck (level III) with no evidence of a fatty hilum.

L. Lamartina, MD • S. Filetti, MD • C. Durante, MD (✉)
Department of Internal Medicine and Medical Specialties, University of Rome "Sapienza", Viale del Policlinico 155, 00161 Rome, Italy
e-mail: cosimo.durante@uniroma1.it

D.S. Cooper, C. Durante (eds.), *Thyroid Cancer*,
DOI 10.1007/978-3-319-22401-5_16

Literature Review

Cervical nodes are the most common sites of persistent/recurrent disease in patients with PTC, and disease of this type occurs in 5–50 % of all patients, depending on their baseline risk level and response to initial therapy [3, 4]. Several diagnostic tools can be used to identify structural disease in the neck during the posttreatment follow-up, each with specific limitations and strengths.

Radioiodine WBS displays an overall accuracy of 90–92 % in this setting, with excellent specificity (up to 100 %) but much more limited sensitivity (51–55 %) [5, 6]. In 25–50 % of patients, single photon emission computed tomography (SPECT)/CT can provide more precise anatomic localization of radioiodine-avid lesions [7–9]. Neither of these methods is capable of differentiating neoplastic lesions from normal residual tissue in the central compartment [5–9], and both are ineffective for detecting radioiodine-refractory metastases.

Ultrasonography is the most accurate tool for exploring the thyroid bed and cervical lymph node compartments, and international guidelines concur in recommending periodic sonography after the primary treatment. The frequency of sonographic surveillance will be dictated by the individual risk for recurrence and the results of serum Tg assays [3, 4, 10, 11]. There are no validated US criteria for distinguishing malignant and benign lesions of the thyroid bed (e.g., tumor recurrence vs. postoperative fibrosis or suture granulomas), but US is much more helpful for classifying cervical lymph nodes [11, 12]. As shown in Table 16.1, foci of punctate hyperechogenicity (reflecting microcalcifications), cystic features,

Table 16.1 Accuracy of ultrasound features in diagnosing malignant involvement of cervical lymph nodes[a]

Features	Sensitivity (%)	Specificity (%)	NPV (%)	PPV (%)	Accuracy (%)	Prevalence (%) in normal LNs
Suspicious for malignancy						
Punctate hyperechogenicity	5–69	93–100	33–60	88–100	56–72	0
Cystic aspect	10–34	91–100	30–66	77–100	48–65	0
Peripheral/Diffuse vascularization	40–86	57–93	31–70	77–80	54–71	1–18
"Thyroid-like" hyperechogenicity	30–87	43–95	38–84	66–96	56–90	4–17
Indeterminate						
Round shape	37	70	45	63	–	4-36
Hilum absent	90.4–100	29–40	67.3	75.9	–	–
Normal						
Hilum present	0.5	–	–	–	–	29–48
Vascularization absent	0	–	–	–	–	33–36

[a]Adapted from Leboulleux et al. [12] and Leenhardt et al. [11]
NPV negative predictive value, *PPV* positive predictive value, *LN* lymph node

peripheral or diffuse increases in vascularity, and the presence of hyperechoic "thyroid-like" tissue are all strongly suggestive of malignancy [11]. The presence of more than one of these features should reinforce the suspicion, but the sole presence of hyperechoic microfoci or cystic features has a positive predictive value for PTC involvement that approaches 100 % [12]. The presence of neoplastic involvement is virtually excluded by visualization of the echogenic lymph node hilum, which can be achieved with either standard gray-scale or color Doppler imaging. Nonvisualization of the hilum and other features, such as a rounded shape, are highly sensitive markers of lymph node malignancy, but they are relatively nonspecific. Therefore, in the absence of other suspicious features, these findings are considered diagnostically indeterminate. The location of a suspicious node can also be informative: positive nodes are most commonly found in neck compartments III, IV, and VI [12]. Nodal metastases are also much more likely in patients whose risk of recurrence has been classified as intermediate to high and in those with abnormal serum Tg values [3, 4]. In the presence of indeterminate findings on ultrasound (especially when they persist over time), either of these factors is usually an indication for second-line testing to determine whether or not the node is indeed malignant.

Cytological assessment of an FNAb specimen is the most common method for confirming metastatic involvement of lymph nodes with indeterminate or suspicious sonographic features. The aspiration should be performed under US guidance by an experienced operator [defined by the European Thyroid Association (ETA) as one who performs at least 150 procedures per year and maintains an inadequate sampling rate below 10 %] [11]. Material is collected with 24- to 27-gauge needles (two or more passes) and smeared on slides or suspended in liquid phase for cytological examination. False-negative results occur in 6–8 % of all cases (due to sampling error), and up to 10 % of samples prove to be inadequate for diagnosis. When cytological and sonographic findings conflict (i.e., normal cytology vs. suspicious sonographic features) or the FNAb sample is inadequate, further diagnostic testing can be undertaken.

The diagnostic yield of an FNAb can be enhanced by assaying Tg levels and/or thyroid-specific gene transcripts in washout fluid from the needle used to collect the cytology aspirate [13] or by another dedicated pass for thyroglobulin or genetic analysis. For the Tg assay, the needle is generally flushed with 1 cc of normal saline. The washout is analyzed using an immunometric assay with a functional sensitivity between 0.1 and 1 mcg/L [11] that has been precalibrated in line with the CRM 457 standard. The results are expressed in nanograms per milliliter, and normal cut-offs vary. The ETA regards levels below 1 ng/mL as normal and those above 10 ng/mL as compatible with thyroid cancer metastasis in a thyroidectomized patient [11]. Values between 1 and 10 ng/mL should be interpreted together with cytology results [11].

Immunometric Tg assays can produce falsely low results in the presence of high Tg concentrations if the excess antigen saturates the binding capacity of the antibodies in the solid-phase support. This so-called hook effect [14] can be excluded by assaying serial dilutions of the sample [15]. The reported sensitivity of washout fluid Tg levels for identifying thyroid cancer lymph node metastases ranges from 88 to 100 % with a specificity from 69 to 100 % [10, 13, 15–18]. This assay can be informative even in the presence of Tg antibodies (AbTg) [16, 19], although false-negative results can also occur in this setting [17]. False negatives are also possible in the presence of anaplastic or poorly differentiated thyroid cancer metastases [16]. False-positive results have also been reported, mainly when a remnant of normal thyroid is mistakenly identified as a suspicious level VI lymph node [13].

When cytology and washout fluid Tg levels are both noninformative, assaying a sample of the FNAb washout for mRNA for thyroid-specific genes (e.g., TSH receptor, Tg) may be useful. The washout in this case is performed with an RNA stabilization solution and the sample frozen for later assay. With polymerase chain reaction amplification, this approach can correctly identify the presence of metastatic tissue, even when the washout fluid contains only a few cells [18]. Its accuracy is substantially better than aspiration cytology or Tg assay of washout (100 % vs. 85 % and 73 %, respectively) [18]. However, this assay is probably available only in tertiary care centers.

It is important to note that the presence of a lymph node with indeterminate or suspicious US findings is not *always* an indication for FNAb: the latter should be offered *only* if the results will have a real impact on patient management [3, 4]. Confirmation of locoregional metastatic involvement is often followed by further treatment, but if this course of action is already precluded by factors like advanced age, comorbidities, or simple patient preferences, an FNAb serves little purpose.

Once the presence of metastatic lymph node involvement has been established, the most effective therapy [20] and the first-line approach recommended by the American Thyroid Association (ATA) Practice Guidelines [3, 4] is surgery. The first reoperation is often (50–70 % of patients), but not invariably, successful in eradicating the disease [20–22]. However, reoperation carries an increased risk of permanent complications [23–25], including nerve resection (e.g., recurrent laryngeal, spinal accessory, and phrenic nerves), hypoparathyroidism, and tracheal or esophageal damage. Decisions have to be based on careful analysis of costs, benefits, and patient preferences. The actual risk of complications depends in part on the skill and experience of the surgeon, so the availability of surgeons specifically trained in neck revision procedures is a critical factor to consider. The proximity of the metastatic node to vital structures in the neck should also be taken into account.

The ATA recommends that surgery should be considered for central neck nodes measuring >8 mm and lateral neck nodes with diameters of >10 mm. For smaller nodes or those that remain stable over time, conservative management based on active surveillance is more appropriate [3, 4]. Only 20 % of all suspicious lymph nodes exhibit volume increases over time [26]. Those posing no threat to vital structures that show no signs of growth can be safely and effectively monitored with periodic (every 6–12 months) US examinations [3, 4, 11]. The patient's wishes and emotional concerns naturally have to be weighed and addressed in all decisions.

Back to the Patient

After the initial therapy, which included total thyroidectomy, central neck dissection, and postoperative radioiodine remnant ablation, the risk of recurrence in this case was rated as intermediate according to the ATA staging system (about 20 %) [4]. At the 1-year follow-up visit, the patient presented with an abnormal rhTSH-stimulated serum Tg level (i.e., >1 ng/mL) and a left lateral neck lymph node that was sonographically indeterminate.

With a small child to care for and a promising new job, the young woman was clearly disconcerted by the possibility (however uncertain) that the disease had spread in spite of the previous treatment and the prospect of a second operation. An FNAb was promptly obtained, and as per routine in our department, aliquots of the needle washout were also collected and retained for assays of Tg levels and thyroid-specific gene expression. The aspirate itself proved to be inadequate for cytological analysis, and the Tg level in the needle washout fluid (10 ng/mL) was in the indeterminate range. However, the presence of metastatic DTC in the suspicious node was confirmed by the presence in the washout fluid of mRNA for the TSH receptor and Tg genes. The pros and cons of a second operation were reviewed in light of this diagnosis, and the patient decided to undergo a selective left lateral neck dissection. The operation was uneventful, and the pathologic examination confirmed metastatic cancer in 2 of the 15 lymph nodes that were removed (pT1b). Six months later, the rhTSH-stimulated serum Tg level was below the detection limit, and no suspicious findings were noted on neck US. Five years have passed since the second operation, and the patient has remained disease-free. She continues to work and care for her family.

Clinical Pearls/Pitfalls

- US is the most accurate tool for identifying metastatic spread to cervical lymph nodes.
- Nodes displaying punctate hyperechogenicity, cystic features, diffuse or peripheral increases in vascularity, or hyperechoic "thyroid-like" tissue on neck US should raise a strong suspicion of malignancy.
- When the suspicious features are limited to a round rather than oval shape and/or the absence of a fatty hilum, the nature of node is indeterminate.
- FNAb for cytology is indicated for most suspicious lymph nodes.
- The diagnostic yield of the FNAb for identification of lymph node metastases can be increased by measuring Tg levels in the FNAb needle washout fluid.
- PCR-based assays can document even low levels of thyroid-specific gene mRNA in the FNAb washout fluid and thereby identify metastatic nodes with 100 % accuracy.
- The first reoperation for persistent/recurrent DTC in the neck is successful in about 50–70 % of cases but carries an increased risk of permanent complications.
- Nonthreatening lymph node metastases that remain stable in size over time can be safely and effectively monitored with periodic (6–12 months) US examinations.

References

1. Cibas ES, Ali SZ. The Bethesda system for reporting thyroid cytopathology. Am J Clin Pathol. 2009;132(5):658–65.
2. Edge SB, Byrd DR, Carducci MA, Compton CC, editors. AJCC cancer staging manual. 7th ed. New York: Springer; 2009.
3. Cooper DS, Doherty GM, Haugen BR, Kloos RT, Lee SL, Mandel SJ, Mazzaferri EL, McIver B, Pacini F, Schlumberger M, Sherman SI, Steward DL, Tuttle RM, American Thyroid Association (ATA) Guidelines Taskforce on Thyroid Nodules and Differentiated Thyroid Cancer. Revised American Thyroid Association management guidelines for patients with thyroid nodules and differentiated thyroid cancer. Thyroid. 2009;19(11):1167–214.
4. Haugen BR, Alexander EK, Bible KC, Doherty GM, Mandel SJ, Nikiforov YE, Pacini F, Randolph GW, Sawka AM, Schlumberger M, Schuff K, Sherman SI, Sosa JA, Steward DL, Tuttle RM, Wartofsky L. American Thyroid Association management guidelines for patients with thyroid nodules and differentiated thyroid cancer. Thyroid. 2015 (in press).
5. Lubin E, Mechlis-Frish S, Zatz S, Shimoni A, Segal K, Avraham A, Levy R, Feinmesser R. Serum thyroglobulin and iodine-131 whole-body scan in the diagnosis and assessment of treatment for metastatic differentiated thyroid carcinoma. J Nucl Med. 1994;35(2):257–62.
6. Franceschi M, Kusić Z, Franceschi D, Lukinac L, Roncević S. Thyroglobulin determination, neck ultrasonography and iodine-131 whole-body scintigraphy in differentiated thyroid carcinoma. J Nucl Med. 1996;37(3):446–51.
7. Tharp K, Israel O, Hausmann J, Bettman L, Martin WH, Daitzchman M, Sandler MP, Delbeke D. Impact of 131I-SPECT/CT images obtained with an integrated system in the follow-up of patients with thyroid carcinoma. Eur J Nucl Med Mol Imaging. 2004;31(10):1435–42.
8. Schmidt D, Szikszai A, Linke R, Bautz W, Kuwert T. Impact of 131I SPECT/spiral CT on nodal staging of differentiated thyroid carcinoma at the first radioablation. J Nucl Med. 2009;50(1):18–23.
9. Grewal RK, Tuttle RM, Fox J, Borkar S, Chou JF, Gonen M, Strauss HW, Larson SM, Schöder H. The effect of posttherapy 131I SPECT/CT on risk classification and management of patients with differentiated thyroid cancer. J Nucl Med. 2010;51(9):1361–7.
10. Pacini F, Schlumberger M, Dralle H, Elisei R, Smit JW, Wiersinga W, European Thyroid Cancer Taskforce. European consensus for the management of patients with differentiated thyroid carcinoma of the follicular epithelium. Eur J Endocrinol. 2006;154(6):787–803.
11. Leenhardt L, Erdogan MF, Hegedus L, Mandel SJ, Paschke R, Rago T, Russ G. European thyroid association guidelines for cervical ultrasound scan and ultrasound-guided techniques in the postoperative management of patients with thyroid cancer. Eur Thyroid J. 2013;2(3):147–59.
12. Leboulleux S, Girard E, Rose M, Travagli JP, Sabbah N, Caillou B, Hartl DM, Lassau N, Baudin E, Schlumberger M. Ultrasound criteria of malignancy for cervical lymph nodes in patients followed up for differentiated thyroid cancer. J Clin Endocrinol Metab. 2007; 92(9):3590–4.
13. Grani G, Fumarola A. Thyroglobulin in lymph node fine-needle aspiration washout: a systematic review and meta-analysis of diagnostic accuracy. J Clin Endocrinol Metab. 2014;99(6):1970–82.
14. Giovanella L. Highly sensitive thyroglobulin measurements in differentiated thyroid carcinoma management. Clin Chem Lab Med. 2008;46(8):1067–73.
15. Giovanella L, Ceriani L, Suriano S, Crippa S. Thyroglobulin measurement on fine-needle washout fluids: influence of sample collection methods. Diagn Cytopathol. 2009;37(1):42–4.
16. Boi F, Baghino G, Atzeni F, Lai ML, Faa G, Mariotti S. The diagnostic value for differentiated thyroid carcinoma metastases of thyroglobulin (Tg) measurement in washout fluid from fine-needle aspiration biopsy of neck lymph nodes is maintained in the presence of circulating anti-Tg antibodies. J Clin Endocrinol Metab. 2006;91(4):1364–9.
17. Jeon MJ, Park JW, Han JM, Yim JH, Song DE, Gong G, Kim TY, Baek JH, Lee JH, Shong YK, Kim WB. Serum antithyroglobulin antibodies interfere with thyroglobulin detection in fine-needle

aspirates of metastatic neck nodes in papillary thyroid carcinoma. J Clin Endocrinol Metab. 2013;98(1):153–60.

18. Arturi F, Russo D, Giuffrida D, Ippolito A, Perrotti N, Vigneri R, Filetti S. Early diagnosis by genetic analysis of differentiated thyroid cancer metastases in small lymph nodes. J Clin Endocrinol Metab. 1997;82(5):1638–41.
19. Latrofa F, Ricci D, Montanelli L, Rocchi R, Piaggi P, Sisti E, Grasso L, Basolo F, Ugolini C, Pinchera A, Vitti P. Thyroglobulin autoantibodies in patients with papillary thyroid carcinoma: comparison of different assays and evaluation of causes of discrepancies. J Clin Endocrinol Metab. 2012;97(11):3974–82. doi:10.1210/jc.2012-2406.
20. Yim JH, Kim WB, Kim EY, Kim WG, Kim TY, Ryu JS, Gong G, Hong SJ, Shong YK. The outcomes of first reoperation for locoregionally recurrent/persistent papillary thyroid carcinoma in patients who initially underwent total thyroidectomy and remnant ablation. J Clin Endocrinol Metab. 2011;96(7):2049–56.
21. Uruno T, Miyauchi A, Shimizu K, Nakano K, Takamura Y, Ito Y, Miya A, Kobayashi K, Yokozawa T, Matsuzuka F, Kuma K. Prognosis after reoperation for local recurrence of papillary thyroid carcinoma. Surg Today. 2004;34(11):891–5.
22. Hughes DT, Laird AM, Miller BS, Gauger PG, Doherty GM. Reoperative lymph node dissection for recurrent papillary thyroid cancer and effect on serum thyroglobulin. Ann Surg Oncol. 2012;19(9):2951–7. doi:10.1245/s10434-012-2380-9. Epub 2012 April 24.
23. Roh JL, Kim JM, Park CI. Central compartment reoperation for recurrent/persistent differentiated thyroid cancer: patterns of recurrence, morbidity, and prediction of postoperative hypocalcemia. Ann Surg Oncol. 2011;18(5):1312–8.
24. Lang BH, Lee GC, Ng CP, Wong KP, Wan KY, Lo CY. Evaluating the morbidity and efficacy of reoperative surgery in the central compartment for persistent/recurrent papillary thyroid carcinoma. World J Surg. 2013;37(12):2853–9.
25. Wierzbicka M, Gurgul E, Wasniewska-Okupniak E, Gryczynska M, Piorunek T, Ruchala M. The feasibility and efficacy of secondary neck dissections in thyroid cancer metastases. Eur Arch Otorhinolaryngol. 2014;271(4):795–9.
26. Robenshtok E, Fish S, Bach A, Domínguez JM, Shaha A, Tuttle RM. Suspicious cervical lymph nodes detected after thyroidectomy for papillary thyroid cancer usually remain stable over years in properly selected patients. J Clin Endocrinol Metab. 2012;97(8):2706–13.

Part IV
Low Risk Differentiated Thyroid Cancer: *Special Issues*

Chapter 17
Papillary Thyroid Carcinoma Diagnosed During Pregnancy

Stephanie Lee and David S. Cooper

Case Presentation

A 46-year-old pregnant female was referred for management of a recently diagnosed papillary thyroid carcinoma. During her initial prenatal visit at 11 weeks of gestation, a nurse midwife detected a right thyroid nodule. Her TSH was normal at 0.96 mU/L. Her primary care doctor arranged for a diagnostic ultrasound that revealed a 4.6 cm right thyroid nodule. She returned the following week for an ultrasound-guided fine-needle aspiration biopsy. The cytology was suspicious for a papillary thyroid carcinoma (Bethesda class V). She was referred for management options. At the time of the endocrine consultation, the patient was para 5 gravida 4 and 19 weeks pregnant. She did not have any other medical conditions. She had no history of head and neck radiation. She had no family history of thyroid disease, including thyroid cancer. She denied neck pressure, voice change, or dysphagia.

An office ultrasound of the thyroid nodule and cervical neck node survey was performed to estimate her stage and direct the extent of surgery. The ultrasound exam revealed a 4.6 × 2.1 × 2 cm solid, hypoechoic, taller-than-wide (anteroposterior/transverse diameter ratio >1) nodule in the upper right thyroid lobe (Fig. 17.1). The nodule contained microcalcifications. An ultrasound node survey of the central and lateral neck revealed two abnormal 1 and 1.5 cm partially cystic, hypervascular nodes inferior to the lower pole of the right thyroid lobe (Fig. 17.2).

S. Lee, MD, PhD
Division of Endocrinology, Boston Medical Center, 732 Harrison Avenue, 2nd Floor, Boston, MA 02118, USA

D.S. Cooper, MD (✉)
Division of Endocrinology, Diabetes, and Metabolism, The Johns Hopkins University School of Medicine, 1830 East Monument St., Suite 333, Baltimore, MD 21287, USA
e-mail: dscooper@jhmi.edu

D.S. Cooper, C. Durante (eds.), *Thyroid Cancer*,
DOI 10.1007/978-3-319-22401-5_17

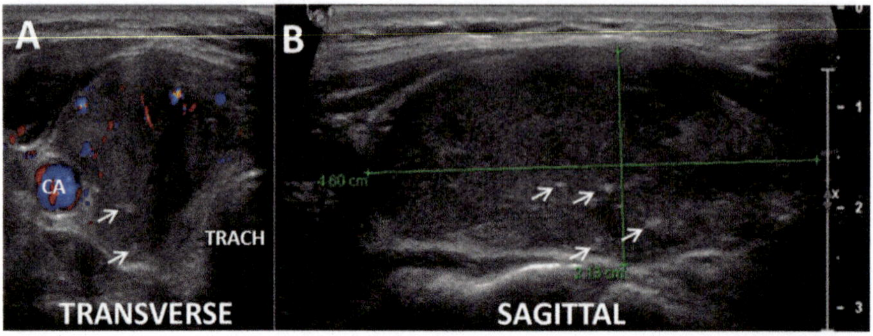

Fig. 17.1 Thyroid ultrasound of the right thyroid lobe shows a 4.6×2.1×2 cm (sagittal×antero-posterior×transverse) solid, hypoechoic nodule. This nodule is hypoechoic with taller-than-wide (anterioposterior/transverse diameter ratio >1) dimensions with microcalcification (*white arrows*) and low intranodular vascular flow by Doppler analysis (grade 3). (**a**) thyroid transverse view with Doppler. (**b**) Thyroid sagittal view. *CA* carotid artery, *TRACH* trachea

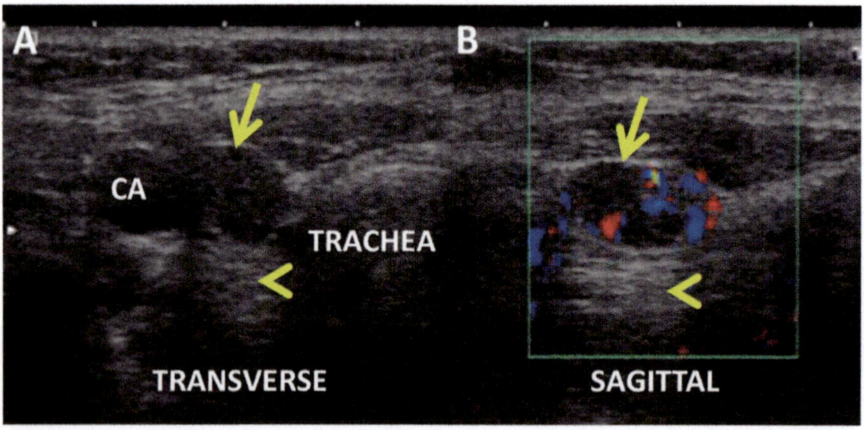

Fig. 17.2 Cervical node ultrasound. A 1.5×0.8×1 cm node (*arrow*) is located inferior to the thyroid in the right thyroid bed, cervical node level VI, between the carotid artery (CA) and the trachea. The node is partially cystic with post-cyst enhancement (*arrowhead*) and peripheral vascular flow in the solid component of the node. (**a**) Node transverse view. (**b**) Node sagittal view with Doppler analysis

Assessment and Literature Review

The risk of malignancy in a thyroid nodule rises with the sonographic appearance of microcalcifications (OR 6.4, 95 % CI 4.9–8.4), blurred margins (OR 4.8, 95 % CI 3.8–6.1), solid hypoechoic appearance (OR 3.8, 95 % CI 2.8–5.1), and taller-than-wide shape in the transverse image [1]. The likelihood of cancer is also very high when a nodal ultrasound survey reveals abnormal lymph nodes [2]. Sonographic features suggestive of metastatic lymph nodes include loss of the fatty hilum, a rounded shape, cystic change, calcifications, and peripheral vascularity [2].

It is recommended that thyroid nodules in pregnant women with euthyroidism and hypothyroidism be evaluated and biopsied with the same criteria as nonpregnant adults [3]. The 4.6 cm hypoechoic nodule was appropriately biopsied based on the high risk of malignancy by ultrasound criteria (solid, hypoechoic, taller-than-wide, microcalcification, abnormal nodes). The ultrasound appearance and a suspicious Bethesda class V cytology are both highly specific for malignancy, with an estimated median risk of malignancy of 70 % based on the meta-analysis reported by Bongiovanni et al. [4]. AJCC/TMN staging is a universal method of communicating extent of disease and correlates with risk of death. A 46-year-old female with a >4 cm papillary thyroid carcinoma with >1 cm metastatic level 6 nodes is at a minimum an AJCC/TMN classification stage 3 patient, but would be stage 1 in a typical young pregnant woman. The decision for surgery during pregnancy requires assessment of the risk of death and recurrence of the differentiated thyroid cancer balanced against the potential harm to the fetus.

There is no consensus to whether surgery for papillary thyroid carcinoma should be performed during pregnancy or postpartum. While most retrospective analyses of patients with differentiated thyroid cancer diagnosed during pregnancy show that delaying surgery does not affect cancer outcomes [5], two other recent studies have shown that thyroid cancer diagnosed in pregnancy has a higher rate of persistence or relapse in the postpartum period [6, 7]. Although one large study showed that surgery performed during pregnancy has greater risk of complications and longer hospital stays [8], but did not provide data on fetal loss, other smaller retrospective studies show that it is safe during pregnancy, with no adverse fetal or maternal outcomes [9, 10]. These studies with fewer than 100 pregnant women show no difference in tumor stage (TMN), recurrence rate, complications of pregnancy, or adverse fetal outcome regardless of whether surgery is performed during or after pregnancy. The general recommendation is to avoid surgery during pregnancy if the tumor remains stable in size or is detected late in pregnancy. On the other hand, if the patient is older as in this case, or if the tumor has been documented to grow significantly or is associated with local or distant metastases, thyroidectomy is appropriate, preferably during the second trimester of pregnancy to avoid miscarriage [10].

Back to the Patient

During this patient's 23rd week of pregnancy, she had an uncomplicated total thyroidectomy and bilateral central neck dissection (level 6). This was done because of her age >45 years, the large size of the mass and the presence of nodal metastases. Her pathology showed a 4 cm partially encapsulated papillary thyroid carcinoma with 9 of 11 nodes containing metastatic papillary thyroid carcinoma. Six weeks after surgery, her thyroglobulin was 0.8 ng/mL with a TSH 0.1 mU/L on levothyroxine therapy. Radioactive iodine therapy was postponed for 1 year to allow her to breast-feed her baby. During the first year after surgery, she was followed with intermittent thyroglobulin levels that were stable and did not rise and neck ultrasound examinations that did not show evidence of residual or recurrent disease.

Clinical Pearls/Pitfalls

- Thyroid cancer diagnosed during pregnancy has a typical indolent course of differentiated thyroid cancer in young adults.
- Thyroid cancer without sonographic evidence of capsular invasion or metastatic nodes may be followed by ultrasound without surgery.
- More advanced disease in a pregnant woman > age 45 years, progression of disease demonstrated by growth of the primary tumor, evidence of invasion, or metastatic nodes are indications for thyroidectomy during pregnancy.
- Thyroidectomy during pregnancy is generally safe but is preferably done during the second trimester.

References

1. Cappelli C, Castellano M, Pirola I, Gandossi E, De Martino E, Cumetti D, Agosti B, Rosei EA. Thyroid nodule shape suggests malignancy. Eur J Endocrinol. 2006;155:27–31.
2. Sohn YM, et al. Diagnostic approach for evaluation of lymph node metastasis from thyroid cancer using ultrasound and fine-needle aspiration biopsy. AJR Am J Roentgenol. 2010;194:38–43.
3. Cooper DS, Doherty G, Haugen BR, Kloos RT, Lee SL, Mandel SJ, Mazzaferri EL, McIver B, Pacini F, Schlumberger M, Sherman SI, Steward DL. Tuttle RM Revised American Thyroid Association management guidelines for patients with thyroid nodules and differentiated thyroid cancer. Thyroid. 2009;19:1167–214.
4. Bongiovanni M, Spitale A, Faquin WC, Mazzucchelli L, Baloch ZW. The Bethesda System for reporting thyroid cytopathology: a meta-analysis. Acta Cytol. 2012;56:333–9.
5. Mazzaferri EL. Approach to the pregnant patient with thyroid cancer. J Clin Endocrinol Metab. 2011;96:265–72.
6. Vannucchi G, Perrino M, Rossi S, Colombo C, Vicentini L, Dazzi D, Beck-Peccoz P, Fugazzola L. Clinical and molecular features of differentiated thyroid cancer diagnosed during pregnancy. Eur J Endocrinol. 2010;162:145–51.
7. Messuti I, Corvisieri S, Bardesono F, Rapa I, Giorcelli J, Pellerito R, Volante M, Orlandi F. Impact of pregnancy on prognosis of differentiated thyroid cancer: clinical and molecular features. Eur J Endocrinol. 2014;170:659–66.
8. Kuy S, Roman SA, Desai R, Sosa JA. Outcomes following thyroid and parathyroid surgery in pregnant women. Arch Surg. 2009;144:399–406.
9. Herzon FS, Morris DM, Segal MN, Rauch G, Parnell T. Coexistent thyroid cancer and pregnancy. Arch Otolaryngol Head Neck Surg. 1994;120:1191–3.
10. Uruno T, Shibuya H, Kitagawa W, Nagahama M, Sugino K, Ito K. Optimal timing of surgery for differentiated thyroid cancer in pregnant women. World J Surg. 2014;38:704–8.

Chapter 18
Risks of Thyroid Hormone Suppression for Differentiated Thyroid Cancer in the Elderly

Swaytha Yalamanchi and David Cooper

Case Presentation

A 91-year-old woman presents for management of papillary thyroid carcinoma (PTC). She underwent a total thyroidectomy 6 years previously. Pathology demonstrated a 1.3 cm focus of PTC with focal tall cell features and metastases in one of four central and two of five left lateral lymph nodes. She was treated with 75 mCi of I-131 and her posttreatment scan showed two foci of radiotracer localization in the thyroid bed and three foci in the anterior lower thorax. The patient underwent resection of a level VI lymph node 4 years later. Pathology showed a 1.5 cm lymph node replaced by PTC and extensive skeletal muscle involvement. Chest CT scan showed multiple pulmonary nodules suspicious for metastatic disease, none of which were iodine-avid on subsequent I-123 scan. The patient also has a history of osteoporosis with a femoral fragility fracture and is being treated with risedronate.

Recent biochemical assessment includes serum thyroid stimulating hormone (TSH) 0.68 mU/L (0.50–4.50), serum free T4 1.6 ng/dl (0.8–1.8), and serum basal thyroglobulin 120 ng/ml with negative serum thyroglobulin antibody titers.

Assessment and Literature Review

PTC is associated with low rates of mortality and recurrence, particularly in patients with low-risk disease. Fully suppressive thyroxine (T4) therapy (serum TSH <0.1 mU/L) does not have a role in the long-term management of low-risk PTC, though

S. Yalamanchi, MD • D. Cooper, MD (✉)
Division of Endocrinology, Diabetes, and Metabolism, Johns Hopkins Hospital,
1830 E. Monument St, Suite 333, Baltimore, MD 21287, USA
e-mail: dscooper@jhmi.edu

D.S. Cooper, C. Durante (eds.), *Thyroid Cancer*,
DOI 10.1007/978-3-319-22401-5_18

may improve survival in patients with high-risk disease. Iatrogenic hyperthyroidism may negatively impact cardiovascular and bone health, particularly in the elderly. Individualized goals regarding T4 suppressive therapy are thus necessary.

Prevalence

The incidence of differentiated thyroid cancer (DTC), particularly low-risk PTC, has increased rapidly over the past 15 years [1]. Although there has been increased detection of incidental subclinical disease on imaging studies, rates of aggressive PTC (tall cell variant histology, tumors with extrathyroidal extension, and distant metastases) and thyroid cancer-specific mortality in the past 10–15 years have also increased [2].

Efficacy of Thyroid Hormone Suppression Therapy

DTC treatment has traditionally included total thyroidectomy, suppression of serum TSH to undetectable levels, and, in selected cases, radioiodine ablation (RAI). Older studies suggested that suppressed TSH levels, regardless of the stage, may be associated with decreased rates of disease progression and recurrence and increased rates of relapse-free survival [3, 4]. Multiple studies since that time, however, have shown that thyroid hormone suppression is beneficial in high-risk, but not low-risk, disease. A prospective study of the National Thyroid Cancer Treatment Cooperative Study Group (NTCTCSG) ($n=617$) found no effect of thyroid hormone suppression in stages I and II disease with minimal effects seen in stages III and IV after adjustment by multivariate analysis [5]. A subsequent study of 4,047 patients in the NTCTCSG demonstrated that T4 suppressive therapy did not modify outcomes in stage I disease. Improved overall survival was seen with moderate suppression in stage II disease and aggressive suppression in stage III and IV disease. T4 suppressive therapy was associated with improved disease-specific survival in high-risk patients, but had no effect on disease-free survival at any stage [6]. Hovens et al. confirmed these findings ($n=366$, mean follow-up=8.85 years) and found that median serum TSH levels >2 mU/L in patients with T1-3, M0 tumors were associated with higher rates of thyroid cancer recurrence (HR 1.41; 95 % CI 1.03–1.95) and death (HR 2.03; 95 % CI 1.22–3.37) as compared to individuals with serum TSH <2 mU/L [7]. Most recently, in a non-inferiority randomized control trial of low-risk DTC patients ($n=433$, mean follow-up=6.9 years), Sugitani et al. demonstrated that disease-free survival in euthyroid patients (mean serum TSH 3.2 mU/L) was similar to that of patients with suppressed serum TSH. Of note, the majority of patients in this cohort underwent central neck dissection and did not receive radioiodine, patterns of care that differ from that seen in North America and Europe [8].

Overall, patients with low-risk DTC have an excellent prognosis, and aggressive TSH suppression is unlikely to be beneficial. In contrast, current evidence suggests that TSH suppression may lower recurrence rates and improve disease-specific survival in patients with more aggressive disease. The appropriate degree of TSH suppression by thyroid hormone suppression therapy remains unknown.

Recommendations for Serum TSH Suppression Goals

The 2015 ATA guidelines recommend initial serum TSH suppression goals for high- and intermediate-risk thyroid cancer patients of <0.1 mU/L and 0.1–0.5 mU/L, respectively. The recommended goal serum TSH for low-risk patients with detectable serum thyroglobulin regardless of remnant ablation status is at or slightly below the lower limit of normal (0.1–0.5 mU/L). Low-risk patients with undetectable serum thyroglobulin levels regardless of whether they have undergone remnant ablation may have serum TSH maintained at the lower end of the reference range (0.5–2 mU/L) [9].

Serum TSH goals at the time of initial assessment should be based on comorbidities (Table 18.1) [9]. TSH targets in the long-term follow-up of DTC depend on comorbidities, the risk of recurrence, and evidence of disease [9] (Table 18.1).

Adverse Effects Associated with Suppressive T4 Therapy in the Elderly

While T4 suppressive therapy may reduce recurrence and mortality rates in individuals with high-risk DTC, there are inherent risks associated with iatrogenic hyperthyroidism. Suppressive thyroxine therapy may negatively impact quality of life [10]. Iatrogenic hyperthyroidism also adversely affects cardiovascular and bone health, particularly in the elderly.

It is unclear if endogenous hyperthyroidism and exogenous hyperthyroidism cause similar adverse event profiles. Serum free T4 levels are high normal or elevated in both situations, but it is uncommon for serum T3 levels to be high

Table 18.1 Suggested long-term serum TSH targets in patients with DTC

	Response to therapy			
Risk from T4 therapy	Excellent (mU/L)	Indeterminate (mU/L)	Biochemically incomplete (mU/L)	Structurally incomplete (mU/L)
Minimal	0.5–2.0[a]	0.1–0.5	<0.1	<0.1
Moderate	0.5–2.0[a]	0.5–2.0[a]	0.1–0.5	<0.1
High	0.5–2.0[a]	0.5–2.0[a]	0.5–2.0[a]	0.1–0.5

Adapted from 2015 ATA guidelines [9]

[a]Serum TSH of 0.5 mU/L represents the lower limit of the reference range for specific TSH assays; this level may be 0.3–0.5 mU/L depending on the assay

normal or elevated in iatrogenic hyperthyroidism, as compared to endogenous hyperthyroidism. The difference in serum T4/T3 ratios in endogenous and exogenous hyperthyroidism may thus result in different end-organ effects [11].

Cardiovascular Disease

Dysrhythmias

Elderly individuals with iatrogenic hyperthyroidism are at increased risk of dysrhythmias and cardiovascular (CV) disease. The elderly also tend to be less symptomatic than their younger counterparts and thus warrant heightened clinical suspicion [12].

The prevalence of atrial fibrillation (AF) in DTC patients 60 years and older has been estimated to be as high as 17.5 %, with paroxysmal AF more common than persistent AF [13]. A Scottish observational study including 17,684 patients (females 85.9 % with mean age of 60.3 years; males with mean age of 61.8 years; median follow-up 4.5 years) on levothyroxine for at least 6 months demonstrated that individuals with exogenously suppressed serum TSH levels of <0.03 mU/L were at increased risk for CV disease (adjusted HR 1.37; 95 % CI 1.17–1.60) and dysrhythmias (adjusted HR 1.6; 95 % CI 1.10–2.33) after adjustment for age, sex, previous thyroid condition, socioeconomic status, and history of diabetes mellitus. The subset of patients with low but non-suppressed serum TSH levels ranging from 0.04 to 0.4 mU/L did not have an increased risk of cardiac events [14].

Cardiovascular Mortality

There has been conflicting data regarding whether exogenous hyperthyroidism results in increased cardiovascular mortality. Bauer et al. found no difference in mortality rates between women on long-term thyroxine therapy and nonusers (relative hazard 1.11, 95 % CI 0.98–1.24, $p \leq 0.09$), even when stratified by serum TSH (<0.5 mU/L vs. >5 mU/L). A prior history of hyperthyroidism, however, was associated with a small increase in all-cause and cardiovascular mortality [15]. In contrast, a population-based observational study (mean age 49 ± 14 years, median follow-up = 8.5 years) demonstrated an increase in CV mortality and all-cause mortality by 3.3- and 4.4-fold, respectively, in patients with DTC independent of age, sex, and CV risk factors. Each tenfold decrease in geometric mean serum TSH was associated with a 3.1-fold increase in CV mortality [16]. Yang et al. similarly observed that among thyroid cancer patients, cardiac disease and cerebrovascular disease were the most frequent causes of non-cancer mortality [17]. The mechanism for increased CV mortality is unclear, but is postulated to be related to an increased risk of AF, impaired diastolic function, and increased left ventricular mass, leading to increased risk of stroke, heart failure, and myocardial infarction, respectively [16].

Bone Health

Bone Mineral Density and Fracture Risk

Data regarding the effect of iatrogenic hyperthyroidism on BMD are conflicting, but largely suggestive of a decrease in BMD and increase in fracture risk in postmenopausal women. The majority of data have not shown compelling evidence of a significant change in bone health in premenopausal women or men treated with T4 suppressive therapy [18–20].

Bauer et al. prospectively followed 686 women at least 65 years of age with subclinical hyperthyroidism (both exogenous and endogenous) and demonstrated that women with a suppressed serum TSH level (≤0.1 mU/L) had a threefold increased risk of hip fracture (relative hazard, 3.6 [95 % CI, 1.0–12.9]) and a fourfold increased risk of vertebral fracture (odds ratio 4.5, 95 % CI 1.3–15.6) as compared to controls (serum TSH 0.5–5.5 mU/L) [21]. The Thyroid Epidemiology Audit and Research Study (TEARS) also demonstrated an increased risk of fractures in both individuals with suppressed serum TSH (<0.03 mU/L) (adjusted HR 2.02, 95 % CI 1.55–2.62) and elevated serum TSH (>4.0 mU/L) (adjusted HR 1.83, 95 % CI 1.41–2.37). Elevated serum TSH levels in the latter group were considered to be a marker for poor compliance with medical therapy. Similar to the pattern seen in cardiovascular events as previously described, individuals with low but non-suppressed serum TSH levels (0.04–0.4 mU/L) did not have an increased risk of fracture [14].

A meta-analysis including five population-based prospective studies demonstrated a nonsignificant increase in the risk of hip fractures (HR 1.38 [CI, 0.92–2.07]) and non-spine fractures when patients with endogenous and exogenous subclinical hyperthyroidism were pooled. The strength of the relationship between subclinical hyperthyroidism and fractures appeared stronger in the setting of a suppressed serum TSH (<0.1 mU/L), but only two studies provided such data [22]. These findings are in keeping with meta-analyses by Faber et al. and Uzzan et al. suggesting that T4 suppressive therapy results in bone loss at an annual rate of 1 % in postmenopausal women [23, 24]. Differences in studies may be partially explained by varying rates of thyroid hormone suppression and calcium intake in the studies [20].

Treatment

Calcium and bisphosphonates are useful in managing bone health in iatrogenic hyperthyroidism. Kung et al. demonstrated that calcium monotherapy (1000 mg/day) was effective in mitigating bone loss, while intranasal calcitonin offered little further benefit [25]. Panico et al. stratified 74 postmenopausal women with DTC and a history of low BMD (T score ≤ −2.5) into three groups based on the duration of T4 suppressive therapy of 3, 6, and 9 years, respectively. All individuals, including controls, were treated with bisphosphonates, calcium, and vitamin D for 2 years, and all demonstrated an increase in lumbar spine BMD. Bisphosphonates were most effective in increasing BMD in the lumbar spine and femoral neck in postmenopausal women receiving T4 suppressive therapy in the short term [26].

Management of Patient

Our patient has recurrent stage IVc PTC with likely pulmonary metastases. Given her persistent high-risk disease, she qualifies for suppressive thyroxine therapy (serum TSH < 0.1 mU/L) by the ATA guidelines. However, the patient is postmenopausal with known osteoporosis. She also is elderly with increased risk of AF and may have underlying cardiac disease that could increase her risk of cardiovascular mortality. In weighing the benefits and risks of suppressive therapy, the patient's goal serum TSH is in the mildly suppressed range (0.1–0.50 mU/L). Given proximity to goal TSH in the low-normal range, the patient's dose of levothyroxine was not adjusted.

Clinical Pearls/Pitfalls

- T4 suppressive therapy does not improve survival in patients with low-risk DTC though it is likely to be beneficial in high-risk patients.
- Serum TSH targets in the long-term follow-up of individuals with DTC depends on the risk of recurrence, evidence of disease, and comorbidities.
- The elderly are at the high risk of developing complications from T4 suppressive therapy, particularly atrial fibrillation and osteoporosis.
- Calcium and bisphosphonates may be useful in mitigating the risk of bone loss in postmenopausal women on suppressive doses of T4.
- Risks of adverse cardiovascular and skeletal effects are minimized by targeting subnormal, rather than fully suppressed serum TSH levels (Table 18.1).

References

1. SEER cancer statistics review, 1975–2011, National Cancer Institute. Bethesda, MD. Based on November 2013 SEER data submission, released April 2014. http://seer.cancer.gov/csr/1975_2011/
2. McLeod DS, Sawka AM, Cooper DS. Controversies in primary treatment of low-risk papillary thyroid cancer. Lancet. 2013;381(9871):1046–57.
3. Pujol P, Daures JP, Nsakala N, Baldet L, Bringer J, Jaffiol C. Degree of thyrotropin suppression as a prognostic determinant in differentiated thyroid cancer. J Clin Endocrinol Metab. 1996;81(12):4318–23.

4. McGriff NJ, Csako G, Gourgiotis L, Lori CG, Pucino F, Sarlis NJ. Effects of thyroid hormone suppression therapy on adverse clinical outcomes in thyroid cancer. Ann Med. 2002;34(7–8): 554–64.
5. Cooper DS, Specker B, Ho M, et al. Thyrotropin suppression and disease progression in patients with differentiated thyroid cancer: results from the national thyroid cancer treatment cooperative registry. Thyroid. 1998;8(9):737–44.
6. Jonklaas J, Sarlis NJ, Litofsky D, et al. Outcomes of patients with differentiated thyroid carcinoma following initial therapy. Thyroid. 2006;16(12):1229–42.
7. Hovens GC, Stokkel MP, Kievit J, et al. Associations of serum thyrotropin concentrations with recurrence and death in differentiated thyroid cancer. J Clin Endocrinol Metab. 2007;92(7): 2610–15.
8. Sugitani I, Fujimoto Y. Does postoperative thyrotropin suppression therapy truly decrease recurrence in papillary thyroid carcinoma? A randomized controlled trial. J Clin Endocrinol Metab. 2010;95(10):4576–83.
9. Haugen BR, Alexander EK, Bible KC, Doherty GM, Mandel SJ, Nikiforov Y, et al. American Thyroid Association Management Guidelines for patients with thyroid nodules and differentiated thyroid cancer. Thyroid. 2015; 24. in press.
10. Giusti M, Melle G, Fenocchio M, et al. Five-year longitudinal evaluation of quality of life in a cohort of patients with differentiated thyroid carcinoma. J Zhejiang Univ Sci B. 2011;12(3): 163–73.
11. Biondi B, Cooper DS. Benefits of thyrotropin suppression versus the risks of adverse effects in differentiated thyroid cancer. Thyroid. 2010;20(2):135–46.
12. Boelaert K, Torlinska B, Holder RL, Franklyn JA. Older subjects with hyperthyroidism present with a paucity of symptoms and signs: a large cross-sectional study. J Clin Endocrinol Metab. 2010;95(6):2715–26.
13. Abonowara A, Quraishi A, Sapp JL, et al. Prevalence of atrial fibrillation in patients taking TSH suppression therapy for management of thyroid cancer. Clin Invest Med. 2012;35(3): E152–6.
14. Flynn RW, Bonellie SR, Jung RT, MacDonald TM, Morris AD, Leese GP. Serum thyroid-stimulating hormone concentration and morbidity from cardiovascular disease and fractures in patients on long-term thyroxine therapy. J Clin Endocrinol Metab. 2010;95(1):186–93.
15. Bauer DC, Rodondi N, Stone KL, Hillier TA, Study of Osteoporotic Fractures Research Group: Universities of California (San Francisco), Pittsburgh, Minnesota (Minneapolis), Kaiser Permanente Center for Health Research, Portland. Thyroid hormone use, hyperthyroidism and mortality in older women. Am J Med. 2007;120(4):343–9.
16. Klein Hesselink EN, Klein Hesselink MS, de Bock GH, et al. Long-term cardiovascular mortality in patients with differentiated thyroid carcinoma: an observational study. J Clin Oncol. 2013;31(32):4046–53.
17. Yang L, Shen W, Sakamoto N. Population-based study evaluating and predicting the probability of death resulting from thyroid cancer and other causes among patients with thyroid cancer. J Clin Oncol. 2013;31(4):468–74.
18. Heemstra KA, Hamdy NA, Romijn JA, Smit JW. The effects of thyrotropin-suppressive therapy on bone metabolism in patients with well-differentiated thyroid carcinoma. Thyroid. 2006;16(6):583–91.
19. Waring AC, Harrison S, Fink HA, et al. A prospective study of thyroid function, bone loss, and fractures in older men: the MrOS study. J Bone Miner Res. 2013;28(3):472–9.
20. Quan ML, Pasieka JL, Rorstad O. Bone mineral density in well-differentiated thyroid cancer patients treated with suppressive thyroxine: a systematic overview of the literature. J Surg Oncol. 2002;79(1):62–9. discussion 69–70.
21. Bauer DC, Ettinger B, Nevitt MC, Stone KL, Study of Osteoporotic Fractures Research Group. Risk for fracture in women with low serum levels of thyroid-stimulating hormone. Ann Intern Med. 2001;134(7):561–8.
22. Wirth CD, Blum MR, da Costa BR, et al. Subclinical thyroid dysfunction and the risk for fractures: a systematic review and meta-analysis. Ann Intern Med. 2014;161(3):189–99.

23. Faber J, Galloe AM. Changes in bone mass during prolonged subclinical hyperthyroidism due to L-thyroxine treatment: a meta-analysis. Eur J Endocrinol. 1994;130(4):350–6.
24. Uzzan B, Campos J, Cucherat M, Nony P, Boissel JP, Perret GY. Effects on bone mass of long term treatment with thyroid hormones: a meta-analysis. J Clin Endocrinol Metab. 1996;81(12):4278–89.
25. Kung AW, Yeung SS. Prevention of bone loss induced by thyroxine suppressive therapy in postmenopausal women: the effect of calcium and calcitonin. J Clin Endocrinol Metab. 1996;81(3):1232–6.
26. Panico A, Lupoli GA, Fonderico F, et al. Osteoporosis and thyrotropin-suppressive therapy: reduced effectiveness of alendronate. Thyroid. 2009;19(5):437–42.

Chapter 19
A Patient in Whom One Pathologist Says She Has Cancer, and Another Says that the Lesion Is Benign

Point of Discussion: Follicular Adenoma Versus Follicular Carcinoma

Justin A. Bishop

Case Presentation

A 53-year-old woman presented to her primary care physician with the complaint of a lump in her neck. Physical examination revealed a discrete, rounded nodule measuring approximately 3 cm, centered in the right lobe of the thyroid gland. The patient was referred for an ultrasound-guided fine-needle aspiration. The ultrasound demonstrated a solitary, smoothly marginated, echogenic 3.0 × 2.1 × 1.3 cm solid thyroid nodule with a well-defined peripheral hypoechoic halo. The fine-needle aspiration diagnosis was "suspicious for a follicular neoplasm," and the patient subsequently underwent a right thyroid lobectomy (Fig. 19.1a). A surgical pathology diagnosis of "minimally invasive follicular carcinoma" was made by the community pathologist on the basis of extensive invasion of the tumor capsule (Fig. 19.1b, c). The patient sought consultation at an academic institution for subsequent completion thyroidectomy and radioactive iodine therapy. Prior to definitive treatment, the pathology slides were re-reviewed by a pathologist with specialist expertise in thyroid pathology. The consultant pathologist made the diagnosis of "follicular adenoma with prominent secondary changes related to fine-needle aspiration" (Fig. 19.1b–d). As a result, the patient required no additional therapy, and after 5 years of follow-up, she has no evidence of disease.

J.A. Bishop, MD (✉)
The Johns Hopkins University School of Medicine, The Harry and Jeannette Weinberg Building, 401 N. Broadway, Room 2249, Baltimore, MD 21231, USA
e-mail: jbishop@jhmi.edu

D.S. Cooper, C. Durante (eds.), *Thyroid Cancer*,
DOI 10.1007/978-3-319-22401-5_19

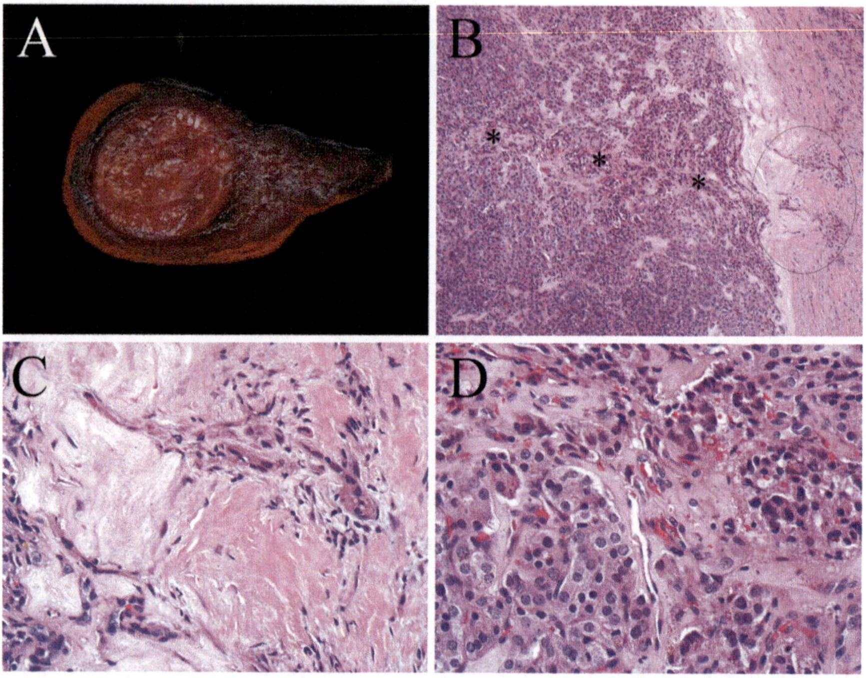

Fig. 19.1 In the presented case, the patient had a solitary, thinly encapsulated 3 cm nodule in her thyroid lobe (**a**, gross photograph). On low power, there is a vague, linear disruption within the tumor (*asterisks*) along with some cellularity within the tumor capsule (*oval*) (**b**, hematoxylin and eosin, ×40). Within the capsule, there were irregular nests of tumor embedded in fibrous stroma (**c**, hematoxylin and eosin, ×400). Within the linear area of tumor disruption, there is evidence of trauma including stromal fibrosis, hemorrhage, and hemosiderin (**d**, hematoxylin and eosin, ×400). In all, the findings are consistent with a benign follicular adenoma with worrisome histologic alterations following fine-needle aspiration of the thyroid gland

Assessment and Literature Review

This case highlights the important differences between the diagnoses of follicular adenoma and follicular carcinoma and the diagnostic difficulties that can arise in making the distinction.

General Considerations

A follicular adenoma is defined as an encapsulated neoplasm of thyroid follicular epithelial differentiation that lacks evidence of invasive growth and does not exhibit the nuclear features of papillary carcinoma [1]. Its malignant counterpart, follicular carcinoma, is actually a diagnosis of exclusion, defined as “a malignant epithelial tumor showing evidence of follicular cell differentiation and not belonging to any other distinctive types of thyroid malignancy" [2]. Follicular carcinoma is subdivided into two general categories: (1) widely invasive tumors that usually lack a capsule and exhibit extensive, clear-cut invasion of surrounding stroma and (2) minimally invasive tumors that invade only into a surrounding capsule. Widely invasive follicular carcinoma is not easily confused with follicular adenoma; as a result, the remainder of this chapter will deal with the differential diagnosis between follicular adenoma and minimally invasive follicular carcinoma.

Clinical Presentation

Both follicular adenomas and minimally invasive follicular carcinomas tend to present similarly as a solitary thyroid nodule, though follicular carcinomas tend to be larger overall. Patients with large tumors may complain of compressive symptoms like dyspnea, coughing, or hoarseness. Almost all patients with these tumors are euthyroid. Because the defining feature of minimally invasive follicular carcinoma is an architectural one (details below), a definitive diagnosis cannot be made by fine-needle aspiration. Both follicular adenoma and follicular carcinoma are likely to be diagnosed as "suspicious for a follicular neoplasm" or "atypical cells of undetermined significance" by fine-needle aspiration [3].

Treatment

Surgical intervention—at minimum, a thyroid lobectomy—is required to make the diagnosis of follicular adenoma or minimally invasive follicular carcinoma. A patient receiving the diagnosis of follicular adenoma requires no additional therapy. In contrast, the treatment of minimally invasive follicular carcinoma is somewhat controversial. Many experts advocate for completion thyroidectomy with subsequent radioactive iodine, although others have argued that a lobectomy alone may be sufficient, particularly in tumors that exhibit only capsular invasion [4]. Because follicular carcinoma only rarely metastasizes to lymph nodes, a prophylactic lymph node dissection is not recommended [4].

Surgical Pathology

Grossly, follicular adenomas and minimally invasive follicular carcinomas have an appearance that is essentially identical: a solitary, well-circumscribed nodule with a well-developed capsule (Fig. 19.2a). At the microscopic level, follicular carcinomas generally tend to be larger; exhibit more hypercellular growth with microfollicular,

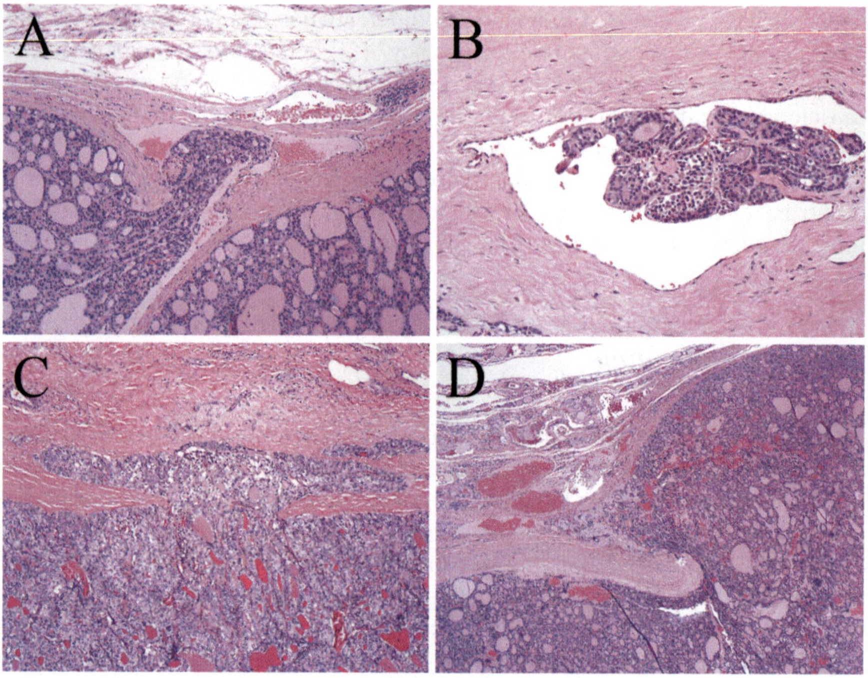

Fig. 19.2 To be regarded as true vascular invasion in an encapsulated follicular carcinoma, the vessel in question must be located within or immediately beyond the tumor capsule (**a**, hematoxylin and eosin, ×40). In addition, the tumor thrombus must extend into the vessel and is usually covered by a layer of endothelial cells (**b**, hematoxylin and eosin, ×200). Foci of capsular invasion in a minimally invasive follicular carcinoma often take the shape of a mushroom cloud (**c**, hematoxylin and eosin, ×100) or a fishhook (**d**, hematoxylin and eosin, ×20)

trabecular, and solid growth patterns; and possess thicker tumor capsules when compared to follicular adenomas. However, the sole histologic feature that distinguishes follicular adenoma from minimally invasive follicular carcinoma is the presence of invasive growth. Specifically, a follicular carcinoma must exhibit capsular and/or vascular invasion. While this may sound relatively straightforward on its face, any practicing pathologist knows that determining the presence of invasive growth in a follicular neoplasm can be very challenging and is fraught with pitfalls.

Vascular invasion is generally regarded as more reliable than capsular invasion for the diagnosis of minimally invasive follicular carcinoma, and the criteria are strict [2]. To qualify as vascular invasion, the vessel in question needs to be either within the capsule or immediately outside of it; vessels inside the tumor itself should not be considered (Fig. 19.2a). The vessel wall must have a clear-cut endothelial lining and a muscle wall. In addition, the focus of tumor must be attached to the vessel wall with protrusion into the lumen (Fig. 19.2b). Tumor that is "free-floating" within a vessel may represent artifactual detachment from surgery or from the grossing station and therefore does not qualify. Similarly, tumor simply "bulging" into a vessel should not be regarded as truly invasive growth. Ideally, the tumor thrombus should be lined by an endothelial layer, though not all authorities agree on the importance of this finding [2, 5]. In addition, some investigators regard the presence of fibrin thrombi as helpful evidence of true vascular invasion [5].

Capsular invasion is defined as contiguous, full-thickness extension of the tumor through its capsule [2]. Very often, this invasion takes the form of a "mushroom cloud" or "fishhook"-like appearance (Fig. 19.2c, d). Mere irregularities of the tumor capsule are not sufficient to qualify as unequivocal invasion. In addition, separate "satellite" nodules immediately outside the tumor capsule are not adequate evidence of invasion. A very specific pitfall in diagnosing capsular invasion involves the artifactual displacement of tumor through the tumor capsule by a fine-needle aspiration, a situation that has been referred to as "worrisome histologic findings following FNA of the thyroid" or "WHAFFT" [6]. The keys to recognizing WHAFFT are noticing (1) the abrupt, linear configuration of the displaced follicles and (2) the secondary reactive changes including hemorrhage, hemosiderin, granulation tissue, and scarring that accompany the displacement. These secondary changes are also typically linear (Fig. 19.1b–d). Moreover, the absence of vascular invasion in this setting is reassuring that the changes are benign.

There are very few ancillary studies that can be utilized to distinguish follicular adenoma from follicular carcinoma. Both tumors frequently harbor *RAS* mutations, and while *PAX8/PPARγ* rearrangements are more common in follicular carcinoma, they can also be seen in follicular adenomas [7]. As a result, there is currently no role for molecular diagnostics in distinguishing the entities. On occasion, immunostaining for vascular endothelial markers (e.g., CD31, ERG) can be helpful in highlighting vessels with tumor thrombi [2]. In the vast majority of cases, however, the diagnosis rests solely on routine light microscopy. As invasion can be a very focal finding, the entire capsule of an encapsulated thyroid neoplasm should be examined for invasive growth. In addition, for a focus suspicious but not diagnostic for invasion, deeper levels into the tissue block are often helpful in resolving the true nature of the area in question. Considering the importance of the distinction, it is reasonable to seek out a second opinion from an experienced thyroid pathologist to confirm the diagnosis for minimally invasive follicular carcinoma [8, 9].

Prognosis

In general, patients with minimally invasive follicular carcinoma have a very good prognosis. However, minimally invasive follicular carcinoma is capable of local recurrence and metastasis [10]. There is increasing evidence that minimally invasive follicular carcinomas that are larger and exhibit extensive vascular invasion are more prone to displaying aggressive behavior [11]. Specifically, tumors with more than 3 foci of vascular invasion seem to be at highest risk of recurrence, and for that reason, it is now recommended that the number of foci of vascular invasion be mentioned in the surgical pathology report [12]. Some authorities have even suggested avoiding the term "minimally invasive" in this tumor subset to avoid confusion and inadequate treatment [13].

Clinical Pearls/Pitfalls

- The significance of making the distinction between follicular adenoma and minimally invasive follicular carcinoma is considerable. While the former is benign and requires only a diagnostic thyroid lobectomy, the latter is capable of aggressive behavior and generally requires further therapy.
- The sole histologic feature that separates follicular adenoma and minimally invasive follicular carcinoma is the presence of invasive tumor growth.
- Mimickers of capsular invasion include capsular irregularities, satellite nodules, and fine-needle aspiration-induced displacement.
- Mimickers of vascular invasion include free-floating displaced tumor, tumor protrusion beneath a vessel, and involvement of an intratumoral vessel.
- The prognosis of follicular carcinoma varies based on the extent of invasion. Follicular carcinomas that exhibit only capsular or minimal (i.e., 3 or fewer) foci of vascular invasion behave indolently. As a result, this information should be included in the pathology report.
- If the diagnosis is in doubt, a second opinion from an expert thyroid pathologist should be sought.

References

1. Rosai J, Carcangiu ML, DeLellis RA. Follicular adenoma. Tumors of the thyroid gland. Washington, DC: ARP; 1992. p. 21–40.
2. Rosai J, Carcangiu ML, DeLellis RA. Follicular carcinoma. Tumors of the thyroid gland. Washington, DC: ARP; 1992. p. 49–64.
3. Cibas ES, Ali SZ. The Bethesda system for reporting thyroid cytopathology. Thyroid. 2009;19(11):1159–65. Epub 2009/11/06.
4. Cooper DS, Doherty GM, Haugen BR, Kloos RT, Lee SL, Mandel SJ, et al. Revised American Thyroid Association management guidelines for patients with thyroid nodules and differentiated thyroid cancer. Thyroid. 2009;19(11):1167–214. Epub 2009/10/29.
5. Mete O, Asa SL. Pathological definition and clinical significance of vascular invasion in thyroid carcinomas of follicular epithelial derivation. Mod Pathol. 2011;24(12):1545–52. Epub 2011/08/02.
6. LiVolsi VA, Merino MJ. Worrisome histologic alterations following fine-needle aspiration of the thyroid (WHAFFT). Pathol Annu. 1994;29(Pt 2):99–120. Epub 1994/01/01.
7. Nikiforov YE. Molecular diagnostics of thyroid tumors. Arch Pathol Lab Med. 2011;135(5):569–77. Epub 2011/04/30.
8. Westra WH, Kronz JD, Eisele DW. The impact of second opinion surgical pathology on the practice of head and neck surgery: a decade experience at a large referral hospital. Head Neck. 2002;24(7):684–93. Epub 2002/07/12.

9. Woolgar JA, Triantafyllou A, Thompson LD, Hunt JL, Lewis Jr JS, Williams MD, et al. Double reporting and second opinion in head and neck pathology. Eur Arch Otorhinolaryngol. 2014;271(5):847–54. Epub 2014/01/18.
10. Thompson LD, Wieneke JA, Paal E, Frommelt RA, Adair CF, Heffess CS. A clinicopathologic study of minimally invasive follicular carcinoma of the thyroid gland with a review of the English literature. Cancer. 2001;91(3):505–24. Epub 2001/02/15.
11. Machens A, Holzhausen HJ, Dralle H. The prognostic value of primary tumor size in papillary and follicular thyroid carcinoma. Cancer. 2005;103(11):2269–73.
12. Ghossein R. Update to the College of American pathologists reporting on thyroid carcinomas. Head Neck Pathol. 2009;3(1):86–93.
13. Ghossein R. Problems and controversies in the histopathology of thyroid carcinomas of follicular cell origin. Arch Pathol Lab Med. 2009;133(5):683–91. Epub 2009/05/07.

Chapter 20
A Case with Postsurgical Hypoparathyroidism

Jessica Pepe and Salvatore Minisola

Case Presentation

A 49-year-old woman complaining of perioral and digital numbness/tingling was referred to our outpatient Mineral Metabolism Unit. One month before, she had a thyroidectomy for a benign multinodular goiter. According to the pathology report, the surgical procedure did not result in the incidental removal of the parathyroid glands. However, 6 h after the thyroidectomy, the patient complained of mild paresthesias and tingling; her serum calcium level was 2.07 mmol/L (normal range 2.2–2.6 mmol/L). The patient was started on intravenous calcium gluconate which provided relief from the symptoms. Two days after surgery, the patient was discharged with a calcium level of 2.19 mmol/L while on oral calcium (1 g a day) and calcitriol (0.25 mcg twice a day) therapy. The patient's symptoms began 3 weeks after discharge from the hospital in conjunction with diarrhea that closely followed food consumption at a banquet. She was still following the prescribed therapy when she came to our Unit 2 days after the acute episode of diarrhea had resolved. Thyroid function was well controlled on oral thyroxine; the patient was also on losartan 50 mg daily for hypertension.

As an outpatient, her initial laboratory tests were as follows: calcium 1.83 mmol/L, phosphorus 2.41 mmol/L (normal range 0.8–1.45 mmol/L), parathyroid hormone 10 ng/L (normal range 14–72 ng/L), and 24-h urinary calcium 12 mmol (normal range 1.25–10 mmol/24 h). On physical examination, she was obese (body mass index of 31 kg/m^2) with no other pathological signs; her blood pressure was 160/95 mmHg. Trousseau and Chvostek signs, which are signs of latent tetany, were positive. Indeed, a tapping of her facial nerve in front of the ear, just below the zygomatic arch, elicited

J. Pepe, MD, PhD (✉) • S. Minisola, MD, Full Professor of Internal Medicine
Department of Internal Medicine and Medical Disciplines, "Sapienza", University of Rome, Viale del Policlinico 155, 00161 Rome, Italy
e-mail: jessica.pepe76@gmail.com

D.S. Cooper, C. Durante (eds.), *Thyroid Cancer*,
DOI 10.1007/978-3-319-22401-5_20

the Chvostek sign, which is a momentary abnormal contraction of the ipsilateral facial muscles. By inflating the sphygmomanometer to a pressure greater than the systolic blood pressure and held in place for three minutes, we caused the Trousseau sign, which includes wrist flexion, interphalangeal joint extension, and thumb adduction. These clinical data were indicative of symptomatic postsurgical hypocalcemia necessitating an adjustment of therapy.

Assessment and Literature Review

Several studies have been published on hypocalcemia following thyroid and other anterior neck surgery; they report the prevalence, duration, severity, potential causes, possible ways to avoid or at least limit permanent hypoparathyroidism, and its medical management [1–3].

Definition and Prevalence

The major biochemical features of hypoparathyroidism are hypocalcemia and absent or low levels of parathyroid hormone (PTH); they also include an increased renal calcium excretion and hyperphosphatemia as a result of the lack of PTH, which physiologically enhances renal tubular calcium reabsorption and increases phosphate excretion. Nowadays, postsurgical hypoparathyroidism is commonly due to thyroidectomy, but it has been reported also after other neck surgical procedures, such as laryngectomy and parathyroidectomy.

The British Association of Endocrine and Thyroid Surgeons audit reported rates of 27.4 and 12.1 %, respectively, for transient (resolving in the first 24–48 h after surgery) and permanent post-thyroidectomy hypocalcemia [4]. Other authors report values of 0.5–10.6 % for permanent hypocalcemia [5, 6]. It is caused by parathyroid devascularization, stunning, or incidental removal of the parathyroid gland(s) during thyroidectomy. In some cases, even when not all the parathyroid tissue has been removed, the remainder can undergo vascular supply compromise secondary to fibrotic changes in the neck after surgery. The surgeon's experience likely influences the risk of postsurgical hypoparathyroidism, with higher-volume surgeons having lower complication rates [7]. Although transient post-thyroidectomy hypocalcemia is self-limited, it can potentially be life-threatening [8]. Hypocalcemic symptoms are uncommon unless serum calcium level is below 2.0 mmol/L (8.0 mg/dL) [9], although it is not known which calcium concentrations will trigger symptoms in any given person and whether the knowledge of this concentration is of clinical importance [10]. Symptoms probably depend on the degree and rapidity of onset of the hypocalcemia, ranging from mild paresthesias and tingling to more severe cramps, tetany, seizures, laryngospasm, congestive heart failure, and arrhythmias due to prolonged QT intervals [3, 11].

The biochemical thresholds used to diagnose hypocalcemia differ across studies. Some protocols required both clinical symptoms and hypocalcemia for the diagnosis, whereas others used either of the two. Clearly, robust definitions are warranted. The incidence of postoperative hypocalcemia for the same cohort ranged widely from 0 to 46 % depending on the definition applied [12]. This probably explains the wide range of hypocalcemia rates after thyroidectomy reported in the literature. However, beyond these uncertain rates, postsurgical hypocalcemia is clearly recognized as very common medical problem worldwide.

Predictors of Post-thyroidectomy Hypocalcemia

To reduce costs, current healthcare practices have led to progressively shorter hospitalizations after thyroidectomy. In this era of cost containment, there has been a great deal of interest in identifying perioperative factors that can predict the development of post-thyroidectomy hypocalcemia soon after operation.

It has been recognized from various studies that no single factor alone can predict the occurrence of hypocalcemia [13–15]. From a recent meta-analysis, preoperative vitamin D, postoperative PTH, and postoperative changes in serum calcium levels are biochemical predictors of post-thyroidectomy hypocalcemia. Clinical predictors include female sex, the presence of Graves' disease, the need for parathyroid autotransplantation, and inadvertent excision of one or more parathyroid glands [2].

It is well known that parathyroid autotransplantation after thyroidectomy predisposes to postoperative hypocalcemia, but it is considered a "prevention" of late parathyroid failure [16, 17]. Some authors, however, have reported no benefit or even worse long-term outcome after parathyroid autotransplantation [18].

It is of interest that vitamin D deficiency is an independent predictor of transient hypocalcemia [19–21]. It can be prevented by performing routine preoperative vitamin D measurement, particularly in high-risk groups such as those with dark skin and malabsorption, the elderly, and obese individuals [22]. However, the cost-effectiveness of such a protocol remains to be established. A recent report provided evidence that the percentage PTH change postoperatively was as a "key predictor" of postoperative hypocalcemia, with vitamin D status, BMI, and thyroid function as additional potential predictors of oral calcium needs [23].

In the absence of reliable or readily applicable predictive tools of post-thyroidectomy hypocalcemia, it is nevertheless of interest to explore the judgments of experienced thyroid surgeons. In this context, a recent prospective study on more than 2500 thyroid operations provided important information: even in a center with more than 1300 thyroidectomies per year carried out by experienced surgeons, the rates of parathyroid complications after surgery differed as did the surgeons' ability to predict hypoparathyroidism; furthermore, an individual risk assessment scored by the surgeons soon after the operation provided useful predictive information [24].

Management of the Case

The patient exhibited symptoms and biochemical features of permanent postsurgical hypoparathyroidism, unresponsive to the prescribed initial therapy. Indeed, after about 30 days following thyroidectomy surgery, her serum PTH level was below the normal range despite low serum calcium values.

In hypoparathyroid patients, blood calcium and phosphate levels can generally be satisfactorily regulated, even though some patients show resistance or a tendency to alternate between hypocalcemia and hypercalcemia. It is important to exclude other potential causes of hypocalcemia. These include poor adherence (denied by this patient) or the concomitant use of medication reducing calcium absorption (excluded in this particular case) that might be potential causes of unsuccessful treatment. Malabsorption is another potential cause, but tests for celiac disease, usually performed to clarify long-lasting hypocalcemia, unresponsive to therapy, were negative in this case. However, this patient reported a lengthy episode of diarrhea which could have caused increased intestinal losses of calcium, magnesium, and calcitriol. In some cases, treatment failure might also be due to the so-called hungry bone syndrome. This is caused by a rapid influx of calcium into the bones due to high bone turnover; it is a recognized cause of hypocalcemia following thyroidectomy for thyrotoxicosis; however, the patient had a preoperative TSH level of 1.17 mUI/L, thus excluding this possibility.

In patients with preserved parathyroid function, hypomagnesemia should be ruled out. The serum magnesium level in our patient was 0.60 mmol/L (normal range 0.7–1.0 mmol/L), probably related to her previous intestinal problems. In physiological conditions, magnesium modulates the function of parathyroid glands through upregulation of the key cellular receptors such as calcium-sensing receptor (CaSR), vitamin D receptor, and fibroblast growth factor 23/Klotho system [25]. In severe hypomagnesemia, a true block of PTH secretion appears to be caused by an effect on the α-subunits of the heterotrimeric G proteins associated with CaSR [26]. Because these proteins have a magnesium-binding site, magnesium deficiency can activate (disinhibit) them, mimicking the effect of CaSR activation and consequently suppressing PTH secretion. A recent paper found a significant correlation between the decrease in serum magnesium from time 0 to 48 h postoperatively and permanent hypocalcemia ($p = 0.015$) [27]. Finally, the patient's vitamin D status was investigated to exclude hypovitaminosis D as a contributor to the lack of response to therapy: vitamin D levels were 17 ng/ml (sufficiency level >20 ng/ml), as can be seen in obese subjects [22].

Therapy

Standard treatment of hypoparathyroidism is oral calcium and vitamin D supplementation, titrated to relieve symptoms but while avoiding side effects such as nephrocalcinosis and nephrolithiasis [28].

At present, there is an ongoing debate concerning the dose and route of supplementation of both calcium and vitamin D, as well as whether supplements should be given to patients preoperatively or postoperatively [29, 30]. In a recent meta-analysis on postsurgical hypocalcemia, obese patients required more calcium and vitamin D to correct their serum calcium than patients with lower body mass index (BMI) [29]. The patient under discussion had a high BMI and therefore could be suspected to have vitamin D deficiency before surgery, even if her vitamin D level was not measured.

Considering the uncertainty of the correct time to start therapy, the "American Thyroid Association Surgical Affairs Committee Writing Task Force" suggests routine postoperative oral calcium administration (e.g., calcium carbonate 1000 mg every 6 to 8-h starting in the recovery room, with or without the addition of calcitriol 0.5–1 mcg daily), because it carries several advantages and relatively little downside [6]. Given the delayed action of these oral agents (1–2 h), dosing may begin immediately upon the discovery of mild symptoms (circumoral and acral paresthesias), to avoid progression to more pronounced symptoms such as muscle twitching and cramping. Since the development of 1α-hydroxylated vitamin D analogues, most patients with hypoparathyroidism have been shifted to treatment with either alfacalcidol or calcitriol, as the plasma half-life of activated vitamin D metabolites is much shorter (approximately 3–6 h) than the biological half-life of vitamin D2 or D3 (approximately 3 weeks). The advantage of the shorter plasma half-life of activated vitamin D metabolites is that a new equilibrium is obtained at a much faster rate.

Only a minority of patients with transient hypoparathyroidism will have permanent hypoparathyroidism (ranging from 0.5 to 10.6 %) (5,6), because the resolution of hypoparathyroidism is most likely related to the recovery of the parathyroid glands from the surgical insult. It is currently difficult to predict which patients will recover, and it is unclear whether any specific intervention will facilitate recovery. Some surgeons do not prescribe calcium supplements in the hope that the resultant mild hypocalcemia will stimulate parathyroid recovery, but recently Sitges-Serra et al. suggested that adequate treatment during the period of transient hypocalcemia may reduce the metabolic stress on the already injured ischemic glands, allowing these glands to "rest and recover," thus possibly reducing the risk of permanent hypoparathyroidism [31]. Routine utilization of calcium and vitamin D supplements after thyroidectomy, or therapy only related to hypocalcemic symptoms, to preserve parathyroid function and avoid permanent hypoparathyroidism, remains a matter of debate. The latest review and meta-analysis identified postoperative calcium and vitamin D supplementation as well as bilateral subtotal thyroidectomy to be effective in preventing transient hypocalcemia compared to the Hartley Dunhill operation (removal of one entire lateral lobe with isthmus and partial/subtotal removal of opposite lateral lobe), but the same meta-analysis did not demonstrate any measure to be significantly associated with a reduction in permanent hypocalcemia [32].

Until recently, hypoparathyroidism was one of the only hormonal insufficiency states that was not treated by hormone replacement therapy. PTH replacement therapy is now approved by the FDA for the treatment of transient and permanent hypoparathyroidism. Available data do suggest an improved quality of life in response to PTH replacement therapy versus calcium and vitamin D analogue therapy [33]. PTH is currently used to treat osteoporosis with a 2-year time limit on therapy. A better understanding of the effects of long-term treatment with PTH in the treatment of hypoparathyroidism is important, because the effect on bone turnover could be different if it is used for a period longer than 2 years [34]. Data in subjects affected by hypoparathyroidism treated with PTH analogues demonstrate a densitometric and histomorphometric improvement in abnormal bone-remodeling dynamics and return of bone metabolism toward normal euparathyroid levels [35, 36].

Long-Term Follow-Up

Patients who develop permanent hypoparathyroidism should receive appropriate follow-up care to monitor for long-term complications related to supplemental therapy. The serum calcium level should be monitored, and soft-tissue calcification and nephrocalcinosis can be prevented by keeping the serum calcium-phosphate product values less than 55 [1, 37]. Not only should calcium level be monitored in these patients, but also other medical aspects because recent epidemiological data have shown that permanent hypoparathyroidism is associated with an increased risk of depression and other neuropsychiatric disease and infections, whereas such patients seem to be protected against fractures of the upper extremities and gastrointestinal malignancies [38].

Management of the Case

In our patient, the acute diarrhea probably worsened an unstable clinical condition so that both calcium (1.5 g daily of calcium as calcium citrate) and calcitriol (0.75 mcg daily) were increased and oral magnesium oxide (400 mg a day) was also added. After 4 weeks, laboratory evaluation showed a calcium level of 2.1 mmol/L, normalization of serum magnesium, and hypercalciuria with a 24 h urinary calcium of 14 mmol (normal range 1.25–10 mmol/24 h). Since her blood pressure was not controlled, a thiazide diuretic was added to mitigate the increased renal calcium excretion. The patient was advised to adhere to a low-sodium diet; magnesium therapy was stopped.

After an additional period of 4 weeks, biochemical parameters were satisfactory [serum calcium, 2.20 mmol/L; serum phosphorus, 1.55 mmol/L (normal range, 0.75–1.45); 24-h urinary calcium, 10 mmol]. The patient was free of symptoms of hypocalcemia; physical examination showed negative Chvostek and Trousseau signs.

Clinical Pearls/Pitfalls

- Hypocalcemia after thyroidectomy is not without cost, as it may lead to a longer postoperative inpatient stay, extra medication, the need for more blood tests, and extra outpatient visits.
- The management of postsurgical hypoparathyroidism is best accomplished by identifying high-risk patients preoperatively.
- Prediction of post-thyroidectomy hypocalcemia still remains a challenge, but postoperative PTH, preoperative vitamin D, and postoperative changes in calcium should be considered predictors of post-thyroidectomy hypocalcemia.
- The aim of treatment with calcium and calcitriol is to keep the level of albumin-adjusted calcium at the lower end of the normal range, to reduce the risk of hypercalcemia and hypercalciuria; PTH therapy may be another therapeutic option for permanent hypoparathyroidism.
- Lack of response to oral therapy in treatment of hypoparathyroidism following thyroidectomy has rarely been reported, and it is mandatory to exclude other potential causes for hypocalcemia.

References

1. Shoback D. Clinical practice. Hypoparathyroidism. N Engl J Med. 2008;359:391–403.
2. Edafe O, Antakia R, Laskar N, Uttley L, Balasubramanian SP. Systematic review and meta-analysis of predictors of post-thyroidectomy hypocalcaemia. Br J Surg. 2014;101:307–20.
3. Khan MI, Waguespack SG, Hu MI. Medical management of postsurgical hypoparathyroidism. Endocr Pract. 2011;17:18–25.
4. Chadwick D, Kinsman R, Walton P, Systems DC. The British Association of Endocrine and Thyroid Surgeon fourth national audit. Henley-on-Thames: Dendrite Clinical Systems Ltd; 2012.
5. Bergenfelz A, Jansson S, Kristoffersson A, Mårtensson H, Reihnér E, Wallin G, et al. Complications to thyroid surgery: results as reported in a database from a multicenter audit comprising 3660 patients. Langenbecks Arch Surg. 2008;393:667–73.
6. Terris DJ, Snyder S, Carneiro-Pla D, Inabnet 3rd WB, Kandil E, Orloff L, American Thyroid Association Surgical Affairs Committee Writing Task Force, et al. American Thyroid Association statement on outpatient thyroidectomy. Thyroid. 2013;23:1193–202.
7. Loyo M, Tufano RP, Gourin CG. National trends in thyroid surgery and the effect of volume on short-term outcomes. Laryngoscope. 2013;123(8):2056–63.
8. Hermann M, Ott J, Promberger R, Kober F, Karik M, Freissmuth M. Kinetics of serum parathyroid hormone during and after thyroid surgery. Br J Surg. 2008;95:1480–7.
9. RohJL PCI. Routine oral calcium and vitamin D supplements for prevention of hypocalcemia after total thyroidectomy. Am J Surg. 2006;192:675–8.
10. Sabour S, Manders E, Steward DL. The role of rapid PACU parathyroid hormone in reducing post thyroidectomy hypocalcemia. Otolaryngology. 2009;141:727–9.
11. Rosato L, Avenia N, Bernante P, De Palma M, Gulino G, Nasi PG, et al. Complications of thyroid surgery: analysis of a multicentric study on 14,934 patients operated on in Italy over 5 years. World J Surg. 2004;28:271–6.
12. Mehanna HM, Jain A, Randeva H, Watkinson J, Shaha A. Postoperative hypocalcemia-the difference a definition makes. Head Neck. 2010;32:279–83.

13. Pradeep PV, Ramalingam K, Jayashree B. Post total thyroidectomy hypocalcemia: a novel multi-factorial scoring system to enable its prediction to facilitate an early discharge. J Postgrad Med. 2013;59:4–8.
14. Pradeep PV, Ramalingam K. Postoperative PTH measurement is not a reliable predictor for hypocalcemia after total thyroidectomy in vitamin D deficiency: prospective study of 203 cases. World J Surg. 2014;38:564–7.
15. Lang BH, Yih PC, Ng KK. A prospective evaluation of quick intraoperative parathyroid hormone assay at the time of skin closure in predicting clinically relevant hypocalcemia after thyroidectomy. World J Surg. 2012;36:1300–6.
16. Lo CY. Parathyroid autotransplantation during thyroidectomy. ANZ J Surg. 2002;72:902–7.
17. Asari R, Passler C, Kaczirek K, Scheuba C, Niederle B. Hypoparathyroidism after total thyroidectomy: a prospective study. Arch Surg. 2008;143:132–7.
18. El-Sharaky MI, Kahalil MR, Sharaky O, Sakr MF, Fadaly GA, El-Hammadi HA, et al. Assessment of parathyroid autotransplantation for preservation of parathyroid function after total thyroidectomy. Head Neck. 2003;25:799–807.
19. Erbil Y, Bozbora A, Ozbey N, Issever H, Aral F, Ozarmagan S, et al. Predictive value of age and serum parathormone and vitamin D3 levels for postoperative hypocalcemia after total thyroidectomy for nontoxic multinodular goiter. Arch Surg. 2007;142:1182–7.
20. Erbil Y, Barbaros U, Temel B, Turkoglu U, Issever H, Bozbora A, et al. The impact of age, vitamin D(3) level, and incidental parathyroidectomy on postoperative hypocalcemia after total or near total thyroidectomy. Am J Surg. 2009;197:439–46.
21. Erbil Y, Ozbey NC, Sari S, Unalp HR, Agcaoglu O, Ersoz F, et al. Determinants of postoperative hypocalcemia in vitamin D-deficient Graves' patients after total thyroidectomy. Am J Surg. 2011;201:685–91.
22. Cipriani C, Pepe J, Piemonte S, Colangelo L, Cilli M, Minisola S. Vitamin d and its relationship with obesity and muscle. Int J Endocrinol. 2014;2014:841248.
23. Al-Dhahri SF, Mubasher M, Al-Muhawas F, Alessa M, Terkawi RS, Terkawi AS. Early prediction of oral calcium and vitamin D requirements in post-thyroidectomy hypocalcaemia. Otolaryngol Head Neck Surg. 2014;151:407–14.
24. Promberger R, Ott J, Bures C, Kober F, Freissmuth M, Seemann R, Hermann M. Can a surgeon predict the risk of postoperative hypoparathyroidism during thyroid surgery? A prospective study on self-assessment by experts. Am J Surg. 2014;208:13–20.
25. Hoorn EJ, Zietse R. Disorders of calcium and magnesium balance: a physiology-based approach. Pediatr Nephrol. 2013;28:1195–206.
26. Vetter T, Lohse MJ. Magnesium and the parathyroid. Curr Opin Nephrol Hypertens. 2002;11:403–10.
27. Hammerstad SS, Norheim I, Paulsen T, Amlie LM, Eriksen EF. Excessive decrease in serum magnesium after total thyroidectomy for Graves' disease is related to development of permanent hypocalcemia. World J Surg. 2013;37:369–75.
28. Bilezikian J, Khan A, Potts Jr J, Brandi M, Clarke B, Shoback D, et al. Hypoparathyroidism in the adult: epidemiology, diagnosis, pathophysiology, target organ involvement, treatment, and challenges for future research. J Bone Miner Res. 2011;26:2317–37.
29. Alhefdhi A, Mazeh H, Chen H. Role of postoperative vitamin D and/or calcium routine supplementation in preventing hypocalcemia after thyroidectomy: a systematic review and meta-analysis. Oncologist. 2013;18:533–42.
30. Romagnoli E, Pepe J, Piemonte S, Cipriani C, Minisola S. Management of endocrine disease: value and limitations of assessing vitamin D nutritional status and advised levels of vitamin D supplementation. Eur J Endocrinol. 2013;169:R59–69.
31. Sitges-Serra A, Ruiz S, Girvent M, Manjon H, Duenas JP, Sancho JJ. Outcome of protracted hypoparathyroidism after total thyroidectomy. Br J Surg. 2010;97:1687–95.
32. Antakia R, Edafe O, Uttley L, Balasubramanian S. Effectiveness of preventative and other surgical measures on hypocalcaemia following bilateral thyroid surgery: a systematic review and meta-analysis. Thyroid. 2015;25:95–106.

33. Rejnmark L, Underbjerg L, Sikjaer T. Therapy of hypoparathyroidism by replacement with parathyroid hormone. Scientifica (Cairo). 2014;2014:765629.
34. Piemonte S, Romagnoli E, Bratengeier C, Woloszczuk W, Tancredi A, Pepe J, et al. Serum sclerostin levels decline in post-menopausal women with osteoporosis following treatment with intermittent parathyroid hormone. J Endocrinol Invest. 2012;35:866–8.
35. Rubin MR, Dempster DW, Sliney Jr J, Zhou H, Nickolas TL, Stein EM, et al. PTH (1-84) administration reverses abnormal bone-remodeling dynamics and structure in hypoparathyroidism. J Bone Miner Res. 2011;26:2727–36.
36. Gafni RI, Brahim JS, Andreopoulou P, Bhattacharyya N, Kelly MH, Brillante BA, et al. Daily parathyroid hormone 1-34 replacement therapy for hypoparathyroidism induces marked changes in bone turnover and structure. J Bone Miner Res. 2012;27:1811–20.
37. National Kidney Foundation. K/DOQI clinical practice guidelines for bone metabolism and disease in chronic kidney disease. Am J Kidney Dis. 2003;42 Suppl 3:S1–201.
38. Underbjerg L, Sikjaer T, Mosekilde L, Rejnmark L. Post-surgical hypoparathyroidism – risk of fractures, psychiatric diseases, cancer, cataract, and infections. J Bone Miner Res. 2014;29:2504–10.

Chapter 21
A Patient with Postsurgical Recurrent Laryngeal Nerve Damage and Nerve Monitoring

David L. Steward and Adam D. Goodale

Case Presentation

A 54-year-old female presented to the clinic for evaluation of a known goiter with worsening compressive symptoms. She had no prior history of radiation exposure or a family history of thyroid cancer. She had been followed by her family physician with previous laboratory evaluation and was euthyroid. An ultrasound exam was performed showing a large goiter with mild substernal extension; no discrete nodules were visualized. A flexible laryngeal exam was performed which revealed symmetric, mobile vocal cords bilaterally. The patient desired a thyroidectomy for treatment of her compressive symptoms. The risks of postoperative hypocalcemia and vocal cord paralysis were explained, and she was scheduled for surgery.

Several weeks later, the patient underwent a total thyroidectomy. Intraoperative nerve monitoring (IONM) was performed using an endotracheal tube-based electrode. Her goiter was largest on the left and this was the initial side of surgery. The nerve stimulator was used to assist in finding the recurrent laryngeal nerve. After removal of the left lobe, the nerve stimulator confirmed the integrity of the recurrent laryngeal nerve. The right lobe was then dissected in a similar fashion. The nerve stimulator had a positive signal at the outset of dissection; however, after the thyroid was removed, there was a loss of nerve signal. The position of the endotracheal tube was checked as well as the setup of the remainder of the system. Despite troubleshooting, the nerve signal from the right recurrent laryngeal nerve (RLN) remained absent. Visually the nerve was grossly intact; however, palpation of the arytenoid failed to confirm nerve integrity with stimulation. The surgery was concluded and the patient was discharged home. She had no obvious voice disturbance immediately following surgery.

D.L. Steward, M.D. (✉) • A.D. Goodale, M.D.
University of Cincinnati College of Medicine, Department of Otolaryngology - Head & Neck Surgery, 231 Albert Sabin Way, MSB Room 6507, Cincinnati, OH 45267, USA
e-mail: david.steward@uc.edu; adam.goodale@uc.edu

D.S. Cooper, C. Durante (eds.), *Thyroid Cancer*,
DOI 10.1007/978-3-319-22401-5_21

Assessment and Literature Review

RLN damage is a potential complication following thyroid surgery. Despite advances in surgical technique, anatomical knowledge, and intraoperative nerve monitoring, the rate of RLN injury remains relatively high. A recent systematic review reported an incidence of temporary RLN palsy in 9.8 % of thyroidectomies and permanent RLN injury in 2.3 % [1]. Injury rates are even higher for cases of secondary thyroidectomy, substernal goiter, and thyroid malignancy [2–5]. Surgeon experience has been shown to influence nerve injury with high-volume thyroid surgeons (those performing more than 100 thyroidectomies a year) having significantly lower nerve injury rates than lower-volume surgeons [6]. Vocal cord paralysis is known to negatively affect both quality of life and work activity with symptoms of breathy dysphonia and dysphagia with unilateral injury and stridor and airway obstruction with bilateral injury.

To accurately assess RLN function, a laryngeal exam is essential. Although some physicians reserve laryngeal exam for symptomatic patients, studies have shown a poor correlation between voice changes and vocal cord paralysis [7, 8]. Often patients will develop progressive paralysis over time with adequate contralateral vocal cord compensation to limit noticeable voice changes. In one study in particular, the authors performed routine laryngeal exam prior to thyroidectomy and noted that one third of patients with preoperative vocal fold motion impairment were asymptomatic [7]. Thus, to accurately determine the presence of iatrogenic vocal cord paralysis, a preoperative baseline exam is necessary. In cases of thyroid malignancy, preoperative RLN paralysis is highly predictive of invasive disease and thus alters surgical management and patient counseling [9]. Although there is variation among physician practices, an accurate assessment of preoperative laryngeal function is beneficial for both planning the extent of surgery and managing patients postoperatively.

Mechanism of Nerve Injury

The intimate relationship between the thyroid and RLN places the nerve at risk for injury during surgical removal. The majority of RLN injuries are secondary to compression, traction, devascularization, or thermal damage during thyroid removal wherein the structural integrity of the nerve remains intact but with damage of its underlying neural elements. The RLN innervates the intrinsic muscles of the larynx and consists of a complement of nerve fibers for both abduction and adduction of the vocal folds. Coordinated laryngeal function is highly dependent on each axon innervating its specific motor unit. When the RLN is damaged, the ultimate effect on laryngeal function, as well as prognosis for recovery, is dependent on the degree of nerve injury which was previously categorized by Sunderland [10]. Neuropraxic injuries are the least severe and are characterized by focal myelin damage without disruption of the axon leading to partial or temporary blockage of nerve conduction with a good prognosis for recovery. More severe damage results in disruption of the nerve axons, or axonotmesis, which leads to significant disruption of nerve conduction; however, the perineurium remains intact which improves the potential for functional recovery. Transection of the nerve, or neurotmesis, results in disruption of the axons, perineurium, and epineurium which is the most severe form of injury and carries the worst prognosis for recovery. The mechanism of injury is important when considering prognosis for recovery and postoperative management.

The superior laryngeal nerve and branches of the RLN must be considered during thyroidectomy. The external branch of the superior laryngeal nerve (EBSLN) traverses in an anteroinferior direction along the inferior constrictor muscle to innervate the cricothyroid muscle. Commonly the EBSLN is closely associated with the blood supply to the superior pole of the thyroid placing it at risk for injury during ligation of these vessels. Damage to the EBSLN often limits the ability to achieve higher pitches as well as increased vocal fatigue. Patients with injury to the EBSLN typically have normal laryngeal exams which limit accurate determination of the incidence of nerve damage. Few studies, all with limited patient populations, have utilized EMG to evaluate postoperative cricothyroid function with incidence of EBSLN injury ranging from 5 to 58 % [11, 12] (Figs. 21.1 and 21.2).

Branches of the RLN prior to entering the larynx are also subject to inadvertent injury. Typically these consist of an anterior and posterior branch and are present in 20–30 % of patients [13, 14]. The anterior branch is primarily responsible for laryngeal muscle function, while the posterior branch contains mainly sensory nerve fibers but may occasionally innervate the posterior cricoarytenoid muscle. If branching is not identified, the posterior branch may be mistaken for the primary RLN with inadvertent transection of the anterior branch resulting in vocal cord paralysis. When present, the branches typically occur distally and are often identifiable at the level of Berry's ligament; however, variation does exist. The presence of these extralaryngeal branches doubles the likelihood of postoperative vocal cord paralysis and should be identified and preserved when present [15]. Branches of the RLN to the esophagus and inferior constrictor may also be present and when injured can impair swallowing postoperatively. Thus, surgeons must maintain a sound knowledge of anatomical variations to limit inadvertent injury to the various nerves in close approximation with the thyroid.

Evaluating Recurrent Laryngeal Nerve Function Intraoperatively

Injury to the RLN is oftentimes difficult to assess intraoperatively. Visually the nerve may appear intact while there can be significant functional damage. Given the inability to assess nerve function, surgeons poorly predict postoperative RLN function with one study reporting as few as 10 % of damaged nerves correctly identified intraoperatively [16]. IONM with nerve stimulation has several key benefits, but its most notable is the ability to assess neural integrity in the operating room and better predict postoperative laryngeal function. Most commonly, IONM is performed using an endotracheal tube-based surface electrode to continuously monitor RLN integrity during thyroidectomy. Manipulation or electrical stimulation of the RLN is recorded by either an audio only system or a system with both audio and visual waveform data to notify the surgeon of evoked neural activity. While continuous nerve monitoring can be useful, nerve stimulation has shown the most promise to improve surgical outcomes. Positive nerve stimulation is very sensitive for intact RLN function. However, a loss of signal is less specific for nerve damage, as this may be secondary to either technical issues or actual nerve damage. Efficient troubleshooting is necessary to limit inappropriate loss of signal. When used by surgeons familiar with IONM, high specificity has been shown to be obtainable [17]. This is particularly valuable when planning a total thyroidectomy to limit the frequency of bilateral RLN paralysis and its associated complications. When the RLN signal is lost on the initial side of surgery during a total thyroidectomy, some surgeons have started to postpone removal of the contralateral lobe. This change in surgical management resulted in a decrease in bilateral RLN paralysis from 17 % to zero percent when the initial side of dissection resulted in a loss of RLN signal [18]. Since most RLN injuries are temporary in nature, a completion thyroidectomy can be performed, if necessary, once nerve function returns.

Although nerve stimulation is a useful tool to protect RLN integrity, visual nerve identification remains the gold standard for nerve protection. Prior to the use of IONM, visual identification of the RLN was shown to decrease RLN injury and remains the gold standard for nerve protection [3, 19]. One of the main hopes of IONM was to further limit the incidence of RLN injury; however, this has yet to be clearly proven. Numerous studies have been published with varying results. A recent meta-analysis of 44 studies showed no statistical difference in RLN injury rates when comparing visual identification of the RLN to IONM [20]. Dralle et al. published a review of approximately 30,000 nerves at risk comparing visual identification versus nerve monitoring with no statistical decrease in RLN injury rates; however, this was thought secondary to lack of statistical power [2]. The only randomized clinical trial evaluating RLN injury rates and IONM did show a statistical benefit [21]. Other studies have shown benefit using IONM in more complex cases. Chan et al. showed decreased RLN injury rates when using IONM for secondary thyroidectomy and thyroidectomy for malignancy [4].

Despite the lack of evidence to support improved patient outcomes, the use of IONM has become increasingly popular over the past two decades. A recent survey of endocrine surgeons showed that approximately 40 % routinely use IONM, and this was most prevalent among high-volume surgeons (greater than 100 cases per year) and younger surgeons (age 35–44) [22].

Clinical Manifestations

A large majority of patients report voice and swallowing complaints after thyroidectomy regardless of RLN function. One study reported that 80 % of patients demonstrated hoarseness and 54 % reported dysphagia 1 week post-thyroidectomy despite normal RLN function [23]. These symptoms typically resolve over the first month postoperatively and are thought secondary to localized swelling, intubation trauma, or muscle injury. On the other hand, patients with RLN injury may not experience voice changes in the immediate postoperative period. Acute laryngeal edema from intubation trauma may create enough bulk for normal voice production; however, once swelling resolves, voice changes will become evident and often present as a "breathy" voice due to insufficient glottal closure. In contrast, bilateral RLN paralysis is often apparent in the immediate postoperative period with acute onset stridor and airway obstruction. Dysphagia is more common in elderly patients with few experiencing severe aspiration. Given the variety of symptoms, a routine laryngeal exam is required to definitively assess RLN function. This is typically performed between 1 and 8 weeks postoperatively and can be done by indirect mirror exam, flexible fiber-optic laryngeal exam, or video laryngoscopy. There can be large variability in laryngeal findings in the setting of RLN injury. Some patients may have persistent voice changes in the setting of normal vocal cord mobility, while other patients will have a flaccid hemilarynx with significant glottic incompetence. The degree of dysfunction is often related to the extent of nerve damage. The use of intraoperative steroids has shown mild benefit in postoperative voice outcomes [24, 25]. In particular, using steroids resulted in a shorter recovery time for temporary RLN paralysis when compared to placebo. The frequency of temporary RLN paralysis was also lower with intraoperative steroids; however, this was not statistically significant. Intraoperative findings should be correlated with laryngeal exam to assist with postoperative management, prognosis, and patient expectations.

Management

The management of RLN injury is dependent on both the nature of injury and the severity of the patient's symptoms. The majority of nerve damage is temporary with approximately 80–90 % of patients experiencing full recovery within 6 months after surgery [17, 26, 27]. Limited improvement in function is expected after that time and more definitive treatment may be necessary. Treatment options of unilateral RLN injury include voice and swallowing therapy, injection laryngoplasty, and laryngeal framework surgery. When the nerve is transected, management begins intraoperatively. For patients with bilateral RLN, paralysis management focuses on maintaining a patent airway, most commonly with a tracheostomy. The appropriate treatment option should be individualized for each patient.

As with all peripheral nerves, the RLN has the ability for regeneration after injury. Post-injury laryngeal function is dependent upon reestablishing pre-injury innervation patterns. Misdirected nerve regeneration results in synkinesis or uncoordinated muscle contractions, leading to impaired laryngeal function. The degree of synkinesis is dependent upon the severity of injury and will dictate the expected return of function. Neuropraxic injuries maintain the integrity of each nerve axon allowing for similar post-injury innervation patterns. With more severe damage, as with axonotmesis and neurotmesis, newly created axons will likely reinnervate motor units dissimilar from pre-injury targets leading to varying degrees of synkinesis. Since laryngeal function and vocal cord motion are dependent upon a highly coordinated series of muscle contractions, synkinesis typically results in absent vocal fold motion. However, due to the predominance of adduction nerve fibers within the RLN, nerve fiber regeneration typically results in medialization of the larynx over time. This results in improved phonation and explains why many patients experience symptomatic improvement without intervention.

Voice and Swallowing Therapy

Patients found to have unilateral vocal cord hypomotility or immotility should be referred to an otolaryngologist or speech pathologist for further evaluation and treatment. Video laryngoscopy can be performed to better characterize vocal cord motility, laryngeal muscle tone, and glottic closure. This initial assessment will establish an objective baseline to evaluate for improvement with various treatment options. In the setting of aspiration, speech pathologist can perform a modified barium swallow (MBS) study or a fiber-optic endoscopic evaluation of swallowing (FEES) to accurately assess the degree of aspiration. Furthermore, these studies can be used to determine an appropriate diet for patients and educate them on certain swallowing maneuvers to limit aspiration. Patients often benefit from swallowing with their head turned toward the affected site to improve glottic closure or tightly holding their breath while swallowing to encourage supraglottic closure and limit aspiration. Patients with persistent aspiration despite swallowing therapy may require additional intervention. When symptoms are limited to voice disturbance, patients should initially be managed conservatively with voice therapy. The goal of voice therapy is to improve glottic closure while avoiding unfavorable compensatory maneuvers, such as supraglottic phonation. Voice therapy is most effective for patients with mild to moderate dysfunction and has been shown to decrease the need for surgical voice intervention [28]. Patients with severe dysfunction are more likely to require surgical intervention; however, voice therapy can still be beneficial. Patients can expect improvement in voice as far as 6 months after surgery; after that time, surgical intervention may be required to further improve voice outcomes.

Surgical Management

Surgical options for unilateral RLN paralysis consist primarily of injection laryngoplasty and laryngeal framework surgery. The goal of surgical augmentation is to improve phonation and glottic closure by medializing the paralyzed vocal cord to abut the contralateral functioning vocal cord during phonation and deglutition. Injection laryngoplasty is a useful tool for voice improvement and has become increasingly popular in the outpatient setting after recent advancements in fiber-optic laryngeal technology and improved injectable materials. Flexible transnasal laryngoscopy with distal chip cameras allows for high-definition laryngeal visualization to ensure accurate injection. There are numerous injectable materials on the market, each with various benefits. Oftentimes, the choice of material is based on the desired duration of effect and surgeon preference. Commonly used materials include the following: carboxymethylcellulose (Radiesse Voice Gel), hyaluronic acid, collagen, calcium hydroxyapatite (Radiesse Voice), micronized dermis (Cymetra), and autologous fat. Injection laryngoplasty was previously reserved for patients who failed conservative voice therapy. However, recent studies have shown that early injection laryngoplasty, deemed within the first year of injury, can decrease the need for future open laryngeal surgery [29]. Injection laryngoplasty remains limited by its isolated effect on the vocal fold as well as its temporary duration of effect; however, in numerous patient populations, its use can be highly beneficial.

Patients with severe vocal cord dysfunction, or who fail injection laryngoplasty, can be treated with open laryngeal framework surgery. Paralysis of the RLN results in anterior, inferior, and lateral displacement of the arytenoid with associated shortening and lateralization of the vocal fold. While injection laryngoplasty is limited to modifying vocal fold volume, open procedures can modify arytenoid and vocal fold position in three dimensions which offers more predictable long-term results. In particular, these procedures can adjust vocal fold height, vocal fold tension, and arytenoid position. These procedures primarily consist of thyroplasty and arytenoid adduction. Other laryngeal framework surgeries that exist, including cricothyroid subluxation and adduction arytenopexy, however, are beyond the scope of this text. Thyroplasty is performed by creating a window within the laryngeal cartilage at the level of the vocal fold and inserting a solid material to medialize the vocal fold. Both Silastic and Gore-Tex are commonly used each with good biocompatibility. Although thyroplasty does not augment arytenoid position, it provides long-term vocal fold medialization with good stability over time. Arytenoid adduction uses a permanent suture to reposition the vocal process of the arytenoid into a more medial phonatory position. This procedure has the benefit of modifying arytenoid position in multiple dimensions to personalize the procedure for each variation in vocal cord position.

Management of a transected recurrent laryngeal nerve, either secondary to iatrogenic injury or removal after malignant invasion, starts within the operating room. In regard to malignant invasion, preference is given to attempted preservation of the RLN when vocal cord function is intact preoperatively and sacrifice of the RLN in the setting of preoperative vocal cord paralysis or encasement by tumor. When a transection injury is identified, reanastomosis should be attempted. Although normal vocal cord function is rare after neurorrhaphy, maintained neural input limits post-injury atrophy with increased bulk and medialization of the arytenoid for improved phonation. Typically the epineurium is reanastomosed using two or three interrupted sutures under microscopic guidance. When a segment of nerve is removed or there is significant retraction of the nerve, a local nerve transfer or cable graft may be required to limit tension at the anastomosis site. Most commonly, the ansa cervicalis is anastomosed to the distal end of the RLN for continued neural input. The ansa cervicalis is primarily active during respiration, deglutition, and phonation which is ideal for laryngeal reinnervation. The ansa cervicalis is also a good candidate for nerve transfer given its similar size to the RLN as well as the limited functional deficit when used. A cable graft can be performed using the great auricular nerve or other cervical sensory donor nerves as a bridge between the proximal and distal ends of the transected RLN. This is less commonly used as it requires two neurorrhaphies which hinder nerve regeneration. Patients with a repaired RLN after transection have the potential for good voice outcomes; however, they are more likely to require static voice augmentation procedures for further improvement.

Although the incidence of bilateral RLN injury is relatively low, patients with post-extubation stridor or airway distress require immediate evaluation. A flexible laryngeal exam should be performed to visually assess the vocal cords. Initial management should focus on establishing a secure airway, typically by either reintubation or tracheostomy. Management of patients with permanent bilateral RLN injury is a balance between maintaining a patent airway and limiting aspiration. Tracheostomy remains the gold standard; however, other procedures, such as arytenoidectomy, cordotomy, and vocal cord lateralization, exist and should be individualized for each patient.

Although care is taken to limit RLN injury, surgeons must be familiar with management options for patients with postoperative injury. The majority of patients will experience spontaneous recovery over time and can be managed with conservative therapy. The remainder of patients may require more invasive therapy to limit aspiration and improve voice outcomes.

Back to the Patient: Outcome

One week after surgery, the patient was seen in the office for postoperative evaluation. She reported having a "breathy" voice since surgery with associated voice fatigue. She denied difficulty with swallowing. A flexible laryngeal exam showed hypomotility of the right vocal cord. The patient was referred to speech pathology for voice therapy. She was seen in follow-up 3 months later with resolution of her voice complaints. A repeat laryngeal exam at that time showed symmetric vocal cord motility with improved phonation time.

Clinical Pearls

- Intraoperative nerve stimulation is a useful tool to assess RLN function intraoperatively.
- A loss of nerve signal may be due to either technical issues or true nerve injury.
- Laryngeal exam is the only way to definitively assess RLN function both before and after surgery.
- The majority of RLN injuries are secondary to compression and traction injuries and are often temporary in duration.

- Neurorrhaphy should be performed in the event of RLN transection.
- Early injection laryngoplasty decreases the need for surgical laryngeal surgery in the setting of RLN injury.

References

1. Jeannon JP, Orabi AA, Bruch GA, Abdalsalam HA, Sima R. Diagnosis of recurrent laryngeal nerve palsy after thyroidectomy: a systematic review. Int J Clin Pract. 2009;63(4):624–9.
2. Dralle H, Sekulla C, Haerting J, Timmermann W, Neumann HJ, Kruse E, et al. Risk factors of paralysis and functional outcome after recurrent laryngeal nerve monitoring in thyroid surgery. Surgery. 2004;136(6):1310–21.
3. Jatzko GR, Lisborg PH, Muller MG, Wette VM. Recurrent nerve palsy after thyroid operations: principal nerve identification and a literature review. Surgery. 1994;115:139–44.
4. Chan W-F, Lang BH, Lo CY. The role of intraoperative neuromonitoring of recurrent laryngeal nerve during thyroidectomy: a comparative study on 1000 nerves at risk. Surgery. 2006;140:866.
5. Martensson H, Terins J. Recurrent laryngeal nerve palsy in thyroid gland surgery related to operations and nerves at risk. Arch Surg. 1985;120:475–7.
6. Sosa JA, Bowman HM, Tielsch JM, Powe NR, Udelsman R. The importance of surgeon experience for clinical and economic outcomes from thyroidectomy. Surgery. 1998;228:320–30.
7. Farrag TY, Samlan RA, Lin FR, Tufano RP. The utility of evaluating true vocal fold motion before thyroid surgery. Laryngoscope. 2006;116:235–8.
8. Steurer M, Passler C, Denk DM, Schneider B, Niederle B, Bigenzahn W. Advantages of recurrent laryngeal nerve identification in thyroidectomy and parathyroidectomy and the importance of preoperative and postoperative laryngoscopic examination in more than 1000 nerves at risk. Laryngoscope. 2002;112:124–33.
9. Randolph GW, Kamani D. The importance of preoperative laryngoscopy in patients undergoing thyroidectomy: voice, vocal cord function, and the preoperative detection of invasive thyroid malignancy. Surgery. 2006;139:357–62.
10. Sunderland S. A classification of peripheral nerve injuries producing loss of unction. Brain. 1951;74:491–516.
11. Furlan JC, Cordeiro AC, Brandao LG. Study of some "intrinsic risk factors" that can enhance an iatrogenic injury of the external branch of the superior laryngeal nerve. Otolaryngol Head Neck Surg. 2003;128:396–400.
12. Jansson S, Tisell LE, Hagne I, Sanner E, Stenborg R, Svensson P. Partial laryngeal nerve lesions before and after thyroid surgery. World J Surg. 1988;12:522.
13. Serpell JW, Yeung MJ, Grodski S. The motor fibers of the recurrent laryngeal nerve are located in the anterior extralaryngeal branch. Ann Surg. 2009;249(4):648–52.
14. Casella C, Pata G, Nascimbeni R, Mittempergher F, Salerni B. Does extralaryngeal branching have an impact on the rate of postoperative transient or permanent recurrent laryngeal nerve palsy? World J Surg. 2009;33:261–5.
15. Sancho JJ, Pascual-Damieta M, Pereira JA, Carrera MJ, Fontane J, Sitges-Serra A. Risk factors for transient vocal cord palsy after thyroidectomy. Br J Surg. 2008;95:961–7.
16. Bergenfelz A, Jansson S, Kristoffersson A, Martensson H, Reihner E, Wallin G, et al. Complications to thyroid surgery: results as reported in a database from a multicenter audit comprising 3660 patients. Langenbecks Arch Surg. 2008;393:667–73.
17. Goretzki PE, Schwarz K, Brinkmann J, Wirowski D, Lammers BJ. The impact of intraoperative neuromonitoring (IONM) on surgical strategy in bilateral thyroid disease: is it worth the effort? World J Surg. 2010;34:1274–84.
18. Randolph GW, Kamani D. Intraoperative neural monitoring in thyroid cancer surgery. Langenbecks Arch Surg. 2014;399:199–207.

19. Chandrasekhar SS, Randolph GW, Seidman MD, Rosenfeld RM, Angelos P, Barkmeier-Kraemer J, et al. Clinical practice guideline: improving voice outcomes after thyroid surgery. Otolaryngol Head Neck Surg. 2013;148:1–37.
20. Higgins TS, Gupta R, Ketcham AS, Sataloff RT, Wadsworth JT, Siancori JT. Recurrent laryngeal nerve monitoring versus identification along on post-thyroidectomy true vocal fold paralysis: a meta-analysis. Laryngoscope. 2011;1212:1009–17.
21. Barczynski M, Konturek A, Stopa M, Honowska A, Nowak W. Randomized controlled trial of visualization versus neuromonitoring of the external branch of the superior laryngeal nerve during thyroidectomy. World J Surg. 2012;36:1340–7.
22. Lombardi CP, Raffaelli M, D'Alatri L, Marchese MR, Rigante M, Paludetti G, et al. Voice and swallowing changes after thyroidectomy in patient without inferior laryngeal nerve injuries. Surgery. 2006;140:1026–34.
23. Sturgeon C, Sturgeon T, Angelos P. Neuromonitoring in thyroid surgery: attitudes, usage patterns, and predictors of use among endocrine surgeons. World J Surg. 2009;33:417–25.
24. Wang LF, Lee KW, Kuo WR, Wu CW, Lu SP, Chiang FY. The efficacy of intraoperative corticosteroids in recurrent laryngeal nerve palsy after thyroid surgery. World J Surg. 2006;30:299–303.
25. Worni M, Schudel HH, Seifert E, Inglin R, Hagemann M, Vorburger SA, Candinas D. Randomized controlled trial on single dose steroids before thyroidectomy for benign disease to improve postoperative nausea, pain, and vocal function. Ann Surg. 2008;248:1060–6.
26. Sadowski SM, Soardo P, Leuchter I, Robert JH, Triponez F. Systematic use of recurrent laryngeal nerve neuromonitoring changes the operative strategy in planned bilateral thyroidectomy. Thyroid. 2013;23:329–33.
27. Dralle H, Sekulla C, Haerting J, Timmermann W, Neumann HJ, Kruse E, et al. Risk factors of paralysis and functional outcome after recurrent laryngeal nerve monitoring in thyroid surgery. Surgery. 2004;136:1310–22.
28. Heuer RJ, Sataloff RT, Emerich K, Rulnick R, Baroody M, Spiegel JR, et al. Unilateral recurrent laryngeal nerve paralysis: the importance of "preoperative" voice therapy. J Voice. 1997;11:88–94.
29. Friedman AD, Burns JA, Heaton JT, Zeitels SM. Early versus late injection medialization for unilateral vocal cord paralysis. Laryngoscope. 2010;120:2042–6.

Part V
High Risk Differentiated Thyroid Cancer:
The Need for Additional Therapy

Chapter 22
A Case of Papillary Thyroid Cancer Without Aggressive Histological Features with Nodal Metastases Detected During Follow-Up in a Younger Patient

Maria Grazia Castagna, Lucia Brilli, and Furio Pacini

The Case

A 19-year-old woman underwent a total thyroidectomy for a suspicious nodule; final pathology described a 1.4 cm papillary cancer, classical variant, with no extra-thyroidal extension. No central neck dissection was performed. After surgery, 30 mCi of radioiodine was administered. The first follow-up visit documented absence of residual disease with undetectable serum Tg and normal neck ultrasound.

During a subsequent follow-up visit (5 years after initial treatment), neck ultrasound showed a 7×7×9 mm thyroid bed nodule suspicious for recurrent disease; Fine-needle aspiration (FNA) biopsy confirmed the presence of recurrent papillary thyroid cancer. At that time, basal Tg was 1.1 ng/ml, rising to 3.4 ng/ml after recombinant human TSH stimulation. A second course of radioiodine was administered using 150 mCi of 131I. The post-therapy scan showed no uptake in the neck. Her endocrinologist recommended surgery in the near future, and she came to our center to discuss whether this was necessary.

Assessment and Literature Review

In differentiated thyroid cancer, structural tumor recurrences in the post-surgery follow-up occur in about 3 % of cases, and they are not different between low-, intermediate-, and high-risk patients [1, 2]. In the case of cervical lymph node

M.G. Castagna, M.D. • L. Brilli, M.D.
Department of Medical, Surgical and Neurological Sciences, University of Siena, Siena, Italy

F. Pacini, M.D. (✉)
Department of Medical, Surgical and Neurological Sciences, University of Siena, Siena, Italy

Policlinico Santa Maria alle Scotte, Viale Bracci 1, 53100 Siena, Italy
e-mail: pacini8@unisi.it

D.S. Cooper, C. Durante (eds.), *Thyroid Cancer*,
DOI 10.1007/978-3-319-22401-5_22

recurrences, the management may include no therapy, compartmental lymph node dissection, radioiodine therapy, ethanol injection, or radiofrequency or laser ablation. The final decision should be made after discussions involving the endocrinologist, the surgeon, and the patient [3]. However, as discussed in the 2009 ATA guidelines, the clinical significance of very small cervical nodal metastases remained to be clarified and no specific recommendation was given [3].

Recent data from retrospective studies have suggested that suspicious but small, stable cervical lymph nodes could be followed with serial ultrasound without intervention. Two recent studies have analyzed the natural history of small thyroid bed nodules or suspicious cervical lymph nodes, demonstrating that cervical lymph nodes and thyroid bed nodules usually remain stable for long periods and could be safely monitored with regular neck ultrasound and biochemical evaluation with Tg measurement [4, 5].

In particular, in a retrospective review of 191 patients with at least one thyroid bed nodule (≤11 mm) over a median follow-up of 5 years, only 9 % of patients had an increase in size of at least one nodule, with a low rate of growth (median 1.3 mm/year) [4]. Suspicious cervical lymph nodes left untreated also revealed a low rate of growth. After a median follow-up of 3.5 years, only 9 % of them (15/166) grew at least 5 mm in the longest diameter, with a rate of growth of 1.5 mm/year with no associated disease-related mortality. Among the fifteen patients, seven underwent FNA biopsy, and cytology was consistent with papillary thyroid cancer in 5 cases [5]. Unfortunately, no prospective and randomized trials with longer follow-up have compared the outcome of recurrent lymph node metastases treated or untreated by surgery.

Based on the most recent studies and reviews, the 2015 ATA guidelines state that smaller lesions (<8 mm in the smallest diameter) probably can be best managed with active surveillance with serial ultrasound complemented by neck CT scans, reserving FNA and subsequent surgical intervention for documented structural disease progression [6]. Size represents one of the main parameters to take into account, and central neck nodes ≥8 mm and lateral neck nodes ≥10 mm in their shortest diameter can be considered for surgical removal. Apart from size, other factors such as the patient's emotional status, lymph node location (near or not to vital structure), the functional status of vocal cords, the patient's comorbidities, histology of primary tumor, and Tg doubling time should be taken into account in the decision to operate. In selected cases, metastatic nodes greater than 8–10 mm in the shortest diameter may be followed without intervention, selecting for surgery those patients in whom there is disease progression during follow-up.

In the case of larger lymph nodes, surgery is the preferred approach. The experience of the surgeon and the risks associated with a second surgery (mostly when the lymph node is localized in a compartment previously dissected) should be taken into account. Compartmental surgery is recommended over "berry picking," due to the high risk of recurrence and higher morbidity in case of re-operative surgery. Careful neck dissection in experienced hands has been associated with short-term decreases in serum Tg levels in 60–90 % of patients, while undetectable serum Tg was obtained in only 30–50 % [7–9]. However, most series suggest that surgery results in the disappearance of structural disease in over 90 % of patients [10].

Back to the Patient

The patient was reassured that her thyroid bed nodules could be closely monitored until there was evidence of progression. Serial neck ultrasound was then performed with a gradual increase in size of the thyroid bed nodule (9 × 11 × 17 mm vs. 7 × 7 × 9 mm). After 5 years, it was decided to perform a compartmental level VI dissection. Final pathology was consistent with papillary thyroid cancer. Six months after the surgery, serum Tg was undetectable and neck ultrasound was negative. She was considered to be in clinical remission and has been followed with annual Tg and neck ultrasound.

Clinical Pearls

- In differentiated thyroid cancer, structural tumor recurrences in the post-surgery follow-up period occur in about 3 % of patients, and the frequency is not different among low-, intermediate-, and high-risk patients.
- Central neck nodes ≥8 mm and lateral neck nodes ≥10 mm in smallest diameter should be considered for surgical removal.
- Suspicious, but small, stable cervical lymph nodes may be followed with serial ultrasound without intervention.

References

1. Castagna MG, Maino F, Cipri C, Belardini V, Theodoropoulou A, Cevenini G, Pacini F. Delayed risk stratification, to include the response to initial treatment (surgery and radioiodine ablation), has better outcome predictivity in differentiated thyroid cancer patients. Eur J Endocrinol. 2011;165(3):441–6.
2. Tuttle RM, Tala H, Shah J, Leboeuf R, Ghossein R, Gonen M, Brokhin M, Omry G, Fagin JA, Shaha A. Estimating risk of recurrence in differentiated thyroid cancer after total thyroidectomy and radioactive iodine remnant ablation: using response to therapy variables to modify the initial risk estimates predicted by the new American Thyroid Association staging system. Thyroid. 2010;20(12):1341–9.
3. Cooper DS, Doherty GM, Haugen BR, Kloos RT, Lee SL, Mandel SJ, Mazzaferri EL, McIver B, Pacini F, Schlumberger M, Sherman SI, Steward DL, Tuttle RM. Revised American Thyroid Association management guidelines for patients with thyroid nodules and differentiated thyroid cancer. Thyroid. 2009;19:1167–214.
4. Rondeau G, Fish S, Hann LE, Fagin JA, Tuttle RM. Ultrasonographically detected small thyroid bed nodules identified after total thyroidectomy for differentiated thyroid cancer seldom show clinically significant structural progression. Thyroid. 2011;21(8):845–53.
5. Robenshtok E, Fish S, Bach A, Domínguez JM, Shaha A, Tuttle RM. Suspicious cervical lymph nodes detected after thyroidectomy for papillary thyroid cancer usually remain stable over years in properly selected patients. J Clin Endocrinol Metab. 2012;97(8):2706–13.
6. Haugen BR, Alexander EK, Bible KC, Doherty GM, Mandel SJ, Nikiforov YE, Pacini F, Randolph GW, Sawka AM, Schlumberger M, Schuff K, Sherman SI, Sosa JA, Steward DL,

Tuttle RM, Wartofsky L. American Thyroid Association Management guidelines for patients with thyroid nodules and differentiated thyroid cancer. Thyroid. 2015.

7. Al-Saif O, Farrar WB, Bloomston M, Porter K, Ringel MD, Kloos RT. Long-term efficacy of lymph node reoperation for persistent papillary thyroid cancer. J Clin Endocrinol Metab. 2010;95(5):2187–94.
8. Schuff KG, Weber SM, Givi B, Samuels MH, Andersen PE, Cohen JI. Efficacy of nodal dissection for treatment of persistent/recurrent papillary thyroid cancer. Laryngoscope. 2008; 118(5):768–75.
9. Yim JH, Kim WB, Kim EY, Kim WG, Kim TY, Ryu JS, Gong G, Hong SJ, Shong YK. The outcomes of first reoperation for locoregionally recurrent/persistent papillary thyroid carcinoma in patients who initially underwent total thyroidectomy and remnant ablation. J Clin Endocrinol Metab. 2011;96(7):2049–56.
10. Tufano RP, Clayman G, Heller KS, Inabnet WB, Kebebew E, Shaha A, Steward DL, Tuttle RM. Management of recurrent/persistent nodal disease in patients with differentiated thyroid cancer: a critical review of the risks and benefits of surgical intervention versus active surveillance. Thyroid. 2015;25(1):15–27.

Chapter 23
A Case of Papillary Thyroid Cancer Without Aggressive Histological Features with Nodal Metastases in an Older Patient

Maria Grazia Castagna, Lucia Brilli, and Furio Pacini

The Case

A 58-year-old woman was found to have a 2 cm right thyroid nodule on routine physical examination. Thyroid ultrasound confirmed a 2.4 cm nodule that was hypoechoic with microcalcifications and internal vascularity. The contralateral lobe showed a hypoechoic 0.8 cm nodule. Fine-needle aspiration (FNA) performed on the right nodule showed a "malignant nodule" (Bethesda class V). No lymph nodes were found in the central and lateral compartments at presurgical neck ultrasound. She underwent a total thyroidectomy and central lymph node dissection. The histological diagnosis was intrathyroidal papillary thyroid carcinoma (2.2 cm in the right lobe) and microscopic nodal metastases in the central neck (4 nodes, <0.2 cm) T2N1aMX, stage III according to the AJCC/UICC system, intermediate risk according to the American Thyroid Association (ATA) risk stratification.

Her surgeon recommended postsurgical radioiodine remnant ablation. The patient came to us to discuss whether this was necessary.

Assessment and Literature Review

For the past 40 years, many clinicians have recommended radioiodine remnant ablation for all differentiated thyroid cancer patients with a primary tumor size greater than 1–1.5 cm. Using this approach, the percentage of patients with differentiated thyroid cancer (DTC) receiving radioiodine remnant ablation as part of

M.G. Castagna, MD • L. Brilli, MD • F. Pacini, MD (✉)
Department of Medical, Surgical and Neurological Sciences, University of Siena, Siena, Italy

Policlinico Santa Maria alle Scotte, Viale Bracci 1, Viale Bracci 1, 53100 Siena, Italy
e-mail: pacini8@unisi.it

D.S. Cooper, C. Durante (eds.), *Thyroid Cancer*,
DOI 10.1007/978-3-319-22401-5_23

the first course of therapy has increased from 6.1 to 48.7 % between 1973 and 2006 [1]. However, the last several years have seen an interest in an individualized risk-adapted management approach to DTC, whereby the intensity of therapy and monitoring is tailored to the expected aggressiveness of the malignancy for each patient [2, 3].

The 2015 American Thyroid Association guidelines [4] state that radioactive iodine (RAI) remnant ablation is not routinely recommended after thyroidectomy for ATA low-risk DTC patients, whereas RAI therapy is routinely recommended after total thyroidectomy for ATA high-risk differentiated thyroid cancer patients. Whether RAI ablation is necessary in patients with ATA intermediate risk is still controversial, and the ATA guidelines state that in this category RAI may be considered on an individual basis.

It is well known that the risk of recurrent disease in N1 patients is related to the number and size of involved lymph nodes [5]. The median risk of nodal recurrence varies significantly by clinical staging, from 2 % in clinical N0 patients to 22 % in clinical N1-positive patients. There is a graded risk of structural disease recurrence, varying from 4 % in patients with fewer than five metastatic lymph nodes to 5 % if all involved lymph nodes are <0.2 cm, to 19 % if more than five lymph nodes are involved, to 21 % if more than ten lymph nodes are involved, to 22 % if macroscopic lymph node metastases are clinically evident (clinical N1 disease), and to as high as 27–32 % if any metastatic lymph node is greater than 3 cm [5]. More recently, the impact of nodal status on outcome has been retrospectively evaluated in 834 patients 45 years or older [6]. A significantly poorer disease-specific survival (DSS) and local or distant recurrence-free survival (RFS) were observed in older patients with pN1b disease at diagnosis (DSS 91 %, regional RFS 90 %, and distant RFS 84 %, respectively) when compared to patients with pN0/NX and pN1a disease (DSS was 100 % for pN0/X and pN1a disease; regional RFR was 99 % for pN0/X and 93 % for pN1a disease; distant RFR was 99 % for pN0/X and pN1a disease). No difference in the clinical outcome was observed between N0/NX and N1a disease [6].

Data about the benefit of RAI ablation in patients with lymph node metastases at diagnosis are not conclusive. There is some evidence that there may be a benefit of adjuvant RAI treatment in improving overall and disease-specific survival as well as disease-free survival in patients with nodal metastases aged ≥45 years [7]. Furthermore, the greatest treatment benefits are observed in patients with N1b disease or lymph nodes >1 cm in diameter [8]. The adjuvant therapeutic efficacy of RAI treatment in improving outcome in patients > age 45 with isolated microscopic central neck disease, in the absence of other adverse features, is unknown. Thus, the relatively good overall prognosis of this group and the uncertainty of RAI therapeutic efficacy for this subgroup are important considerations in decision-making.

Several studies have shown that postoperative/pre-RAI ablation nonstimulated or stimulated Tg can predict disease-free remission and mortality in DTC patients [9–14]. Based on this observation, several authors have suggested that postoperative/pre-ablative Tg, performed approximately 3–6 months after total thyroidectomy, can be used for planning RAI ablation therapy in low-/intermediate-risk DTC patients [14–16]. Specifically, in intermediate DTC patients, an unstimulated postoperative Tg <1.0 ng/ml was associated with excellent clinical outcome and recurrence rate <1 % [16] in patients that did not receive RAI ablation. The negative predictive value of stimulated serum Tg <2.0 pg/ml was 94.1 % for intermediate-risk patients, and it increased to 97 % when stimulated serum Tg values were combined with negative neck ultrasound [17]. A similar significant decrease of recurrences is reported in intermediate-risk patients with negative postsurgical neck ultrasonography [18].

A selective approach of RAI ablation in intermediate-risk patients has been recently evaluated in 193 DTC patients with N1 disease [19]. RAI ablation was performed on 172 patients (74 %). In the total group, the 5-year DSS and RFS were 100 % and 92 %, respectively. Stratifying by RAI ablation, the 5-year regional RFS and distant RFS for patients who did not have RAI ablation were 100 %, not significantly different from that observed in patients who had RAI ablation (93 %, $p=0.26$ and 0.27, respectively). In conclusion, in patients with N1 disease at diagnosis classified as being at low risk of recurrent disease, postoperative Tg levels and neck ultrasound could be helpful in identifying patients that may not benefit from RAI ablation.

Back to the Patient

Based on the above considerations, the patient was scheduled to have serum Tg measurement on levothyroxine therapy using an ultrasensitive assay plus neck ultrasound 3 months after surgery. At this time, serum Tg was <01 ng/ml (TSH 03 mU/l) with negative antiTg antibodies, and neck ultrasound was unremarkable. RAI ablation was not performed, and annual monitoring of serum Tg and neck ultrasound was recommended. Serum TSH was maintained in the low normal range (0.1–0.5 mU/l). She has now been followed for 3 years without any evidence of recurrent disease.

Clinical Pearls

- Despite limitations in the studies reported in the literature, especially the lack of randomized trials, it is likely that RAI ablation is not needed for all patients with locoregional node metastases.
- In patients with lymph node metastases at diagnosis, the greatest potential for benefit of RAI ablation is in patients with a high volume of nodal disease, lymph node disease outside the central neck, and advanced patient age.
- The efficacy of adjuvant RAI treatment in improving long-term thyroid cancer outcomes in patients with isolated microscopic central neck nodal disease in the absence of other adverse features is unknown. In this group of patients, the decision must be individualized, considering additional parameters such as the levels of serum Tg after surgery, the results of neck ultrasound, and the preferences of the patient.

References

1. Iyer NG, Morris LG, Tuttle RM, Shaha AR, Ganly I. Rising incidence of second cancers in patients with low-risk (T1N0) thyroid cancer who receive radioactive iodine therapy. Cancer. 2011;117:4439–46.
2. Tuttle RM, Sabra MM. Selective use of RAI for ablation and adjuvant therapy after total thyroidectomy for differentiated thyroid cancer: a practical approach to clinical decision making. Oral Oncol. 2013;49:676–83.
3. Tuttle RM, Leboeuf R. Follow up approaches in thyroid cancer: a risk adapted paradigm. Endocrinol Metab Clin North Am. 2008;37:419–35.
4. Haugen BR, Alexander EK, Bible KC, Doherty GM, Mandel SJ, Nikiforov YE, Pacini F, Randolph GW, Sawka AM, Schlumberger M, Schuff K, Sherman SI, Sosa JA, Steward DL, Tuttle RM, Wartofsky L. American thyroid association management guidelines for patients with thyroid nodules and differentiated thyroid cancer. Thyroid. 2015.
5. Randolph GW, Duh QY, Heller KS, LiVolsi VA, Mandel SJ, Steward DL, Tufano RP, Tuttle RM, American Thyroid Association Surgical Affairs Committee's Taskforce on Thyroid Cancer Nodal Surgery. The prognostic significance of nodal metastases from papillary thyroid carcinoma can be stratified based on the size and number of metastatic lymph nodes, as well as the presence of extranodal extension. Thyroid. 2012;22:1144–52.
6. Nixon IJ, Wang LY, Palmer FL, Tuttle RM, Shaha AR, Shah JP, Patel SG, Ganly I. The impact of nodal status on outcome in older patients with papillary thyroid cancer. Surgery. 2014; 156:137–46.
7. Jonklaas J, Sarlis NJ, Litofsky D, Ain KB, Bigos ST, Brierley JD, Cooper DS, Haugen BR, Ladenson PW, Magner J, Robbins J, Ross DS, Skarulis M, Maxon HR, Sherman SI. Outcomes of patients with differentiated thyroid carcinoma following initial therapy. Thyroid. 2006;16: 1229–42.
8. Chow SM, Yau S, Kwan CK, Poon PC, Law SC. Local and regional control in patients with papillary thyroid carcinoma: specific indications of external radiotherapy and radioactive iodine according to T and N categories in AJCC 6th edition. Endocr Relat Cancer. 2006;13: 1159–72.
9. Heemstra KA, Liu YY, Stokkel M, Kievit J, Corssmit E, Pereira AM, Romijn JA, Smit JW. Serum thyroglobulin concentrations predict disease-free remission and death in differentiated thyroid carcinoma. Clin Endocrinol. 2007;66:58–64.
10. Kim TY, Kim WB, Kim ES, Ryu JS, Yeo JS, Kim SC, Hong SJ, Shong YK. Serum thyroglobulin levels at the time of 131I remnant ablation just after thyroidectomy are useful for early prediction of clinical recurrence in low-risk patients with differentiated thyroid carcinoma. J Clin Endocrinol Metab. 2005;90:1440–5.
11. Lin JD, Huang MJ, Hsu BR, Chao TC, Hsueh C, Liu FH, Liou MJ, Weng HF. Significance of postoperative serum thyroglobulin levels in patients with papillary and follicular thyroid carcinomas. J Surg Oncol. 2002;80:45–51.
12. Ronga G, Filesi M, Ventroni G, Vestri AR, Signore A. Value of the first serum thyroglobulin level after total thyroidectomy for the diagnosis of metastases from differentiated thyroid carcinoma. Eur J Nucl Med. 1999;26:1448–52.
13. Sawka AM, Orlov S, Gelberg J, Stork B, Dowar M, Shaytzag M, Tabatabaie V, Freeman JL, Walfish PG. Prognostic value of postsurgical stimulated thyroglobulin levels after initial radioactive iodine therapy in well-differentiated thyroid carcinoma. Head Neck. 2008;30: 693–700.
14. Toubeau M, Touzery C, Arveux P, Chaplain G, Vaillant G, Berriolo A, Riedinger JM, Boichot C, Cochet A, Brunotte F. Predictive value for disease progression of serum thyroglobulin levels measured in the postoperative period and after (131)I ablation therapy in patients with differentiated thyroid cancer. J Nucl Med. 2004;45:988–94.
15. Bernier MO, Morel O, Rodien P, Muratet JP, Giraud P, Rohmer V, Jeanguillaume C, Bigorgne JC, Jallet P. Prognostic value of an increase in the serum thyroglobulin level at the time of the

first ablative radioiodine treatment in patients with differentiated thyroid cancer. Eur J Nucl Med Mol Imaging. 2005;32:1418–21.

16. Ibrahimpasic T, Nixon IJ, Palmer FL, Whitcher MM, Tuttle RM, Shaha A, Patel SG, Shah JP, Ganly I. Undetectable thyroglobulin after total thyroidectomy in patients with low- and intermediate-risk papillary thyroid cancer--is there a need for radioactive iodine therapy? Surgery. 2012;152:1096–105.
17. Lee JI, Chung YJ, Cho BY, Chong S, Seok JW, Park SJ. Postoperative-stimulated serum thyroglobulin measured at the time of 131I ablation is useful for the prediction of disease status in patients with differentiated thyroid carcinoma. Surgery. 2013;153:828–35.
18. Lepoutre-Lussey C, Maddah D, Golmard JL, Russ G, Tissier F, Trésallet C, Menegaux F, Aurengo A, Leenhardt L. Post-operative neck ultrasound and risk stratification in differentiated thyroid cancer patients with initial lymph node involvement. Eur J Endocrinol. 2014; 170:837–46.
19. Nixon IJ, Ganly I, Patel SG, Palmer FL, Di Lorenzo MM, Grewal RK, Larson SM, Tuttle RM, Shaha A, Shah JP. The results of selective use of radioactive iodine on survival and on recurrence in the management of papillary thyroid cancer, based on Memorial Sloan-Kettering Cancer Center risk group stratification. Thyroid. 2013;23:683–94.

Chapter 24
A Patient with a Large Hürthle Cell Carcinoma of the Thyroid and Nodal Metastases

Leonard Wartofsky

Case

A 67-year-old man was referred to our endocrine clinic by his primary care physician for the management of a 5.6 cm thyroid nodule in the left lobe with a recent fine-needle aspiration (FNA) cytology interpreted as an indeterminate diagnosis favoring a follicular neoplasm (Bethesda class IV). A repeat FNA was sent for mutational analysis and was positive for the *RAS* oncogene, and the patient was referred for thyroidectomy. Preoperative ultrasonography confirmed the left lobe nodule which was hypoechoic with irregular margins and lacked any calcification, and there was suspicion for involved lateral neck lymph nodes. Fine-needle aspiration of the suspicious lymph node confirmed thyroid cancer, and he underwent a total thyroidectomy and central and modified left neck dissection. The surgical pathology described a 6 cm poorly encapsulated tumor with both local invasiveness with extrathyroidal extension and vascular invasion at 8 identified sites. The predominant cell type was oncocytic or oxyphilic with microfollicle formation consistent with a Hürthle cell follicular carcinoma. Extrathyroidal extension was evident with several implants of tumor ranging from 2 to 11 mm in the lateral neck; 6/12 lymph nodes from Level VI and 12/31 lymph nodes from left Levels II and III were positive for metastatic tumor [Stage 4A (T3, N1B, MX)] (Fig. 24.1).

L. Wartofsky, MD (✉)
MedStar Washington Hospital Center, 110 Irvig St., NW, Washington, DC 20010, USA

Georgetown University School of Medicine, Washington, DC, USA

D.S. Cooper, C. Durante (eds.), *Thyroid Cancer*,
DOI 10.1007/978-3-319-22401-5_24

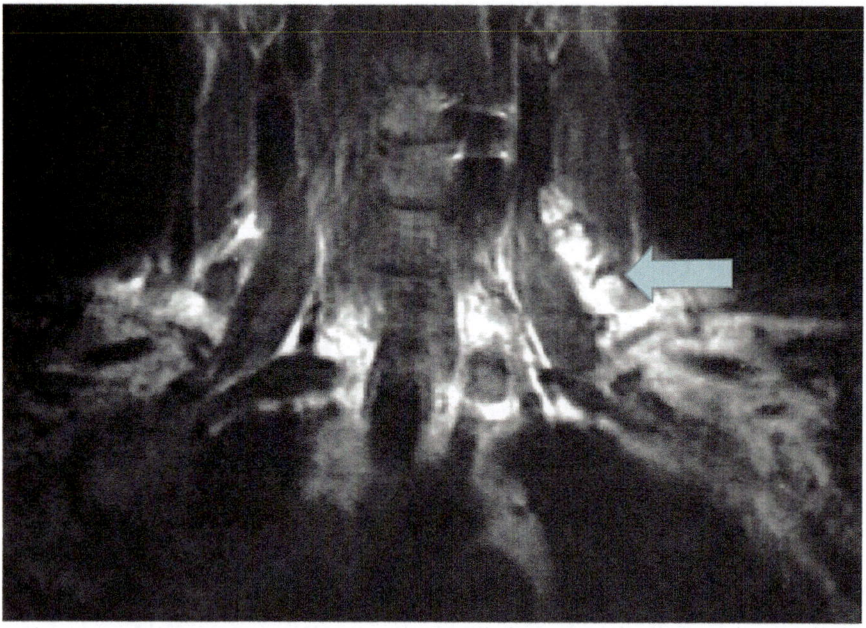

Fig. 24.1 Magnetic resonance imaging (MRI) of patient's neck demonstrating lymph node metastases in left neck (*arrow*)

Hürthle Cell Carcinoma: Literature Review

Some thyroid tumors with predominant oncocytic cytology may be benign or so-called Hürthle cell adenomas [1]. Based upon postoperative surgical pathology, the risk of carcinoma in a nodule with FNA cytology read as Hürthle cell neoplasm ranges from 10 to 45 % in various series [2]. The likelihood that such a nodule is a carcinoma increases with nodule size [3] with approximately 50 % of tumors >4 cm and 100 % of tumors >6 cm being malignant [4]. In addition to tumor size, other factors associated with malignancy are male sex, age>65, and highly elevated serum levels of thyroglobulin (Tg) [5], but cancer is still common but less frequent when Tg levels are <500 ng/mL [6].

In this patient, the finding of a RAS mutation on the fine-needle-aspirated material constituted an additional motivation for proceeding to total thyroidectomy [7]. Although a reading of follicular lesion of uncertain significance (FLUS) carries a low risk of malignancy of 5–20 %, in this patient the interpretation as follicular neoplasm (FN; Bethesda Class IV) carries a somewhat higher risk of 20–30 %, and the large size of the nodule implies an even higher risk [8]. In one study, 87/513 (17 %) of indeterminate nodules on FNA had a positive mutation, and 70 % of these were RAS point mutations as in our patient [9]. In contrast to our patient who had a Hürthle cell carcinoma, most RAS-positive thyroid cancers are papillary thyroid cancers and tend to have a good prognosis [10].

Sonography cannot reliably predict which nodules may be carcinoma as these lesions may present a wide variety of sonographic findings [11], but typically will lack calcification. Current guidelines of the American Thyroid Association [12] do not recommend screening thyroid nodules with FDG-PET scans, but thyroid nodules found incidentally to be positive on PET scan warrant FNA cytology to rule out malignancy. Because there is a correlation between PET positivity and clinical aggressiveness of tumors, Hürthle cell carcinoma is likely to be positive on FDG-PET [13] and was recently also found to be positive on an 18-F DOPA PET scan [14].

Hürthle cells are often present in Hashimoto's thyroiditis, and the presence of a Hürthle cell lesion in a thyroid gland involved with Hashimoto's thyroiditis can present a difficult challenge [15]. The Hürthle cell variant of follicular thyroid cancer was first described in 1928 on the basis of the distinctive cellular features of oxyphilic cells with abundant cytoplasm that lack any of the typical cytologic features of papillary thyroid carcinoma such as nuclear pseudoinclusions. Like classic follicular thyroid carcinoma, Hürthle cell cancers may be classified as either minimally invasive with less than four foci of capsular invasion or widely invasive [16]. In general, follicular thyroid cancer is more likely to metastasize to distant sites like lung and bone *via* vascular invasion and hematogenous spread and typically does not spread to local or regional lymph nodes as is typical of papillary thyroid cancer. Thus, it is less common for the Hürthle cell variant of follicular carcinoma to spread to lymph nodes as it did in this case, and the presence of involved lymph nodes is an independent predictor of reduced disease-free survival [17]. Bishop et al. [18] noted that locoregional soft tissue metastases may be more characteristic of this tumor than lymph node metastases. Whether the prognosis of fully encapsulated minimally invasive small Hürthle cell cancers may be excellent is controversial, with one recent study indicating significant risk of residual or recurrent disease [19]. However, the more invasive types such as the solid or trabecular subtypes are more aggressive, and their course is often marked by both locoregional and distant metastases [20–22]. Identification and classification of the degree of invasiveness is critical to the determination of how aggressively therapy is to be implemented. Unfortunately, a large proportion of Hürthle cell cancers do not trap radioiodine, and even those that may demonstrate 131-I uptake tend to be less radiosensitive than are papillary thyroid cancers. Nevertheless, in contrast to the general consensus and based on an analysis of clinical outcomes in 485 patients with follicular thyroid cancer and 73 patients with Hürthle cell cancer, Sugino et al. [23] concluded that the Hürthle cell patients fared no worse in regard to prognosis.

Management of the Patient

Postoperatively, the patient was started on levothyroxine 0.15 mg/day and placed on a low iodine diet in preparation for diagnostic radioiodine scanning and potential ablation. At 4 weeks postsurgery when his serum TSH level was 0.38, his serum

Tg measured 1224 ng/mL, and after preparation with recombinant human thyrotropin (rhTSH; Thyrogen®), an iodine-123 scan indicated moderate uptake in the right thyroid bed and faint uptake in 3 foci in the left lateral neck and one focus in the anterior mediastinum. The scan results prompted repeat ultrasonography of the neck which indicated either nodules or suspicious lymph nodes in the left neck. Magnetic resonance imaging (MRI) [24, 25] confirmed the lesions which appeared to correlate with the foci of radioiodine uptake on the isotopic scan, and the patient was referred back to his surgeon. A repeat left lateral neck compartmental node dissection was performed with removal of 18 additional lymph nodes, 9 of which were positive for metastatic tumor. At 3 months after his original surgery, his serum Tg was 88 ng/mL with a TSH of 0.03. He was again placed on a low iodine diet and after 2 weeks was treated with an activity of 175 mCi radioiodine facilitated by rhTSH preparation. His posttreatment total body scan revealed only modest uptake of iodine-131, and it is anticipated that he may need to be treated with external radiotherapy [26] or local interventional ablation [27, 28] should persistent locoregional disease be documented.

Clinical Pearls/Pitfalls

1. While the majority of Hürthle cell neoplasms based on cytologic examination may be benign, tumors larger than 4 cm and advanced age are worrisome for an increased likelihood of Hürthle cell carcinoma.
2. Hürthle cell carcinomas can present with locoregional lymph node or soft tissue metastasis and hence are an exception to the general teaching that follicular cancers are angioinvasive and present with distant metastases.
3. Finding 4 or more sites of invasion through the capsule classifies these tumors as highly invasive and associated with greater risk, thereby warranting more aggressive therapy.
4. Hürthle cell carcinoma frequently will not take up sufficient radioiodine to result in effective therapy, and external radiation or targeted chemotherapy may be required. However, radioiodine remnant ablation is always recommended.

References

1. Rossi ED, Martini M, Straccia P, Raffaelli M, Pennacchia I, Marrucci E, Lombardi CP, Pontecorvi A, Fadda G. The cytologic category of oncocytic (Hürthle) cell neoplasm mostly includes low-risk lesions at histology: an institutional experience. Eur J Endocrinol. 2013; 169(5):649–55.
2. Auger M. Hürthle cells in fine-needle aspirates of the thyroid: a review of their diagnostic criteria and significance. Cancer Cytopathol. 2014;122(4):241–9.
3. Lee KH, Shin JH, Ko ES, Hahn SY, Kim JS, Kim JH, Oh YL. Predictive factors of malignancy in patients with cytologically suspicious for Hürthle cell neoplasm of thyroid nodules. Int J Surg. 2013;11(9):898–902.

4. Sippel RS, Elaraj DM, Khanafshar E, Zarnegar R, Kebebew E, Duh QY, Clark OH. Tumor size predicts malignant potential in Hürthle cell neoplasms of the thyroid. World J Surg. 2008; 32(5):702–7.
5. Strazisar B, Petric R, Sesek M, Zgajnar J, Hocevar M, Besic N. Predictive factors of carcinoma in 279 patients with Hürthle cell neoplasm of the thyroid gland. J Surg Oncol. 2010;101(7): 582–6.
6. Suh I, Vriens MR, Guerrero MA, Griffin A, Shen WT, Duh QY, Clark OH, Kebebew E. Serum thyroglobulin is a poor diagnostic biomarker of malignancy in follicular and Hürthle-cell neoplasms of the thyroid. Am J Surg. 2010;200:41–6.
7. Yip L, Wharry LI, Armstrong MJ, Silbermann A, McCoy KL, Stang MT, et al. A clinical algorithm for fine-needle aspiration molecular testing effectively guides the appropriate extent of initial thyroidectomy. Ann Surg. 2014;260:163–7.
8. McCoy KL, Carty SE, Armstrong MJ, Seethala RR, Ohori NP, Kabaker AS, et al. Intraoperative pathologic examination in the era of molecular testing for differentiated thyroid cancer. J Am Coll Surg. 2012;215:546–54.
9. Nikiforov YE, Nikiforova MN. Molecular genetics and diagnosis of thyroid cancer. Nat Rev Endocrinol. 2011;7:569–80.
10. Gupta N, Dasyam AK, Carty SE, Nikiforova MN, Ohori NP, Armstrong M, et al. RAS mutations in thyroid FNA specimens are highly predictive of predominantly low-risk follicular pattern cancers. J Clin Endocrinol Metab. 2013;98:E914–22.
11. Maizlin ZV, Wiseman SM, Vora P, Kirby JM, Mason AC, Filipenko D, Brown JA. Hürthle cell neoplasms of the thyroid: sonographic appearance and histologic characteristics. J Ultrasound Med. 2008;27(5):751–7.
12. Haugen BR, Alexander EK, Bible KC, Doherty GM, Mandel SJ, Nikiforov Y, et al. American Thyroid Association Management Guidelines for patients with thyroid nodules and differentiated thyroid cancer. Thyroid. 2015; 24.
13. Riemann B, Uhrhan K, Dietlein M, Schmidt D, Kuwert T, et al. Diagnostic value and therapeutic impact of (18)F-FDG-PEET-CT in differentiated thyroid cancer. Results of a German multicentre study. Nuklearmedizin. 2013;53:1–6.
14. Pauleau G, Palazzo FF, Essamet W, Sebag F, Taieb D. Hürthle cell neoplasms: a new differential diagnosis of 18F-FDOPA-avid thyroid nodules? J Clin Endocrinol Metab. 2013;98: 865–6.
15. Lee J, Hasteh F. Oncocytic variant of papillary thyroid carcinoma associated with Hashimoto's thyroiditis: a case report and review of the literature. Diagn Cytopathol. 2009;37(8):600–6.
16. Mai KT, Khanna P, Yazdi HM, Perkins DG, Veinot JP, Thomas J, Lamba M, Nair BD. Differentiated thyroid carcinomas with vascular invasion: a comparative study of follicular. Hürthle cell and papillary thyroid carcinoma. Pathology. 2002;34:239–44.
17. Mills SC, Haq M, Smellie WJ, Harmer C. Hürthle cell carcinoma of the thyroid: retrospective review of 62 patients treated at the Royal Marsden Hospital between 1946 and 2003. Eur J Surg Oncol. 2009;35(3):230–4.
18. Bishop JA, Wu G, Tufano RP, Westra WH. Histological patterns of locoregional recurrence in Hürthle cell carcinoma of the thyroid gland. Thyroid. 2012;22(7):690–4.
19. Kuo EJ, Roman SA, Sosa JA. Patients with follicular and Hürthle cell microcarcinomas have compromised survival: a population level study of 22,738 patients. Surgery. 2013;154: 1246–53.
20. Haigh PI, Urbach DR. The treatment and prognosis of Hürthle cell follicular thyroid carcinoma compared with its non-Hürthle cell counterpart. Surgery. 2005;138:1152–7.
21. Ganly I, Ricarte FJ, Eng S, Ghossein R, Morris LG, Liang Y, Socci N, Kannan K, Mo Q, Fagin JA, Chan TA. Genomic dissection of Hürthle cell carcinoma reveals a unique class of thyroid malignancy. J Clin Endocrinol Metab. 2013;98:E962–72.
22. Ghossein RA, Hiltzik DH, Carlson DL, Patel S, Shaha A, Shah JP, Tuttle RM, Singh B. Prognostic factors of recurrence in encapsulated Hürthle cell carcinoma of the thyroid gland: a clinicopathologic study of 50 cases. Cancer. 2006;106:1669–76.

23. Sugino K, Kameyama K, Ito K, Nagahama M, Kitagawa W, Shibuya H, Ohkuwa K, et al. Does Hürthle cell carcinoma of the thyroid have a poorer prognosis than ordinary follicular thyroid carcinoma? Ann Surg Oncol. 2013;20(9):2944–50.
24. Takashima S, Sone S, Takayama F, Wang Q, Kobayashi T, Horii A, Yoshida JI. Papillary thyroid carcinoma: MR diagnosis of lymph node metastasis. AJNR Am J Neuroradiol. 1998; 19:509–13.
25. Gross ND, Weissman JL, Talbot JM, Andersen PE, Wax MK, Cohen JI. MRI detection of cervical metastasis from differentiated thyroid carcinoma. Laryngoscope. 2001;111:1905–9.
26. Foote RL, Brown PD, Garces YI, McIver B, Kasperbauer JL. Is there a role for radiation therapy in the management of Hürthle cell carcinoma? Int J Radiat Oncol Biol Phys. 2003; 56:1067–72.
27. Lewis BD, Hay ID, Charboneau JW, McIver B, Reading CC, Goellner JR. Percutaneous ethanol injection for treatment of cervical lymph node metastases in patients with papillary thyroid carcinoma. Am J Roentgenol. 2002;178:699–704.
28. Dupuy DE, Monchik JM, Decrea C, Pisharodi L. Radiofrequency ablation of regional recurrence from well-differentiated thyroid malignancy. Surgery. 2001;130:971–7.

Chapter 25
A Case of a Large, Invasive PTC with Gross Residual Disease (pT4) After Surgery

Meredith Giuliani and James Brierley

Case Presentation

A 62-year-old, previously healthy, man presented with a slowly enlarging mass in his right neck associated with progressive hoarseness over a 3-month period, but he had no complaints of pain, difficulty in swallowing, or difficulty in breathing. The family physician palpated a non-tender mass in the right mid neck that measured about 4 cm. He organized an ultrasound that confirmed a 4 cm mass in the right thyroid lobe and he referred the patient to a head and neck surgeon. An iodinated contrast-enhanced computed tomography (CT) scan of the neck confirmed a 4 cm mass in the right thyroid gland with possible extrathyroidal extension posteriorly toward the tracheal-esophageal groove and several suspicious right-sided lymph nodes (See Fig. 25.1). A fine-needle biopsy was performed which was compatible with papillary thyroid cancer.

Literature Review

Most patients with differentiated thyroid carcinoma (DTC) are treated by complete surgical excision (thyroidectomy or hemithyroidectomy) and, depending on the risk of recurrence, may receive postoperative radioiodine(^{131}I) combined with TSH suppressive therapy both of which have been reported to reduce locoregional recurrence and improve survival in higher risk patients [1].

M. Giuliani, MB • J. Brierley, MB (✉)
Department of Radiation Oncology, University of Toronto, Toronto, ON, Canada

Department of Radiation Oncology, Princess Margaret Cancer Centre, 610 University Ave, Toronto, ON M5G2M9, Canada
e-mail: James.Brierley@rmp.uhn.on.ca

D.S. Cooper, C. Durante (eds.), *Thyroid Cancer*,
DOI 10.1007/978-3-319-22401-5_25

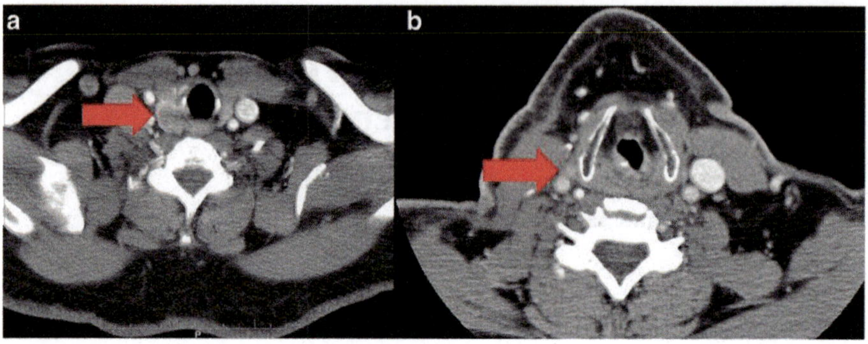

Fig. 25.1 Staging CT images. (**a**) Preoperative CT, the *red arrow* indicated the mass in the right lobe of the thyroid. (**b**) A postoperative CT, the *red arrow* indicated the area of gross residual disease

Locally advanced DTC with clinical extrathyroid extension is an uncommon clinical scenario, although more frequent in older patients, especially men. It can be a significant challenge if it recurs, as uncontrolled cancer in the neck can be devastating with laryngeal, tracheal, and esophageal obstruction, skin ulceration and necrosis, and even carotid artery rupture. Following extensive surgery, the disrupted blood flow to the thyroid bed may result in poor distribution of ^{131}I to residual tumor foci. Further, patients in this group often have less well-differentiated tumors that may not take up iodine as avidly as those that are more well differentiated, and therefore, surgery and postoperative ^{131}I may not adequately control persistent cervical disease. Consequently, additional treatment with external beam radiotherapy (EBRT) may be beneficial. However, there is a lack of randomized evidence to guide its use and confirm its benefit. The only randomized trial comparing observation with EBRT was in patients with pT3/4 pN0/1 with DTC, and it closed early due to poor accrual [2]. The study randomized patients without distant metastasis following an R0 (no residual disease) or R1 (microscopic residual disease) resection and TSH suppression therapy. The dose of EBRT was 59.4 Gy if an R0 resection had been performed and 66.6 Gy if R1 resection had been performed. The data were subsequently reported as a prospective cohort study which showed EBRT was well tolerated and there were no recurrences; however, there was only a 3 % recurrence rate in the observation group. Many patients did not meet the American Thyroid Association (ATA) guideline criteria [3] on the use of EBRT and had relatively low risk disease; therefore, a benefit from EBRT may not have been expected [4].

With the lack of randomized data, institutional series are used to inform management. In a typical series of high-risk, (pT2-T4, N0/1) DTC patients who received EBRT (median dose 62Gy), the 4-year locoregional control was 72 %. EBRT however can cause significant side effects, and in this series 5 % remained dependent on a feeding tube [5]. The extent of disease following surgery remains an important prognostic factor despite treatment with EBRT. In another report of high-risk patients who received EBRT, the 5-year locoregional control rate for patients with clear or microscopic margins was 89 %, compared to a 69 % rate of control in those with macroscopic residual or unresectable disease [6]. Our own data have shown that EBRT in older patients (age >60) with extrathyroidal extension (ETE) has significantly improved 5-year local relapse-free rate. In addition, in patients with post-operative gross residual disease treated with radiotherapy, the 10-year cause-specific survival and local recurrence-free rate were 48 and 90 %, respectively. This demonstrates clearly that even though local disease can be controlled with EBRT, patients continue to die from metastatic disease [7].

The ATA guidelines recommend consideration of EBRT in patients older than 45 years with gross extrathyroidal extension and high likelihood of microscopic residual disease [3]. EBRT should also be considered in patients with gross residual disease. It is our policy to recommend EBRT in patients over age 50 with gross residual disease after surgery or with extrathyroid extension that invades posteriorly into the tracheal-esophageal groove that is unlikely to be controlled by ^{131}I, and in whom salvage surgery may require an ablative surgical procedure such as laryngectomy (T4a or T4b). Patients with minimal ETE (T3) with positive margins or ETE that invades anteriorly into the strap muscles can usually be resected with clear margins and do not require EBRT. Similarly as ^{131}I is more likely to be effective, we rarely recommend EBRT in younger patients unless they have T4b disease.

Minimizing toxicity from EBRT is a critical consideration in DTC. Toxicity is related to both dose and the volume of tissue that is irradiated. The optimal target volume for EBRT is controversial. Larger elective target volumes have the potential to reduce recurrence, but are associated with increased toxicity. The late effects following EBRT to the head and neck region are also dependent on the volumes radiated as well as the dose to normal structures. Structures of particular concern include the parotid glands [8] radiation to which potentiates the risk of xerostomia, which may already be of concern if high activities of ^{131}I have already been administered; the pharyngeal constrictors [9], which can result in feeding tube dependence; and, although more of a risk in other head and neck cancers, the mandible [10], which can be associated with a risk of osteo-radionecrosis. Our usual radiation volume includes the surgical thyroidectomy bed and nodal levels III, IV, VI, and part of level V, extending from the hyoid bone superiorly to the aortic arch inferiorly. Other centers use larger volumes. Two reports have recently concluded that larger volumes result in fewer recurrences and that larger volumes should be used. In one study, limited field EBRT was compared to extended radiotherapy volumes. They had no out of field recurrences in the larger volume patients in contrast to those with smaller volume irradiation. There was also an improved relapse-free rate of 89 % compared to a perhaps surprisingly low 40 % with the smaller volume [11]. The second report recommended extending the treatment volumes to the level of the carina to avoid upper mediastinal failures [6]. If radiotherapy is extended into the mediastinum, the simulation CT scan should include the whole lungs so the dose to the lungs can be ascertained and the radiation planning technique chosen to ensure a safe radiation dose is given and that risk of pneumonitis is minimized. As we reported 90 % local relapse-free rate in our series [7], we do not think that volumes need to be extended.

Intensity-modulated radiotherapy (IMRT) which allows modulation of the intensity of the radiotherapy beam ensures better distribution of radiation dose to the intended treatment volumes and is especially suitable for treating complex volumes such as the thyroid bed. It results in a more homogenous dose distribution and sparing of normal tissues than other radiation techniques. In randomized studies in squamous cell carcinomas of the head and neck, IMRT reduced side effects and improve quality of life [12]. The MD Anderson group, in a study of high-risk patients given EBRT, also reported that IMRT was associated with less frequent late toxicity in DTC [13]. The local relapse-free rate was high at 79 % at 4 years.

It is our institutional policy to deliver 60Gy in 30 fractions to the thyroid bed and areas of surgical dissection if there is concern for microscopic residual disease and a lower dose of 54Gy in 30 fractions to undissected areas at risk of microscopic disease. In the case of gross residual disease, a dose of 66Gy in 33 fractions is given to the residual disease plus a margin for uncertainty with 56Gy in 33 fractions to the areas at risk of microscopic disease. A preoperative CT scan with contrast is a great aid in planning any postoperative radiation therapy, as well as being helpful to the surgeon in planning the operation. In our institution, surgeons routinely perform CT scans with contrast in any patient with a potential T4 tumor (a large mass, pain, or hoarseness). Previously, concern that the use of iodinated contrast may interfere with the effectiveness of ^{131}I by reducing uptake has been expressed. However, with modern water-soluble contrast media, only a 1- or 2-month delay is required for the urinary iodine levels to fall, which is not an undue delay. Other centers have a preference for cervical MRI, but identification of lymph nodes and laryngeal cartilage involvement may be inferior when compared to a contrast-enhanced CT scan. Although in theory EBRT could reduce the effectiveness of ^{131}I, there is no good evidence to support this; however, our preference is usually to give ^{131}I, then perform postoperative CT scans after the post ^{131}I therapy scan, and reassess the extent of disease after surgery as seen on all imaging modalities. A PET scan if available may provide additional information. If however there is concern about the extent of local disease that may cause an oncological emergency without control of that disease, such as gross residual disease after spinal cord decompression, then we will give EBRT before ^{131}I.

The use of chemotherapy concurrent with EBRT in patients with DTC is another area of controversy. In a report from Memorial Sloan Kettering Cancer Center, there was no major difference in acute or late toxicity between the two, but there was a nonstatistically different improvement in local progression-free survival (90.0 % with chemoradiation and 73.0 % with radiation alone). However, the numbers were small and the local progression-free rate with the addition of chemotherapy was similar to our own experience without chemotherapy. Similar to the report from our institution, despite local control in the neck, there was a high distant relapse rate of 47 % [14].

Management

The patient was treated with a total thyroidectomy and neck dissection. The tumor involved the right cricothyroid joint, and gross disease was left *in situ* as it was not resectable without significant functional impairment. This was biopsied at the time of surgery and confirmed to be residual carcinoma. The final pathology was a 4.0 cm angioinvasive papillary carcinoma with 30 % warthin-like and 25 % tall cell changes. There was extrathyroidal extension and positive margins; 4 of 51 lymph nodes were involved: 3 from level VI and 1 from level IV. The final stage was pT4a N1b. Postoperatively, he received 125 mCi (4.62 GBq) of ^{131}I and was placed on suppressive doses of levothyroxine. His post-therapy radioiodine scan showed two foci of uptake in the thyroid bed, possibly representing residual disease. There was no evidence of distant disease. A post-radioiodine CT scan confirmed the location of the residual disease in the thyroid bed.

He was then considered for EBRT. On examination, he had a healed surgical scar but no palpable residual disease. Flexible nasopharyngoscopy demonstrated a paralyzed right vocal cord. His postoperative CT scan showed a 5 mm area of likely residual disease in the right thyroid bed (See Fig. 25.1b). He was treated with 66 Gy in 33 fractions of radiotherapy to the area of gross residual disease as identified on postoperative imaging and 60Gy in 33 fractions to the thyroid bed and bilateral necks with an IMRT plan (See Fig. 25.2).

Outcome

The patient experienced 7.4 % weight loss during radiotherapy and Radiotherapy Oncology Group (RTOG) grade 2 mucositis, esophagitis, laryngitis, and skin reactions. He was supported throughout treatment without a feeding tube. He has subsequently made a full recovery and is able to tolerate a normal diet. He does not experience xerostomia and remains free of recurrence 5 years later.

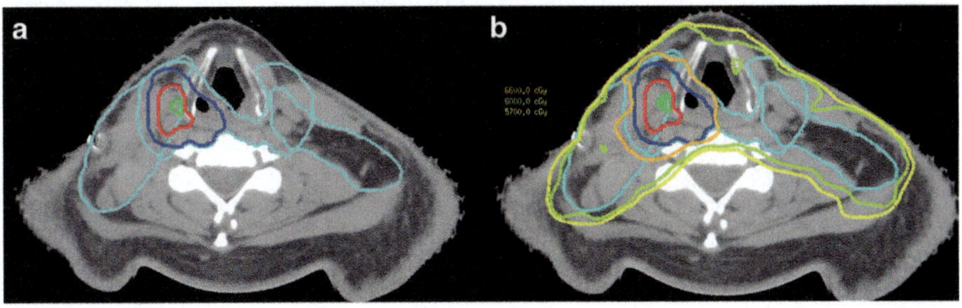

Fig. 25.2 Radiotherapy plan. (**a**) *Green* represents the GTV, *red* the HTV, *dark blue* the CTV66, and *light blue* the CTVs60. (**b**) The addition of the radiotherapy isodose lines 66Gy in *light orange*, 60Gy in *green yellow*, and 57Gy in *yellow*

Clinical Pearls/Pitfalls

- Gross residual disease following surgery for differentiated thyroid cancer is a complex clinical situation requiring multidisciplinary input and management.
- EBRT can increase locoregional control and possibly survival in older patients with extrathyroidal extension and with gross residual disease
- The ideal dose and treatment volumes remain uncertain.
- IMRT likely conveys an improvement in the toxicity profile.

References

1. Brierley J, Tsang R, Panzarella T, Bana N. Prognostic factors and the effect of treatment with radioactive iodine and external beam radiation on patients with differentiated thyroid cancer seen at a single institution over 40 years. Clin Endocrinol (Oxf). 2005;63:418–27.
2. Biermann M, Pixberg M, Riemann B, Schuck A, Heinecke A, Schmid KW, Willich N, Dralle H, Schober O, MSDS Study Group. Clinical outcomes of adjuvant external-beam radiotherapy for differentiated thyroid cancer - results after 874 patient-years of follow-up in the MSDS-trial. Nuklearmedizin. 2009;48:89–98; quiz N15.
3. American Thyroid Association Guidelines Taskforce on Thyroid N, Differentiated Thyroid Cancer, Cooper DS, Doherty GM, Haugen BR, Kloos RT, Lee SL, Mandel SJ, et al. Revised American Thyroid Association management guidelines for patients with thyroid nodules and differentiated thyroid cancer. Thyroid. 2009;19:1167–214.
4. Brierley JD. Update on external beam radiation therapy in thyroid cancer. J Clin Endocrinol Metab. 2011;96:2289–95.
5. Terezakis SA, Lee KS, Ghossein RA, Rivera M, Tuttle RM, Wolden SL, Zelefsky MJ, Wong RJ, Patel SG, Pfister DG, Shaha AR, Lee NY. Role of external beam radiotherapy in patients with advanced or recurrent nonanaplastic thyroid cancer: memorial sloan-kettering cancer center experience. Int J Radiat Oncol Biol Phys. 2009;73:795–801.
6. Azrif M, Slevin NJ, Sykes AJ, Swindell R, Yap BK. Patterns of relapse following radiotherapy for differentiated thyroid cancer: implication for target volume delineation. Radiother Oncol. 2008;89:105–13.
7. Sia MA, Tsang RW, Panzarella T, Brierley JD. Differentiated thyroid cancer with extrathyroidal extension: prognosis and the role of external beam radiotherapy. J Thyroid Res. 2010;2010:183461.
8. Eisbruch A, Ten Haken RK, Kim HM, Marsh LH, Ship JA. Dose, volume, and function relationships in parotid salivary glands following conformal and intensity-modulated irradiation of head and neck cancer. Int J Radiat Oncol Biol Phys. 1999;45:577–87.
9. Feng FY, Kim HM, Lyden TH, Haxer MJ, Feng M, Worden FP, Chepeha DB, Eisbruch A. Intensity-modulated radiotherapy of head and neck cancer aiming to reduce dysphagia: early dose-effect relationships for the swallowing structures. Int J Radiat Oncol Biol Phys. 2007;68:1289–98.
10. O'Sullivan B, Rumble RB, Warde P, Members of the IIEP. Intensity-modulated radiotherapy in the treatment of head and neck cancer. Clin Oncol. 2012;24:474–87.
11. Kim TH, Chung KW, Lee YJ, Park CS, Lee EK, Kim TS, Kim SK, Jung YS, Ryu JS, Kim SS, Cho KH, Shin KH. The effect of external beam radiotherapy volume on locoregional control in patients with locoregionally advanced or recurrent nonanaplastic thyroid cancer. Radiat Oncol. 2010;5:69.

12. Kam MK, Leung SF, Zee B, Chau RM, Suen JJ, Mo F, Lai M, Ho R, Cheung KY, Yu BK, Chiu SK, Choi PH, Teo PM, Kwan WH, Chan AT. Prospective randomized study of intensity-modulated radiotherapy on salivary gland function in early-stage nasopharyngeal carcinoma patients. J Clin Oncol. 2007;25:4873–9.
13. Schwartz DL, Lobo MJ, Ang KK, Morrison WH, Rosenthal DI, Ahamad A, Evans DB, Clayman G, Sherman SI, Garden AS. Postoperative external beam radiotherapy for differentiated thyroid cancer: outcomes and morbidity with conformal treatment. Int J Radiat Oncol Biol Phys. 2009;74:1083–91.
14. Romesser PB, Sherman EJ, Shaha AR, Lian M, Wong RJ, Sabra M, Rao SS, Fagin JA, Tuttle RM, Lee NY. External beam radiotherapy with or without concurrent chemotherapy in advanced or recurrent non-anaplastic non-medullary thyroid cancer. J Surg Oncol. 2014;110:375–82.

Suggested Readings

Giuliani M, Brierley J. Indications for the use of external beam radiation in thyroid cancer. Curr Opin Oncol. 2014;26(1):45–50.

Brierley JD, Schwartz DL, Tsang RW. External beam radiotherapy for thyroid malignancy. In: Randolph GW, editor. Surgery of the thyroid and parathyroid gland. Philadelphia: Elsevier; 2013. Chapter 52.

Part VI
High Risk Differentiated Thyroid Cancer: *The Use of Radioiodine*

Chapter 26
A Patient with Papillary Carcinoma of the Thyroid with Elevated Serum Thyroglobulin but Negative Imaging Studies

Leonard Wartofsky

Case

A 39-year-old woman presented to our office for a first visit having recently moved to the area. She had a history of presentation in late 2008 with a neck mass which on FNA biopsy was suspicious for papillary thyroid carcinoma (Bethesda class V), leading to a total thyroidectomy in early 2009. The surgical pathology revealed a 3.5 cm classic papillary cancer, and there were 2/6 central compartment nodes and 5/11 right lateral lymph nodes that were positive for metastasis, with report of tumor to the surgical margin and minimal extrathyroidal extension (pT3, N1b, Mx—Stage I according to AJCC/UICC TNM staging system, 7th edition). She received 90 mCi of radioiodine in April 2009. Her course until the present time had been one of the repeatedly measurable serum thyroglobulin (Tg) ranging from 8 to 20 ng/mL on TSH suppression without any success in localizing the source of the Tg by imaging studies. Since 2009, she had undergone annual ultrasonography of the neck, neck and chest CT on two occasions, MRI of the neck on two occasions, and recombinant human TSH (rhTSH; Thyrogen®)-stimulated iodine-131 scans on two occasions, all without identification of tumor. On two occasions, mildly suspicious lymph nodes in both the right and left neck underwent ultrasound-guided FNA for cytology and Tg measurement of the aspirate, but both were negative. She is well educated, well read on her disease, concerned about the continuing measurable levels of Tg, and asked if there are any other diagnostic or therapeutic options.

L. Wartofsky, M.D. (✉)
MedStar Washington Hospital Center, 110 Irvig St., NW, Washington, DC 20010, USA

Georgetown University School of Medicine, Washington, DC 20010, USA
e-mail: Leonard.Wartofsky@Medstar.net

D.S. Cooper, C. Durante (eds.), *Thyroid Cancer*,
DOI 10.1007/978-3-319-22401-5_26

Assessment

The case is illustrative of a patient with a biochemically incomplete response to treatment (i.e., persistent measurable Tg levels) but no evidence of structural disease. Ruling out the possibility of stable iodine contamination negating radioiodine uptake, we can explain the fact that her residual tumor is not seen on ultrasound, CT, MRI, or iodine-131 scans because the tumor deposits are small and below the detection sensitivity of the imaging modality, or because the tumor has dedifferentiated and is no longer taking up iodine. She is anti-Tg antibody negative, and there presumably should be no reason for an artifactually or falsely elevated serum Tg.

Relevant Literature

The current Guidelines of the American Thyroid Association (ATA) [1] suggest that imaging with ^{18}F-fluorodeoxyglucose (FDG) positron emission tomography (PET) coupled with a CT scan should be considered in patients in whom the serum Tg is elevated to >10 ng/ml and the usual iodine-131 scan is negative. Studies have confirmed the efficacy of FDG-PET scanning when radioiodine uptake is absent [2, 3]. Leboulleux et al. [4] performed a meta-analysis of a total of 789 patients in 25 separate studies without radioiodine uptake for whom the sensitivity of FDG-PET/CT was found to be 83 % and the specificity was 84 %. FDG-PET/CT imaging may be enhanced with TSH stimulation [5] and is most likely to be helpful with larger tumors that have dedifferentiated, i.e., lost ability to trap radioiodine. Similarly, FDG-PET-positive tumors tend to have a significantly worse prognosis due in large part to the absence of RAI uptake that precludes therapy with radioiodine [6]. Given the situation of measurable Tg but negative imaging, obtaining a FDG-PET/CT scan would be advisable and consistent with the recommendations in the Guidelines. Should the latter imaging disclose a locoregional metastasis or any localizable lesion, the therapeutic options to be considered include surgical excision, local ablative therapy such as radiofrequency or thermal ablation under CT guidance [7], or empiric radioiodine therapy (in spite of the likelihood of little uptake). RAI has been given in this clinical scenario [8] in patients with ostensibly no RAI uptake on preliminary diagnostic scans with a demonstrable salutary effect in perhaps a third of patients who demonstrate positive uptake on a post-therapy scan and a subsequent fall in serum Tg, but such empiric therapy has not been shown to be successful in the majority of studies [9–12]. The sensitivity of FDG-PET/CT scanning may be improved by TSH stimulation (either by rhTSH or thyroid hormone withdrawal) [5], and sensitivity is greatest when Tg levels are elevated to >10 ng/ml [1]. Because iodine-124 emits a positron and can be imaged by PET scanning and shares the same radio pharmacokinetics as iodine-131, studies have suggested that iodine-124 PET may be more useful for the identification of metastatic lesions than FDG-PET and, moreover when positive, demonstrates radioiodine avidity suggesting opportunity for RAI therapy with iodine-131 [13, 14]. When the iodine-124 is given in low doses (~2 mCi), stunning of the subsequent iodine-131 treatment dose has not been considered a problem [15]. It should be emphasized that just because tumor deposits take up RAI does not mean that the tumor is radiosensitive and will be destroyed by therapy [16], especially in those tumors that are FDG avid. Finally, should the iodine-124 scan show no uptake, as was seen with iodine-123 in the case presented, or should the tumor be noted to progress after therapy, then a repeat therapeutic dose of iodine-131 would not be recommended [1].

Subsequent Management

When next seen, the patient had a serum Tg of 7.5 on levothyroxine suppression and underwent rhTSH stimulation with a poststimulation Tg of 94 ng/ml and a negative iodine-123 scan (1.2 mCi; 444 MBq). She then underwent iodine-124 PET/CT (1.7 mCi;63 MBq) and iodine-131 dosimetry (2 mCi; 74 MBq) [17–19] (see Figs. 26.1 and 26.2). The iodine-131 scan (Fig. 26.1a) was largely negative, whereas the iodine-124 PET revealed a focus of uptake posteriorly (Fig. 26.1b) that

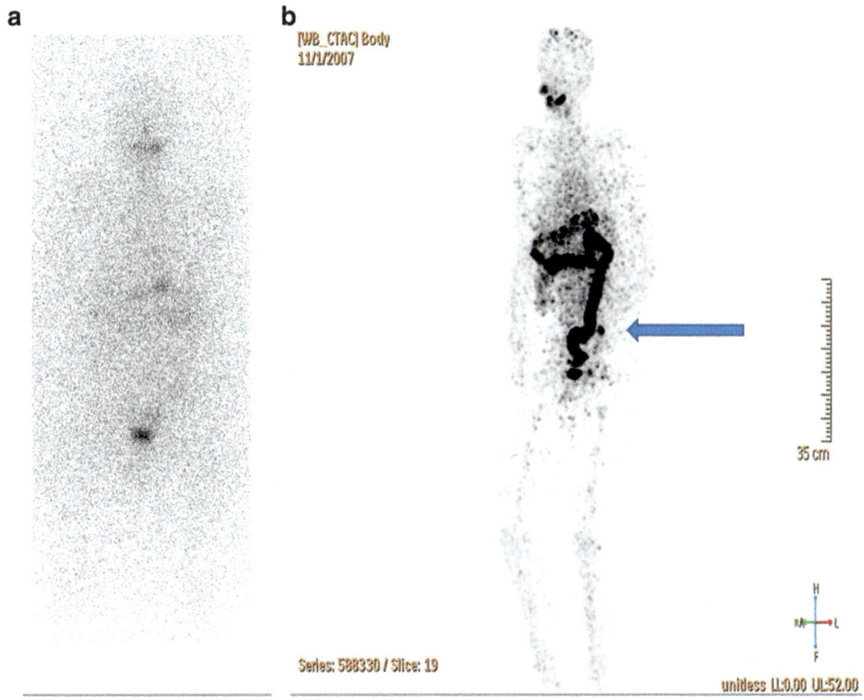

Fig. 26.1 (**a**) Iodine-123 scan (1.2 mCi; 444 MBq) indicating little detectable uptake. (**b**) Iodine-124 PET/CT (1.7 mCi;63 MBq) revealing a focus of uptake posteriorly

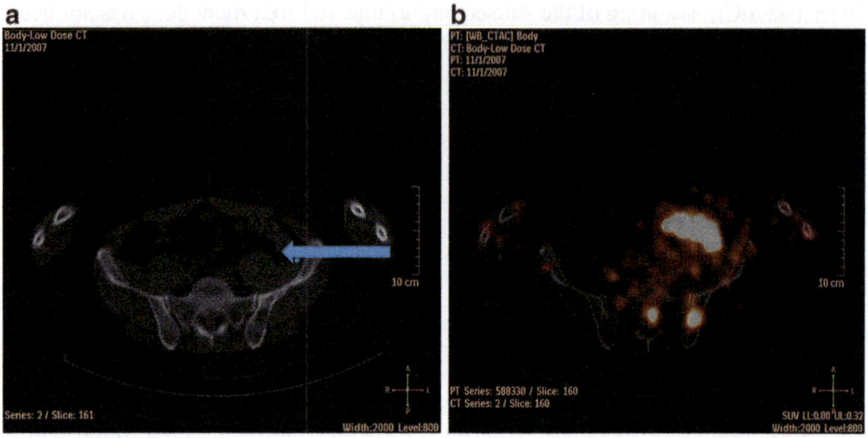

Fig. 26.2 (**a**) Computerized tomographic scan of pelvis indicating that the focus positive on PET scan was located in the *left* pelvic bone (*arrow*). (**b**) Fusion of the transverse CT image of the pelvis with the corresponding transverse iodine-124 PET image demonstrating localization of the lesion. The fused images demonstrated that the abnormal iodine-124 uptake corresponded precisely to the abnormality on the CT scan. In addition to localizing this abnormality, the 124I images demonstrated a second focus of abnormal iodine-124 uptake that correlated with another abnormality in the sacrum on the CT image suggesting an additional metastasis

was identified by CT (Fig. 26.2a) as being in the left pelvic bone (arrow). Figure 26.2b indicates fusion of the transverse CT image of the pelvis with the corresponding transverse iodine-124 PET image, which demonstrates the utility of fusing the iodine-124 PET image with the CT image. The fused images demonstrated that the abnormal iodine-124 uptake corresponded precisely to the abnormality on the CT scan. In addition to the identification of this abnormality, the iodine-124 images demonstrated a second focus of abnormal iodine-124 uptake that correlated with another abnormality in the sacrum on the CT image suggesting an additional metastasis. The dosimetry estimated that she could receive a 440 mCi dose of iodine-131 safely with less than 72 mCi retained at 48 h. Although the patient was advised of the small likelihood of cure or significant improvement with another dose of radioiodine in the face of negative diagnostic radioiodine scans [9–12], she nevertheless was desirous of one more therapy. She was treated with 392 mCi, and the findings on the post-therapy iodine-131 scan were consistent with those seen on the iodine-124 PET scan, i.e., positive uptake in the identified metastases. At 4 months post-therapy, her blood neutrophil and platelet counts were normal, and her serum Tg has fallen to 1.9 ng/ml on suppression therapy. The follow-up plan is to continue twice yearly monitoring with serum Tg measurements, and a repeat iodine-124 PET/CT scan will be considered in 12–18 months unless her serum Tg becomes undetectable with time. She would be declared refractory to radioiodine and not considered for additional therapy should there be evidence of progressive disease as indicated by a rising Tg level and/or increased structural disease. In the latter circumstance, we will consider external radiation therapy or other attempts at local ablation.

Clinical Pearls/Pitfalls

1. It is useful to tailor therapeutic interventions by risk stratification of patients according to 2014 ATA Guidelines on outcome status after initial treatment, which in this case indicated a biochemically incomplete response that was subsequently shown after iodine-124 PET scanning to be structurally incomplete.
2. Iodine-124 is associated with improved imaging over iodine-123 and lower radiation dose than iodine-131, thereby avoiding stunning. Although iodine-124 availability is currently confined to larger academic centers (because it is not an FDA-approved radioisotope and an IND is required), iodine-124 PET/CT scan should be considered in patients in whom the serum Tg is elevated to >10 ng/ml and the traditional iodine-131 scan is negative.
3. Another difference between iodine-124 and iodine-123 or iodine-131 is that iodine-124 emits a positron and can be imaged with a positron emission tomography (PET) scanner. The positron-emitting iodine-124 in combination with PET/CT makes it possible to measure the spatial distribution of radioiodine in tumors and normal organs at high resolution and sensitivity. Thus, iodine-124 PET/CT may provide improved delineation of the extent of metastases in well-differentiated thyroid cancer.
4. Radioiodine refractory tumors or those that fail to take up radioiodine should not be given additional doses of iodine-131.

References

1. Haugen BR, Alexander EK, Bible KC, Doherty GM, Mandel SJ, Nikiforov Y, et al. American Thyroid Association Management Guidelines for patients with thyroid nodules and differentiated thyroid cancer. Thyroid. 2015; 24.
2. Marcus C, Whitworth PW, Surasi DS, Pai SI, Subramaniam RM. PET/CT in the management of thyroid cancers. Am J Roentgenol. 2014;202(6):1316–29.
3. Riemann B, Uhrhan K, Dietlein M, Schmidt D, Kuwert T, Dorn R, et al. Diagnostic value and therapeutic impact of (18)F-FDG-PET/CT in differentiated thyroid cancer. Results of a German multicentre study. Nucl Med. 2013;52(1):1–6.
4. Leboulleux S, Schroeder PR, Schlumberger M, Ladenson PW. The role of PET in follow-up of patients treated for differentiated epithelial thyroid cancers. Nat Clin Pract Endocrinol Metab. 2007;3:112–21.
5. Leboulleux S, Schroeder PR, Busaidy NL, Auperin A, Corone C, Jacene HA, Ewertz ME, Bournaud C, Wahl RL, Sherman SI, Ladenson PW, Schlumberger M. Assessment of the incremental value of recombinant thyrotropin stimulation before 2-[18F]-Fluoro-2-deoxy-D-glucose positron emission tomography/computed tomography imaging to localize residual differentiated thyroid cancer. J Clin Endocrinol Metab. 2009;94:1310–6.
6. Robbins RJ, Wan Q, Grewal RK, Reibke R, Gonen M, Strauss HW, Tuttle RM, Drucker W, Larson SM. Real-time prognosis for metastatic thyroid carcinoma based on 2-[18F]fluoro-2-deoxy-D-glucose-positron emission tomography scanning. J Clin Endocrinol Metab. 2006;91: 498–505.
7. Wartofsky L. Adjunctive local approaches to metastatic thyroid cancer. In: Thyroid cancer: a comprehensive guide to clinical management. 2nd ed. New York: Humana/Springer; 2006. p. 509–13.

8. Mazzaferri EL. Empirically treating high serum thyroglobulin levels. J Nucl Med. 2005;46:1079–88.
9. Kim WG, Ryu JS, Kim EY, Lee JH, Baek JH, Yoon JH, et al. Empiric high-dose 131-iodine therapy lacks efficacy for treated papillary thyroid cancer patients with detectable serum thyroglobulin but negative cervical sonography and 18F-fluorodeoxy-glucose positron emission tomography scan. J Clin Endocrinol Metab. 2010;95:1169–73.
10. Leboulleux S, El Bez I, Borget I, Elleuch M, Deandreis D, Al Ghuzlan A, et al. Postradioiodine treatment whole-body scan in the era of 18-florodeoxyglucose positron emission tomography for differentiated thyroid carcinoma with elevated serum thyroglublin levels. Thyroid. 2012;22:832–8.
11. Rosario PW, Mourao GF, dos Santos JB, Calsolari MR. Is empirical radioactive iodine therapy still a valid approach to patients with thyroid cancer and elevated thyroglobulin? Thyroid. 2014;24:533–6.
12. Sabra MM, Grewal RK, Tala H, Larson SM, Tuttle RM. Clinical outcomes following empiric radioiodine therapy in patients with structurally identified metastatic follicular cell-derived thyroid carcinoma with negative diagnostic but positive post-therapy 131-I whole-body scans. Thyroid. 2012;22:877–83.
13. Phan HT, Jager PL, Paans AM, Plukker JT, Sturkenboom MG, Sluiter WJ, Wolffenbuttel BH, Dierckx RA, Links TP. The diagnostic value of 124I-PET in patients with differentiated thyroid cancer. Eur J Nucl Med Mol Imaging. 2008;35:958–65.
14. Freudenberg LS, Jentzen W, Stahl A, Bockisch A, Rosenbaum-Krumme SJ. Clinical applications of 124I-PET/CT in patients with differentiated thyroid cancer. Eur J Nucl Med Mol Imaging. 2011;38 Suppl 1:S48–56.
15. Van Nostrand D, Moreau S, Bandaru VV, Atkins F, Chennupati S, Mete M, Burman K, Wartofsky L. (124)I positron emission tomography versus (131)I planar imaging in the identification of residual thyroid tissue and/or metastasis in patients who have well-differentiated thyroid cancer. Thyroid. 2010;20:879–83.
16. Deandreis D, Al GA, Leboulleux S, Lacroix L, Garsi JP, Talbot M, Lumbroso J, Baudin E, Caillou B, Bidart JM, Schlumberger M. Do histological, immunohistochemical, and metabolic (radioiodine and fluorodeoxyglucose uptakes) patterns of metastatic thyroid cancer correlate with patient outcome? Endocr Relat Cancer. 2011;18:159–69.
17. Eschmann SM, Reischl G, Bilger K, Kuperferschlager J, Thelen MH, Dohmen BM, Bares R. Evaluation of dosimetry of radioiodine therapy in benign and malignant thyroid disorders by means of iodine-124 and PET. Eur J Nucl Med Mol Imaging. 2002;29:760–7.
18. Barth A, Robbins RJ, Larson SM. Patient-specific dosimetry for 131-I thyroid cancer therapy using 124-I PET and 3-dimensional-internal dosimetry (3D-ID) software. J Nucl Med. 2004;45:1366–72.
19. Freudenberg LS, Jentzen W, Gorges R, Petrich T, Marlowe RJ, Knust J, Bockrish A. 124-I PET dosimetry in advanced differentiated thyroid cancer: therapeutic impact. Nuclearmedizin. 2007;46:121–8.

Chapter 27
A Young Child with Papillary Thyroid Cancer and Metastatic Pulmonary Disease: Role of Radioactive Iodine Therapy in Children

Monica L. Arango and Steven G. Waguespack

Introduction

Papillary thyroid carcinoma is rare in the pediatric population and is treated with surgery by a high-volume thyroid surgeon followed by possible radioactive iodine (RAI) therapy, which is given in the context of postoperative staging (a diagnostic thyroid scan and a stimulated thyroglobulin (Tg) level) [1, 2], especially in cases of known or suspected distant metastases. Children with PTC and metastatic pulmonary disease typically respond satisfactorily to ^{131}I therapy and demonstrate a continuous improvement of Tg levels years beyond treatment [3, 4]. However, some patients may need more than one treatment with ^{131}I, and the optimal approach to the evaluation and treatment of children with pulmonary metastases from PTC remains unresolved [5]. Given the excellent prognosis of children with PTC and pulmonary metastases as well as the possible risk for second malignancies [4, 6, 7] and increased overall mortality among pediatric PTC survivors [8], the risks of multiple RAI doses must be constantly weighed against the potential benefits.

M.L. Arango, MD, FAAP (✉)
Division of Pediatric Endocrinology, The University of Texas, Health Science Center at Houston, 6431 Fannin Street, MSB 3.020, Houston, TX 77030, USA
e-mail: monica.L.Arango@uth.tmc.edu

S.G. Waguespack, MD, FAAP, FACE
Department of Endocrine Neoplasia and Hormonal Disorders, MD Anderson Cancer Center, University of Texas, Unit 1461, 301402, Houston, TX 77230, USA
e-mail: swagues@mdanderson.org

D.S. Cooper, C. Durante (eds.), *Thyroid Cancer*,
DOI 10.1007/978-3-319-22401-5_27

Case Presentation

A 9-year-old Hispanic male with a historyof multiple upper respiratory infections but no risk factors for thyroid cancer presented to an otolaryngologist with an enlarged cervical lymph node, which had been present for at least a year. He underwent an excisional lymph node biopsy, which revealed metastatic PTC, follicular variant. Initial comprehensive staging included a TSH of 3.46 mIU/L and Tg 354 ng/ml (normal <55 for an intact thyroid) with negative Tg antibodies; a neck ultrasound and contrast-enhanced computed tomography (CT) scan of the neck that revealed a diffusely infiltrating carcinoma with clinical N1b disease; and a chest X-ray (CXR) negative for pulmonary metastases. The patient had a total thyroidectomy and bilateral central and lateral neck dissections with final pathologic staging revealing a multifocal, bilateral T3N1bMx PTC, conventional type; tumor was negative for the *BRAF* V600E mutation. Postoperative staging 2 months after surgery (after ensuring a normal 24-h urine iodine level) included a withdrawal ^{123}I thyroid scan and a stimulated Tg level (concomitant TSH 191 mIU/L). There was no uptake identified on the diagnostic scan, but the stimulated Tg was 145 ng/ml (<0.9 post-thyroidectomy), suggesting residual metastatic disease. Given the high Tg level and risk for metastatic disease, he was treated empirically with 45 mCi of ^{131}I (weight-adjusted dose equivalent to a 150 mCi dose in a 70 kg adult; ^{131}I dose = 150 mCi X weight of patient (kg)/70). Posttreatment scan showed minimal diffuse bilateral pulmonary uptake as well as uptake bilaterally in the nodes of Rouviere (retropharyngeal lymph nodes), best seen with SPECT-CT imaging (Fig. 27.1).

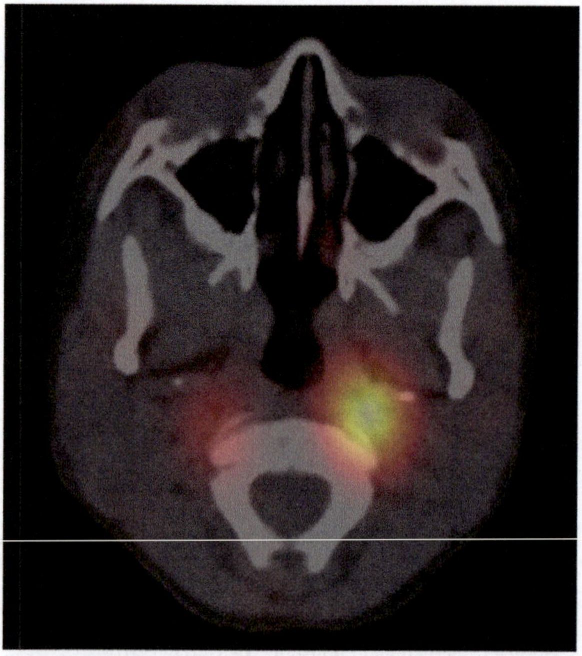

Fig. 27.1 Posttreatment ^{131}I SPECT-CT reveals intense uptake in a left retropharyngeal LN (node of Rouviere) and to a lesser extent in a right retropharyngeal LN

Assessment and Literature Review

Thyroid cancer is rare in the pediatric population, but the incidence appears to be increasing, especially in adolescents. PTC is the most common variant and accounts for 90 % or more of childhood thyroid cancers. Pediatric PTC is frequently multifocal and bilateral. Regional lymph node metastases occur in >80 % of cases and are often the reason a child with PTC comes to clinical attention [9, 10]. Children with a significant cervical disease burden are at the highest risk of hematogenous metastases to the lungs, which occur in up to 25 % of cases [5, 9, 11–13]. Despite the apparent aggressive clinical presentation of PTC when diagnosed during childhood and a higher rate of pulmonary metastases compared with adults, disease-specific mortality in pediatric PTC is extremely low (~2 % or less decades after diagnosis) [5, 7, 8, 14, 15]. This excellent long-term prognosis, coupled with unique concerns regarding the potential late sequelae related to overzealous treatment at a young age (e.g., second malignancies [4, 6–8] and pulmonary fibrosis [16]), makes the management of pediatric PTC with lung metastases challenging. Furthermore, there have been no prospective clinical trials to guide decision-making, and our understanding of pediatric PTC primarily comes from adult PTC, in addition to clinical reviews, pediatric PTC case series, and expert opinion. It is only recently that formal guidelines for the management of pediatric PTC have been developed by the American Thyroid Association (ATA) [1].

In most cases, it is recommended that the initial evaluation of children with PTC includes a preoperative CXR to assess for macroscopic lung metastases; the finding of which may alter plans for subsequent RAI therapy [2]. However, a CXR is not sensitive enough to identify small-volume micronodular pulmonary metastases [13], and for that reason, some centers also consider chest CT scanning at diagnosis, especially in children with bulky cervical disease, who are at the highest risk for distant metastases [11]. Current pediatric guidelines do not advocate routine chest CT in all patients [1], with the additional understanding that postoperative staging with RAI, if indicated, will effectively identify most children with pulmonary metastases, even those with negative baseline radiographic imaging [13]. In the end, knowledge regarding the presence or absence of pulmonary metastases does not alter the plan for initial therapy, which is the appropriate oncologic surgery (total thyroidectomy ± compartment-oriented neck dissection) by a high-volume thyroid surgeon.

The inaugural pediatric ATA guidelines introduced a postoperative risk categorization (ATA pediatric low, intermediate, and high risk) based upon TNM staging that helps to identify patients at risk of distant metastases and thereby determine which children should undergo routine postoperative staging with RAI [1]. Using this novel classification, children with significant central or lateral neck lymph node involvement are considered intermediate or high risk, depending on the extent and volume of disease. In most intermediate- (clinical N1a or microscopic N1b disease) and in all high-risk (clinical N1b disease) patients, including patients already known to have distant metastases, postoperative staging with a diagnostic RAI scan and a TSH-stimulated Tg is recommended [1, 2].

In some children, the diagnostic whole-body scan may be negative for lung uptake (Fig. 27.2a), but the Tg may be significantly elevated, thereby suggesting the presence of distant metastases. The absolute value of hyper-thyroglobulinemia that predicts lung metastases in children remains largely unstudied, but empiric RAI therapy is usually administered to a child who is high risk for distant metastases (based upon the ATA Pediatric risk categories) and whose stimulated Tg is >10 ng/ml [1]. Although the empiric use of ^{131}I is not associated with cure in adults with negative diagnostic RAI scans and known structural disease [17], this issue remains unstudied in children, who may be more prone to benefit from RAI in this setting due to the inherent differences in tumor biology. In all cases, after ^{131}I therapy, a post-therapy scan is recommended 4–7 days in order to identify iodine-avid disease that may not have been readily visible on the diagnostic whole-body scan and also to help determine iodine avidity in known or suspected metastatic disease previously seen on radiographic imaging (Fig. 27.2b).

The goal of^{131}I therapy in children with pulmonary metastases is to decrease the risk of thyroid cancer progression and theoretically to improve mortality by eliminating iodine-avid disease while reducing the risk of late complications, such as pulmonary fibrosis [16]. The intent of therapy is no longer to render every patient with a negative thyroglobulin, since that is achievable in only about 50 % of pediatric patients with pulmonary metastases [1, 5].

Those children identified to have iodine-avid distant disease will likely benefit from ^{131}I therapy. Therefore, ^{131}I is typically administered at an empiric activity that is proportionately equivalent to a 150–200 mCi dose in an adult (sometimes less, if significant diffuse pulmonary uptake is present). Dosimetry is considered in children with diffuse pulmonary metastases but is not readily available in all centers. In these cases, the goal is to ensure that the whole-body retention 48 h after ^{131}I administration does not exceed 2.96 GBq (80 mCi) in the presence of iodine-avid diffuse lung metastases [18], which should minimize the very real concern of pulmonary fibrosis in this population [16].

Children with small-volume, iodine-avid micronodular (<1 cm) lung disease are the most likely to respond to treatment [19], and they may ultimately become disease-free, whereas others, especially those with a more extensive metastatic disease burden, may never become cancer-free as assessed by Tg levels [3–5, 19]. The nadir response to RAI can take 1–2 years or more [3], and because of this, current recommendations are to wait until the disease either progresses or unequivocally remains persistent before proceeding to subsequent evaluation and treatment with ^{131}I [1, 2]. The thought is that such a cautious approach to repeated ^{131}I therapy may help to mitigate long-term sequelae of RAI, while also ensuring durable control of disease. Further studies are required regarding the optimal dosing and timing of ^{131}I for children with PTC and iodine-avid pulmonary metastases. In all cases, the decision to treat a child with RAI should be individualized [1, 2], preferably by clinicians experienced in the management of advanced pediatric PTC.

After initial ^{131}I therapy, children with PTC and lung metastases should be monitored while continuing TSH suppression (goal TSH <0.1 mIU/L). In addition to monitoring the TSH-suppressed Tg, intermittent imaging with CXR or CT chest

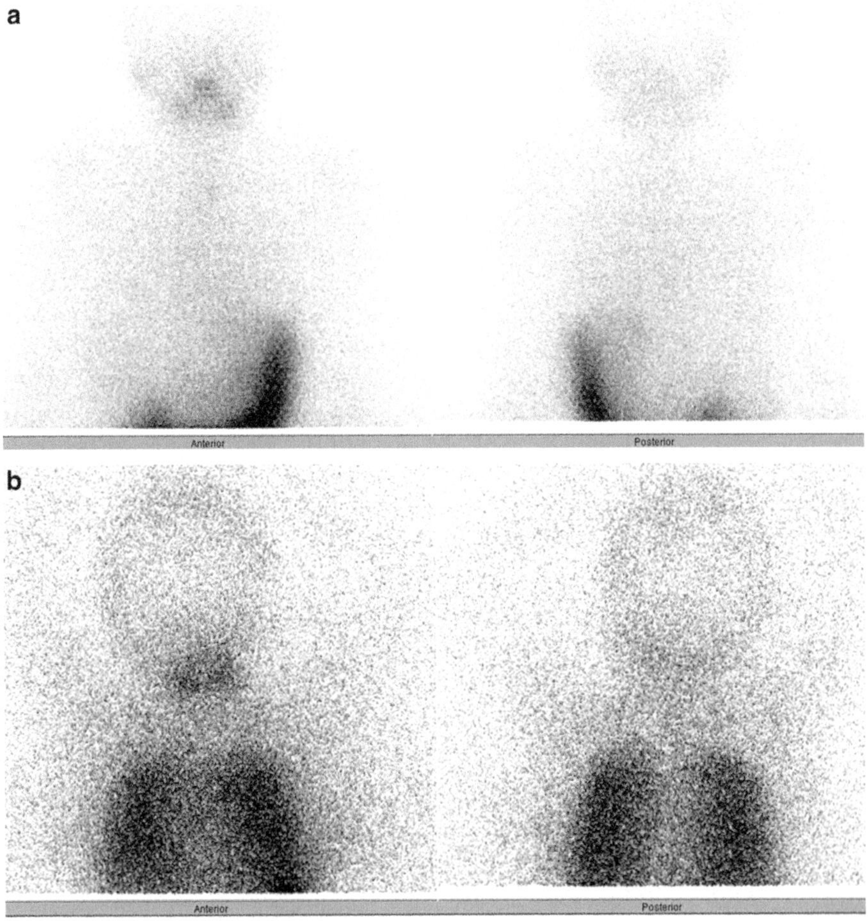

Fig. 27.2 Diagnostic (**a**) and posttreatment (**b**) ^{131}I scans in a 12-year-old boy with stage II PTC. The diagnostic study revealed no evidence of iodine-avid pulmonary metastases, but he was treated empirically with ^{131}I due to a stimulated Tg of 767 ng/ml and known pulmonary metastases that previously demonstrated iodine avidity. The posttreatment scan 7 days after ^{131}I clearly demonstrates diffuse pulmonary metastases

should be done to assess for structural disease progression. Once the nadir radiographic and biochemical Tg response is reached, repeat evaluation with a diagnostic WBS should be considered in those with documented iodine-avid disease, but retreatment with RAI should be limited to those children who still have evidence of disease and who also benefited from prior ^{131}I therapy. In children who develop iodine non-avid or nonresponsive PTC, continued observation and TSH suppression are indicated, with systemic therapies considered at referral centers if iodine-refractory disease significantly progresses or becomes clinically symptomatic.

Back to the Case

Following RAI therapy, expectant monitoring and TSH suppressive therapy commenced, and the patient's suppressed Tg over the following 2 years never reached a nadir; instead, it slowly rose from 13.5 to 29.5 ng/ml. Cross-sectional imaging revealed no overt evidence for cervical disease (outside of prominent nodes of Rouviere) and multiple tiny pulmonary nodules measuring up to 3 mm (noting that this was an initial diagnostic CT chest and that the pulmonary nodules were not as clearly seen on SPECT-CT previously obtained after initial RAI therapy). At the age of 12, he had a hypothyroid ^{131}I thyroid scan (2.4 mCi) and a stimulated Tg that revealed no evidence of pathologic RAI uptake (Fig. 27.2a) and a value of 767 ng/ml, respectively. A second empiric ^{131}I dose of 58 mCi (weight-adjusted dose equivalent to a 156 mCi dose in a 70 kg adult) was administered, and posttreatment scan obtained 7 days after high-dose RAI revealed diffuse bilateral lung uptake (Fig. 27.2b). A year later, CT neck and chest and cervical US revealed no evidence of progression, and a non-suppressed Tg (TSH 2.4 mIU/L) was 60 ng/ml. He continues to be monitored expectantly while continuing TSH suppression.

Clinical Pearls

- Young children with PTC often present with extensive locoregional and pulmonary metastatic disease.
- The risk for pulmonary metastases is highest in children with extensive cervical disease.
- Despite the presence of pulmonary metastases, disease-specific mortality is low with survival over decades anticipated.
- RAI is indicated for children with known or suspected pulmonary metastases. A diagnostic whole-body scan may fail to reveal iodine-avid pulmonary metastases, and so a delayed posttreatment scan obtained 4–7 days after RAI is critical for identifying iodine-avid disease.
- Use of dosimetry (if available) in children with diffuse pulmonary metastases can ensure that the administered activity of ^{131}I is below that which would place the child at risk for pulmonary fibrosis.
- The clinical response of pulmonary metastases to ^{131}I may take years to fully appreciate, and given the long-term risks of RAI in children, the current approach is to retreat with ^{131}I only if there is evidence of disease beyond 1 year or if there is disease progression in a patient who was previously felt to respond/benefit to therapeutic RAI; RAI therapy every 6–12 months until the patient becomes Tg and/or diagnostic scan negative is no longer the approach to treatment.
- It remains unclear how to define iodine non-avid/nonresponsive disease in children, although there will be a subset of children who do not respond to ^{131}I as anticipated.
- TSH suppression is indicated as an adjunct to RAI, and the goal of TSH is <0.1 mIU/L in a child with pulmonary metastatic disease.

References

1. Francis GL, Waguespack SG, Bauer AJ, Angelos P, Benvenga S, Cerutti JM, Dinauer CA, Hamilton J, Hay ID, Luster M, Parisi MT, Rachmiel M, Thompson GB, Yamashita S. Management guidelines for children with thyroid nodules and differentiated thyroid cancer: The American Thyroid Association guidelines task force on pediatric thyroid cancer. Thyroid. 2015;25(7):716–59.
2. Waguespack SG, Francis G. Initial management and follow-up of differentiated thyroid cancer in children. J Natl Compr Canc Netw. 2010;8:1289–300.
3. Biko J, Reiners C, Kreissl MC, Verburg FA, Demidchik Y, Drozd V. Favourable course of disease after incomplete remission on (131)I therapy in children with pulmonary metastases of papillary thyroid carcinoma: 10 years follow-up. Eur J Nucl Med Mol Imaging. 2011;38:651–5.
4. Dottorini ME, Vignati A, Mazzucchelli L, Lomuscio G, Colombo L. Differentiated thyroid carcinoma in children and adolescents: a 37-year experience in 85 patients. J Nucl Med. 1997;38:669–75.
5. Pawelczak M, David R, Franklin B, Kessler M, Lam L, Shah B. Outcomes of children and adolescents with well-differentiated thyroid carcinoma and pulmonary metastases following (1)(3)(1)I treatment: a systematic review. Thyroid. 2010;20:1095–101.
6. Iyer NG, Morris LG, Tuttle RM, Shaha AR, Ganly I. Rising incidence of second cancers in patients with low-risk (T1N0) thyroid cancer who receive radioactive iodine therapy. Cancer. 2011;117:4439–46.
7. Vassilopoulou-Sellin R, Goepfert H, Raney B, Schultz PN. Differentiated thyroid cancer in children and adolescents: clinical outcome and mortality after long-term follow-up. Head Neck. 1998;20:549–55.
8. Hay ID, Gonzalez-Losada T, Reinalda MS, Honetschlager JA, Richards ML, Thompson GB. Long-term outcome in 215 children and adolescents with papillary thyroid cancer treated during 1940 through 2008. World J Surg. 2010;34:1192–202.
9. Zimmerman D, Hay ID, Gough IR, Goellner JR, Ryan JJ, Grant CS, McConahey WM. Papillary thyroid carcinoma in children and adults: long-term follow-up of 1039 patients conservatively treated at one institution during three decades. Surgery. 1988;104:1157–66.
10. Frankenthaler RA, Sellin RV, Cangir A, Goepfert H. Lymph node metastasis from papillary-follicular thyroid carcinoma in young patients. Am J Surg. 1990;160:341–3.
11. Wada N, Sugino K, Mimura T, Nagahama M, Kitagawa W, Shibuya H, Ohkuwa K, Nakayama H, Hirakawa S, Yukawa N, Rino Y, Masuda M, Ito K. Treatment strategy of papillary thyroid carcinoma in children and adolescents: clinical significance of the initial nodal manifestation. Ann Surg Oncol. 2009;16:3442–9.
12. Vassilopoulou-Sellin R, Klein MJ, Smith TH, Samaan NA, Frankenthaler RA, Goepfert H, Cangir A, Haynie TP. Pulmonary metastases in children and young adults with differentiated thyroid cancer. Cancer. 1993;71:1348–52.
13. Bal CS, Kumar A, Chandra P, Dwivedi SN, Mukhopadhyaya S. Is chest x-ray or high-resolution computed tomography scan of the chest sufficient investigation to detect pulmonary metastasis in pediatric differentiated thyroid cancer? Thyroid. 2004;14:217–25.
14. Hogan AR, Zhuge Y, Perez EA, Koniaris LG, Lew JI, Sola JE. Pediatric thyroid carcinoma: incidence and outcomes in 1753 patients. J Surg Res. 2009;156:167–72.
15. Demidchik YE, Demidchik EP, Reiners C, Biko J, Mine M, Saenko VA, Yamashita S. Comprehensive clinical assessment of 740 cases of surgically treated thyroid cancer in children of Belarus. Ann Surg. 2006;243:525–32.
16. Hebestreit H, Biko J, Drozd V, Demidchik Y, Burkhardt A, Trusen A, Beer M, Reiners C. Pulmonary fibrosis in youth treated with radioiodine for juvenile thyroid cancer and lung metastases after Chernobyl. Eur J Nucl Med Mol Imaging. 2011;38:1683–90.

17. Sabra MM, Grewal RK, Tala H, Larson SM, Tuttle RM. Clinical outcomes following empiric radioiodine therapy in patients with structurally identifiable metastatic follicular cell-derived thyroid carcinoma with negative diagnostic but positive post-therapy 131I whole-body scans. Thyroid. 2012;22:877–83.
18. Verburg FA, Reiners C, Hanscheid H. Approach to the patient: role of dosimetric RAI Rx in children with DTC. J Clin Endocrinol Metab. 2013;98:3912–9.
19. Bal CS, Garg A, Chopra S, Ballal S, Soundararajan R. Prognostic factors in pediatric differentiated thyroid cancer patients with pulmonary metastases. J Pediatr Endocrinol Metab. 2014;28(7-8):745–51.

Chapter 28
A Patient with Bone Metastases from Follicular Carcinoma of the Thyroid

Leonard Wartofsky

Case

The patient is a 55-year-old man referred to us from his endocrinologist in Morgantown, West Virginia. He had originally presented in West Virginia during August 2013 complaining of numbness in his right leg extending up to his abdomen. He was found to have tumor involving the thoracic spine on CT scan. Emergency surgery in late August 2013 included a corpectomy of the T8 vertebral body with decompression of T8-T11 with a laminectomy and debulking of the tumor. The surgical pathology of the spine tumor suggested thyroid cancer, and at that evaluation, he was noted to complain of hoarseness and have a neck mass. He underwent thyroidectomy in early September 2013, and the surgical pathology revealed his tumor to be a follicular thyroid cancer. The right recurrent laryngeal nerve was sacrificed due to its being encased in tumor, and he remained hoarse postoperatively. A follow-up MRI of the thoracic spine in November 2013 disclosed probable metastasis to the first rib on the left as well as tumor involving the right pedicle of T12 with additional metastases to L1, L3, L4, and L5. He underwent external radiation therapy for ten treatments (dosage unknown) in late November 2013. A CT scan of the head (without contrast) done in late November 2013 described a lytic lesion in the left anteroparietal calvarium. In addition, CT scan of the chest and abdomen with contrast in December 2013 described a lesion in the right lung, some hypodensities in the liver, and a 1.7×1.5 cm nodule in the adrenal gland. In the other facility, he was treated with 120 mCi radioactive iodine. His tumor was apparently producing sufficient thyroid hormone that his serum TSH level failed to elevate post thyroidectomy, and he was prepared for scanning and

L. Wartofsky, MD (✉)
MedStar Washington Hospital Center, Washington, DC 20010, USA

Georgetown University School of Medicine, Washington, DC 20007, USA
e-mail: leonard.wartofsky@medstar.net

D.S. Cooper, C. Durante (eds.), *Thyroid Cancer*,
DOI 10.1007/978-3-319-22401-5_28

Table 28.1 Laboratory values

Date	TSH (mIU/L)	Tg (ng/ml)	ANTI-Tg-AB (IU/ml)	Course
10/04/13	4.18	16,340	<2	Thyroidectomy 9/7/13
10/26/13	1.09	12,503	<2	IMRT to lumbar spine 11/13
12/22/13	0.36	9517	<2	120 mCi 131-I (12/23/13)
01/13/14	2.99	3303	<2	
02/23/14	3.72	1662	<20 (different assay)	
03/12/14	54	2840	<2	360 mCi 131-I (3/17/14)
06/02/14	1.92	142	<2	
08/22/14	0.09	64	<2	

TSH thyrotropin, *Tg* thyroglobulin, *TgAb* antithyroglobulin antibodies

radioiodine therapy with recombinant human TSH. The posttreatment scan disclosed foci of uptake in the head, neck, chest, shoulders, abdomen, and pelvis. Plain films of the lumbar spine in January 2014 again described metastasis at L4 and L5 and in his left rib. His physical examination was totally unremarkable except for the thyroidectomy scar and subjective numbness in the right lower extremity (Table 28.1).

Assessment

This 55-year-old man presented with widespread metastases to multiple bones which were subsequently confirmed to be from a follicular carcinoma of the thyroid. According to his medical record notes, his serum thyroglobulin levels were quite high and fell after surgery and radioiodine ablation (Values not available Table 28.1), but remained markedly elevated. His post-therapy scan indicates fairly good radioiodine uptake suggesting potential benefit from additional radioactive iodine treatment. Our approach will be to do additional imaging to assess the current extent and location of residual disease in order to determine possible therapeutic approaches.

Relevant Literature

In general, distant metastases from thyroid cancer can be seen in 4–6 % of patients at initial presentation [1, 2]. Distant metastatic disease can subsequently develop in 10–30 % of patients [3, 4], depending on the histology (about 10 % in papillary cancer and 20–30 % in follicular and Hurthle cell cancers), most commonly to the lung and bones. The presence of distant metastases may be heralded by an extremely elevated serum thyroglobulin, with the findings confirmed by plain radiography, 131-I whole body scan, CT, MRI, PET/CT, or bone scan. Radioiodine uptake in a bone lesion will indicate that it is derived from thyroid cancer, but absent that, a bone biopsy is advisable to confirm the diagnosis. Other imaging modalities for bone lesions may include thallium-201, technetium-99m, or iodine-124 PET. Survival with metastatic disease will depend upon the site of the metastases, the age of the patient, and whether or not the lesions are radioiodine avid. Other factors influencing prognosis and statistically significant by univariate analysis include gender, extent of surgery, and histologic type [1, 3]. Clinically, patients will present with bone pain or fracture, swelling at the site, or spinal metastases with symptoms of cord compression. The more common bony sites for metastases are the spine, pelvis, ribs, femur, and skull. Bone metastases connote a significantly poorer prognosis than that noted in the majority of thyroid cancer patients. In a retrospective analysis by Shoup et al. [5] of 242 patients, 40 % had metastases on presentation and they had a 10-year survival of 26 % with a median survival of 4.1 years. The importance of age is apparent as seen with a 10-year survival in those patients <45 years old of 58 % compared to only 13 % in those >45 years old.

The treatment of bone metastases typically involves radioiodine, assuming that the lesions are RAI avid, and it is the younger patients who are more likely to have RAI uptake, a fact that likely is linked to their better survival statistics. This may account for why some studies show clear benefit of RAI therapy [6, 7], while others do not [8, 9]. Preparation for radioiodine therapy requires an elevated serum TSH level which may be achieved by either thyroid hormone withdrawal or administration of recombinant human TSH [10, 11]. Those lesions that are FDG/PET avid tend to be less differentiated and more resistant to RAI treatment [12, 13]. RAI may be administered as either a standard or "empiric" dose or activity based upon consensus guidelines and physician experience, or as a "dosimetric" activity based on how the patient's body handles (retains and excretes) a given activity of radioiodine. When there is RAI uptake, arguments have been made for administering the highest dose feasible that is within safe limits as can be determined by dosimetry [14], and dosimetric approaches have been shown to be potentially more efficacious than empiric dosage [15]. However, relatively lower doses appear to be appropriate in older patients [16]. In the absence of RAI uptake, other therapeutic modalities may be tried but will be associated with less salutary effect. There is hope that redifferentiating agents such as selumetinib might prove useful for these patients in the future [17]. When feasible, particularly for isolated and/or symptomatic bone metastasis, other approaches to management could include surgical resection with or without cementoplasty, radiofrequency ablation, external radiation, arterial embolization, or targeted chemotherapy, along with adjunctive use of bisphosphonates [18]. Pak et al. [19] reviewed a 32-year experience with surgical metastasectomy with 51 metastases excised in 29 patients who had a variety of types of thyroid cancer. Many of the patients received adjunctive therapy with XRT and RAI as well with a resultant 78 % survival at 5 years that dropped to 50 % at 10 years, with age >45 a poor prognostic factor.

External beam radiation is employed for pain relief and for lesions in critical or weight-bearing areas, as well as for those lesions not amenable to surgery or RAI treatment. It is typically given in doses of 50 Gy in 25 fractions for solitary bone lesions and 40 Gy in 20 fractions for vertebral lesions. Arterial embolization has been employed by Eustatia-Rutten and colleagues [20] with 41 embolizations in

16 patients resulting in clinical improvement in 60 % of subjects. The procedure requires visualization of the artery feeding the metastasis by selective catheterization, and then particles of isobutyl, Gelfoam, or polyvinyl alcohol are injected with relief of pain and improvement in neurologic symptoms. The best results are seen in those patients who also have had RAI, XRT, or surgical treatment. Radiofrequency ablation (RFA) [21, 22] uses probes inserted under CT guidance to generate thermal energy to achieve local tissue temperatures >50 °C inducing cell death. RFA has rarely been applied to bone lesions and has found greater application to lesions in the liver, kidney, or bone. While planar radioiodine scanning with iodine-131 is the primary imaging procedure for differentiated thyroid cancer, scanning with iodine-124 PET offers advantages of detecting both positron emission as well as the spatial distribution of radioiodine uptake and allows improved detection of the extent of residual disease [23–27].

Subsequent Management

The degree of thyroglobulin elevation indicated persistent residual disease. Given that his earlier post-therapy radioiodine scan showed significant uptake and the actual activity administered (120 mCi) was relatively low, the patient was deemed a good candidate for higher-dose radioiodine therapy to be determined by dosimetry [14]. He was withdrawn from his levothyroxine therapy, and after 3 weeks, his serum TSH level had risen to 42 mU/L. He then underwent routine total body scanning with iodine-131 (Fig. 28.1) as well as iodine-124 PET scanning which again clearly delineated good isotope uptake, with particularly better visualization of the extent of bone metastases by the iodine-124 PET images (Fig. 28.2). Regional lesional dosimetry afforded by iodine-124 indicated that sufficient uptake of activity in specific lesions could be achieved for therapeutic benefit based on earlier data on locoregional dosimetry [25, 28]. The dosimetry calculations predicted that he could receive as much as 410 mCi of iodine-131 safely and have less than 100 mCi retained in total body at 48 h. He was treated with 360 mCi iodine-131 in late March 2014 at a time that his TSH measured 54 mU/L; the post-therapy scan was essentially identical to the pretreatment diagnostic scan demonstrating good uptake in multiple sites estimated to approximate 72 Gy or 7200 rads. Follow-up studies by his physicians in West Virginia on June 2, 2014, included a serum thyroglobulin of 142 ng/ml and a TSH of 1.92 mU/L. His dose of levothyroxine was increased, and the last studies recorded to date on August 22, 2014 included a thyroglobulin of 64 ng/ml and a TSH of 0.09 mU/L. His total white blood cell, absolute neutrophil, and platelet counts have remained within normal limits. Recommendations to his physicians included continuing suppressive dosage of levothyroxine, adjunctive therapy with bisphosphonates or denosumab, monitoring serum thyroglobulin every 6 months, considering local intervention on selective lesions by XRT or RFA as warranted, and a potential additional dosimetric radioiodine dose based upon demonstrated progressive disease, persistent iodine uptake, and relatively normal blood counts.

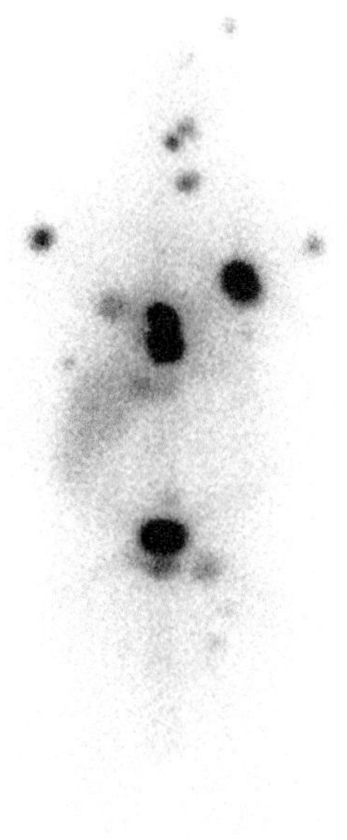

Anterior

Fig. 28.1 Post-thyroid hormone withdrawal total body scan after 4 mCi iodine-131

Clinical Pearls/Pitfalls

1. Lesions positive on FDG/PET scanning are likely to represent poorly differentiated thyroid cancer, not demonstrate radioiodine uptake, and have a poor prognosis.
2. Follicular thyroid carcinoma metastatic to bone heralds a poor prognosis for cure especially in older patients with extensive disease that does not take up radioiodine.
3. While several therapeutic approaches to bone metastases exist, the best opportunity for palliative stabilization of progression or remission rests with a combination of surgical resection when feasible, radioactive iodine and external radiation therapy. Radioiodine uptake by lesions does not necessarily indicate radiosensitivity.
4. Although the current ATA Guidelines [29] indicate that no recommendation can be made about the superiority of dosimetric RAI administration over empiric dosage, they do acknowledge that there are theoretical advantages to dosimetric approaches to the treatment of both locoregional and metastatic diseases.

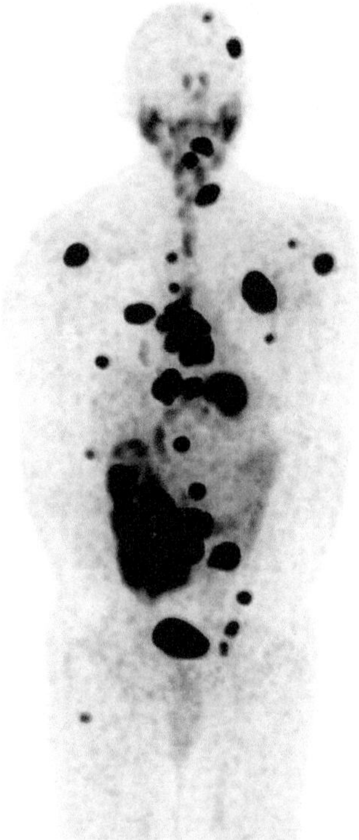

Fig. 28.2 Total body iodine-124 PET/CT scan with 1.7 mCi iodine-124

5. While currently available only in major academic centers, iodine-124 PET/CT scans are superior to either traditional iodine-131 scans or FDG/PET scans for more definitive imaging of metastases from thyroid cancer.
6. High dosage radioiodine therapy by dosimetry can be administered safely and has proven effective in at least one study.

References

1. Verburg FA, Mader U, Tanase K, Thies E-D, Diessl S, Buck AK, Luster M, Reiners C. Life expectancy is reduced in differentiated thyroid cancer patients>45 years old with extensive local tumor invasion, lateral lymph node, or distant metastases at diagnosis and normal in all other DTC patients. J Clin Endocrinol Metab. 2013;98:172–80.
2. Klubo-Gwiezdzinska J, Morowitz D, Van Nostrand D, Burman KD, Vasko V, Soberman M, Wartofsky L. Metastases of well-differentiated thyroid cancer to the gastrointestinal system. Thyroid. 2010;20:381–7.
3. Schlumberger MJ. Papillary and follicular thyroid carcinoma. N Engl J Med. 1998;338:297–306.
4. Shaha AR, Ferlito A, Rinaldo A. Distant metastases from thyroid and parathyroid cancer. ORL J Otorhinolaryngol Relat Spec. 2001;63:243–9.

5. Shoup M, Stojadinovic A, Nissan A, Ghossein RA, Freedman S, Brennan MF, et al. Prognostic indicators of outcomes in patients with distant metastases from differentiated thyroid carcinoma. J Am Coll Surg. 2003;197(2):191–7.
6. Hindie E, Melliere D, Lange F, Hallaj I, de Labriolle-Vaylet C, Jeanguillaume C, et al. Functioning pulmonary metastases of thyroid cancer: does radioiodine influence the prognosis? Eur J Nucl Med Mol Imaging. 2003;30(7):974–81.
7. Bernier MO, Leenhardt L, Hoang C, Aurengo A, Mary JY, Menegaux F, et al. Survival and therapeutic modalities in patients with bone metastases of differentiated thyroid carcinomas. J Clin Endocrinol Metab. 2001;86(4):1568–73.
8. Dinneen SF, Valimaki MJ, Bergstralh EJ, Goellner JR, Gorman CA, Hay ID. Distant metastases in papillary thyroid carcinoma: 100 cases observed at one institution during 5 decades. J Clin Endocrinol Metab. 1995;80(7):2041–5.
9. Pittas AG, Adler M, Fazzari M, Tickoo S, Rosai J, Larson SM, Robbins RJ. Bone metastases from thyroid carcinoma: clinical characteristics and prognostic variables in one hundred forty-six patients. Thyroid. 2000;10(3):261–8.
10. Van Nostrand D, Khorjekar G, O'Neil J, Moreau S, Atkins F, Kharazi P, Mete M, Chennupati S, Burman KD, Wartofsky L. Recombinant human thyroid stimulating hormone versus thyroid hormone withdrawal in the identification of metastasis in differentiated thyroid cancer with 131I planar whole body and 124I PET. J Nucl Med. 2012;53:359–62.
11. Klubo-Gwiezdzinska J, Burman KD, Van Nostrand D, Mete M, Jonklaas J, Wartofsky L. Radioiodine treatment of metastatic thyroid cancer: relative efficacy and side effect profile after preparation by thyroid hormone withdrawal vs. recombinant human TSH. Thyroid. 2012;22:310–7.
12. Wang W, Larson SM, Tuttle RM, Kalaigian H, Kolbert K, Sonenberg M, Robbins RJ. Resistance of [18f]-fluorodeoxyglucose-avid metastatic thyroid cancer lesions to treatment with high-dose radioactive iodine. Thyroid. 2001;11(12):1169–75.
13. Robbins RJ, Wan Q, Grewal RK, Reibke R, Gonen M, Strauss HW, Tuttle RM, Drucker W, Larson SM. Real-time prognosis for metastatic thyroid carcinoma based on 2-[18F]fluoro-2-deoxy-D-glucose-positron emission tomography scanning. J Clin Endocrinol Metab. 2006; 91:498–505.
14. Van Nostrand D, Atkins F, Yeganeh F, Acio E, Bursaw R, Wartofsky L. Dosimetrically-determined doses of radioiodine for the treatment of metastatic thyroid carcinoma. Thyroid. 2002;12(2):121–34.
15. Klubo-Gwiezdzinska J, Van Nostrand D, Atkins FB, Burman KD, Jonklaas J, Mete M, Wartofsky L. Efficacy of dosimetric versus empirically determined prescribed activity of 131-I for therapy of differentiated thyroid Cancer. J Clin Endocrinol Metab. 2011;96:3217–25.
16. Kulkarni K, Van Nostrand D, Atkins F, Aiken M, Burman K, Wartofsky L. The relative frequency in which empiric dosages of radioiodine would potentially "over-" or "under-" treat patients who have metastatic well-differentiated thyroid cancer. Thyroid. 2006;16:1019–51.
17. Ho AL, Grewal RK, Leboeuf R, Sherman EJ, Pfister DG, Deandreis D, et al. Selumetinib-enhanced radioiodine uptake in advanced thyroid cancer. N Engl J Med. 2013;368(7): 623–32.
18. Vitale G, Fonderico F, Martignetti A, Caraglia M, Ciccarelli A, Nuzzo V, et al. Pamidronate improves the quality of life and induces clinical remission of bone metastases in patients with thyroid cancer. Br J Cancer. 2001;84(12):1586–90.
19. Pak H, Gourgiotis L, Chang WI, Guthrie LC, Skarulis MC, et al. Role of metastasectomy in the management of thyroid carcinoma: the NIH experience. J Surg Oncol. 2003;82(1):10–8.
20. Eustatia-Rutten CF, Romijn JA, Guijt MJ, Vielvoye GJ, van den Berg R, Corssmit EP, et al. Outcome of palliative embolization of bone metastases in differentiated thyroid carcinoma. J Clin Endocrinol Metab. 2003;88(7):3184–9.
21. Dupuy DE, Monchik JM, Decrea C, Pisharodi L. Radiofrequency ablation of regional recurrence from well-differentiated thyroid malignancy. Surgery. 2001;130:971–7.
22. Wartofsky L. Adjunctive local approaches to metastatic thyroid cancer. In: Wartofsky L, Van Nostrand D, editors. Thyroid cancer: a comprehensive guide to clinical management. 2nd ed. Totowa, NJ: Humana/Springer; 2006. p. 509–13.

23. Eschmann SM, Reischl G, Bilger K, Kuperferschlager J, Thelen MH, Dohmen BM, Bares R. Evaluation of dosimetry of radioiodine therapy in benign and malignant thyroid disorders by means of iodine-124 and PET. Eur J Nucl Med Mol Imaging. 2002;29:760–7.
24. Van Nostrand D, Moreau S, Bandaru VV, Atkins F, Chennupati S, et al. (124)I positron emission tomography versus (131)I planar imaging in the identification of residual thyroid tissue and/or metastasis in patients who have well-differentiated thyroid cancer. Thyroid. 2010; 20:879–83.
25. Sgouros G, Kolbert KS, Sheikh A, Pentlow KS, Mun EF, Barth A, et al. Patient-specific dosimetry for 131-I thyroid cancer therapy using 124-I PET and 3-dimensional-internal dosimetry (3D-ID) software. J Nucl Med. 2004;45:1366–72.
26. Phan HT, Jager PL, Paans AM, Plukker JT, Sturkenboom MG, Sluiter WJ, Wolffenbuttel BH, Dierckx RA, Links TP. The diagnostic value of 124I-PET in patients with differentiated thyroid cancer. Eur J Nucl Med Mol Imaging. 2008;35:958–65.
27. Maxon HR, Thomas SR, Samaratunga RC. Dosimetric considerations in the radioiodine treatment of macrometastases and micrometastases from differentiated thyroid cancer. Thyroid. 1997;7(2):183–7.
28. Hobbs RF, Wahl RL, Lodge MA, Javadi MS, Cho SY, Chien DT, et al. 124-I PET-based 3D-RD dosimetry for a pediatric thyroid cancer patient: real=time treatment planning and methodologic comparison. J Nucl Med. 2009;50:1844–7.
29. Haugen BR, Alexander EK, Bible KC, Doherty GM, Mandel SJ, Nikiforov Y, et al. American Thyroid Association Management guidelines for patients with thyroid nodules and differentiated thyroid cancer. Thyroid. 2015; 24.

Chapter 29
Radioiodine Therapy in Lactating Women with Higher-Risk Differentiated Thyroid Cancer

Swaytha Yalamanchi and David S. Cooper

Case Presentation

A 30-year-old woman presents 1 month status post total thyroidectomy with left and central neck dissection for management of papillary thyroid carcinoma (PTC). Pathology demonstrated multifocal and BRAF-positive PTC with the largest tumor focus being 6 cm in diameter. Six of fourteen central lymph nodes and seven of thirty-three lateral lymph nodes were positive for disease. The patient gave birth approximately 5 months earlier and stopped breastfeeding 2 weeks prior to presenting to endocrinology clinic.

Assessment and Literature Review

Both lactating and non-lactating women may have breast uptake on scintigraphy. In the former group, uptake may persist up to 32 weeks following cessation of lactation. Dopamine agonists may shorten the time interval between cessation of breastfeeding and initiation of radioiodine therapy in patients with differentiated thyroid cancer. Regardless of the use of dopamine agonist therapy, it is imperative to perform a pretreatment I-123 scan in women with recent lactation or galactorrhea to confirm that breast uptake is absent prior to proceeding with I-131 radioiodine therapy.

S. Yalamanchi, MD
Division of Endocrinology, Diabetes, and Metabolism, Johns Hopkins Hospital,
1830 E. Monument St, Suite 333, Baltimore, MD 21287, USA

D.S. Cooper, MD (✉)
Division of Endocrinology, Diabetes, and Metabolism,
The Johns Hopkins University School of Medicine,
1830 East Monument Street, Suite 333, Baltimore, MD 21287, USA
e-mail: dscooper@jhmi.edu

D.S. Cooper, C. Durante (eds.), *Thyroid Cancer*,
DOI 10.1007/978-3-319-22401-5_29

Definitions/Background

The incidence of thyroid cancer has increased more rapidly than other malignancies in recent years, independent of age and ethnicity. This growth is likely partly due to a rise in subclinical disease detected on imaging studies performed for alternate reasons, though large tumors, including those >4 cm, have also increased [1, 2].

DTC includes papillary and follicular subtypes and is by far the most common form of thyroid cancer. Surgery is the primary therapy for DTC with the approach dictated by the extent of disease, age, and comorbidities.

Radioiodine Ablation

Postoperative radioactive iodine (RAI) ablationtherapy is used in specific cases to achieve the following interrelated goals: (1) remnant ablation to facilitate initial staging and subsequent detection of recurrent disease via serum thyroglobulin and I-131 scan, (2) adjuvant therapy to decrease the risk of recurrence and mortality by eliminating suspected disease, and (3) documentation and treatment of known persistent disease [3]. Guidelines from the American Thyroid Association (ATA) recommend RAI therapy in all patients with known distant metastases, gross extrathyroidal extension, or primary tumor size greater than 4 cm. RAI is also recommended for selected patients with a thyroid cancer focus 1–4 cm in size without extrathyroidal extension if lymph node metastases and/or other high-risk features (e.g., age greater than 45, certain histological subtypes, intrathyroidal vascular invasion, multifocal disease) exist that would place individuals into the category of intermediate to high risk of recurrence or death [3].

Relative and Absolute Contraindications to RAI Therapy

Both relative and absolute contraindications to radioiodine therapy exist. Radioiodine is concentrated in thyroid follicular cells via the membrane sodium-iodide symporter (NIS) [4]. Pregnancy is an absolute contraindication to therapeutic I-131 administration due to risk of fetal exposure. Thyroid fetal tissue, which begins to form at 10–12 weeks, may be destroyed, potentially resulting in cretinism [5]. In a series of 237 women, 55 of whom ultimately underwent a therapeutic abortion, six infants developed hypothyroidism with four having intellectual disabilities. Three of these six women received radioiodine in the second trimester. The rates of fetal and neonatal complications were otherwise similar to that of uncomplicated pregnancies [6]. Women who were either recently or are actively breastfeeding should not receive radioiodine therapy for the following additional reasons: (1) risk of exposure to I-131 to the child and (2) risk of breast tissue exposure to radiation secondary to high levels of the NIS in breast tissue during lactation [5].

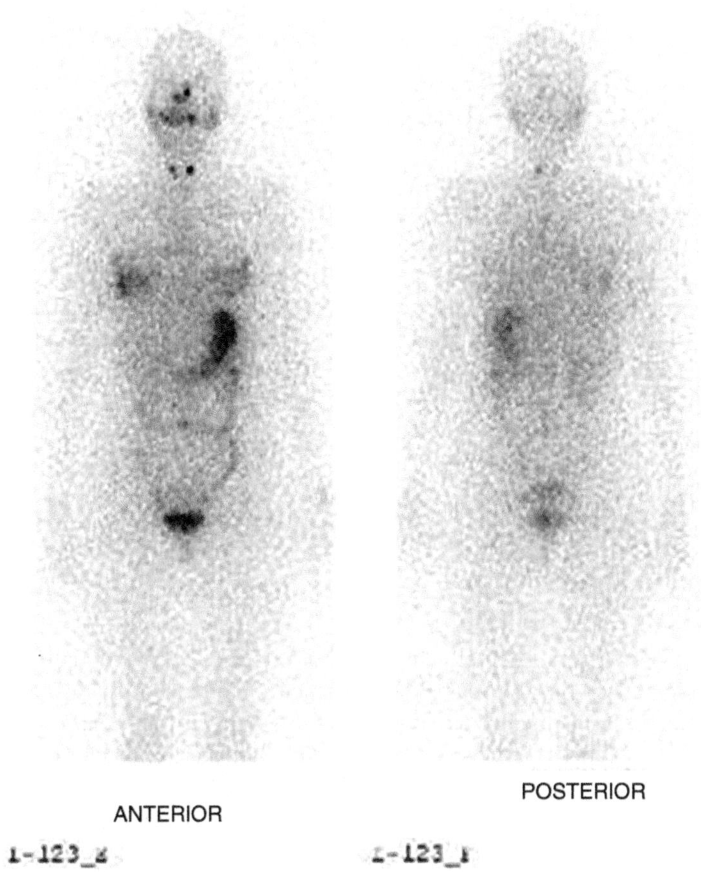

Fig. 29.1 Pretreatment I-123 scan in a patient with low-risk papillary thyroid cancer, idiopathic hyperprolactinemia, and mild galactorrhea demonstrating bilateral breast uptake. The decision was made not to treat this patient with radioiodine based on the scan

Women may have breast uptake on pretreatment scintigraphy for a multitude of other reasons including hyperprolactinemia [7, 8], breast cancer/tumor [9], and mastitis [10] (Fig. 29.1). False positive uptake may also occur due to contamination or uptake in the ribs, lung, liver, and soft tissue.

Risk of Secondary Malignancy Associated with RAI Therapy

The risk of second primary malignancy (SPM)after administration of RAI is well documented, but generally thought to be low. Although the risk of both leukemia and salivary gland malignancies is increased, there is no evidence of greater risk of breast cancer [11–13]. The risk of breast cancer among women with increased breast radioiodine uptake has not been examined.

Prevalence

A retrospective study performed from 2000 to 2006 to examine the utility of radioiodine scans prior to RAI therapy in patients with DTC showed that 6 % of non-lactating women had evidence of breast uptake on pretreatment scans [14]. Similarly, Hammami et al. demonstrated that approximately 6 % of all nonpregnant and non-lactating women (23 had not breastfed for an average of 11.4 months; four were nulliparous; three were postmenopausal) with iatrogenic hypothyroidism following thyroid hormone withdrawal also had breast uptake on radioiodine scans. The authors noted four different patterns of radioiodine breast uptake: “full,” “focal,” “crescentic,” and “irregular.” No association, however, could be made between scintigraphy patterns and etiology of breast uptake. The majority of women did not have expressible galactorrhea (52 %) and were normoprolactinemic (76 %; the remainder had prolactin levels <2.5 times the upper limit of normal, likely due to iatrogenic hypothyroidism) [15].

Pathophysiology

Iodide is an essential component of thyroid hormones tri-iodothyronine (T3) and thyroxine (T4). Intracellular iodide stores are maintained by NIS, located on the basolateral plasma membrane of thyroid follicular cells. NIS expression facilitates the use of radioiodine for both diagnostic and therapeutic purposes in the management of thyroid cancer. Active iodide transport also occurs in extrathyroidal tissues, including the lactating breasts, salivary glands, small intestine, and stomach [4]. In lactating breast tissue, expression of NIS allows iodide to be concentrated and secreted into breast milk for neonatal nutrition. NIS is generally present in breast tissue only during gestation and lactation. This is likely due in part to a threshold level of estrogen necessary for both direct effects on mammary gland NIS transcription, as well as effects via oxytocin and prolactin [16]. Expression of NIS has also been found to be high in fibroadenomas and, to a lesser extent, malignant breast tissue [9].

Role of Prolactin

Hyperprolactinemia, even in the postmenopausal woman with baseline atrophic breast tissue, may also result in increased breast uptake on scintigraphy that is reversible with normalization of prolactin levels [7, 17]. Both animal models and cultured human breast cancer cells respond to prolactin stimulation with increased expression of NIS and thus radioiodine uptake [7].

Medical Therapy

False positive breast uptake should first be ruled out by taking a focused history with consideration of lateral radiographic views and SPECT imaging. Subsequently, if the decision is made to proceed with radioiodine therapy, breastfeeding should be discontinued, and/or offending agents resulting in hyperprolactinemia should be stopped if medically feasible. Little data exist regarding therapeutic options. Hsiao et al. published a case report of a single postpartum woman treated with bromocriptine with subsequent minimal breast uptake on scintigraphy 8 weeks after cessation of breastfeeding [18]. Brzozowska et al. reported an observational case series of eight postpartum women who were followed by I-123 scintigraphy; five women received dopamine agonist therapy (cabergoline or bromocriptine) and three women received no therapy. The duration of ongoing breast uptake on scintigraphy was quite variable, but lasted up to 32 weeks in women who did not receive dopamine agonist therapy. In contrast, women who received dopamine agonist therapy had negative uptake studies sooner (3–10 weeks in four of the five women in the treatment group) [19]. Although data are limited in this clinical setting, cabergoline is generally regarded to be more efficacious in the normalization of prolactin levels as compared to bromocriptine [20]. Thus, patients may be initiated on cabergoline 0.25 mg twice/week (titrated up to 1 mg twice/week) or bromocriptine 7.5 mg twice/day based on existing data. Although dopamine agonists may shorten the time interval between cessation of breastfeeding and radioiodine therapy, it is unlikely that a delay in the administration of I-131 will change the final outcome of patient. Diagnostic scintigraphy with an I-123 scan should be performed prior to administration of therapeutic I-131 to confirm absence of breast uptake [14, 19].

Management of the Case

Our patient qualifies for RAI therapy on the basis of her bulky primary tumor focus and metastatic disease. As she had stopped breastfeeding only 2 weeks prior, she was initiated on cabergoline 0.5 mg twice/week. Six weeks later, she underwent a pretreatment scan that showed no evidence of breast uptake. The patient was treated with 75 mCi of radioiodine and had a posttreatment scan showing two foci of uptake in the thyroid bed. She has done well subsequently without clinical, sonographic, or biochemical evidence of recurrent disease including a negative total body scan and an undetectable serum thyroglobulin after recombinant TSH nine months later.

Clinical Pearls/Pitfalls

- Breast uptake on I-123 scintigraphy is possible in the setting of recent cessation of breastfeeding or in non-lactating women with hyperprolactinemia, breast cancer/tumor, or mastitis.

- Breast uptake of radioiodine is likely mediated by hormonal control of mammary gland NIS with interplay between estrogen, oxytocin, and prolactin.
- The 2015 ATA guidelines recommend deferring RAI for at least 6–8 weeks after women have stopped breastfeeding [3]]. The ATA guidelines on Radiation Safety after RAI recommend waiting 3 months after cessation of lactation before administration of therapeutic RAI with a 123-I scan if treatment is urgent or if there is concern regarding residual breast uptake [5]. However, breast uptake has been reported to persist for up to 8 months after cessation of lactation. In contrast with both of the aforementioned guidelines, we thus recommend a pretreatment scan prior to radioiodine administration in all women with a history of recent lactation, galactorrhea, breast cancer/tumor, and mastitis.
- Dopamine agonists may shorten the time interval between cessation of breastfeeding and radioiodine therapy.

References

1. SEER Cancer Statistics Review, 1975–2011. National Cancer Institute. Bethesda, MD. Based on November 2013 SEER data submission, released, April 2014. http://Seer.cancer.gov/csr/1975_2011/
2. Pellegriti G, Frasca F, Regalbuto C, Squatrito S, Vigneri R. Worldwide increasing incidence of thyroid cancer: update on epidemiology and risk factors. J Cancer Epidemiol. 2013;2013, 965212.
3. Haugen B, Alexander E, Bible K, Doherty G, Mandel S, Nikiforov Y, Pacini F, Randolph G, Sawka A, Schuff K, Schlumberger M, Sherman S, Sosa JA, Steward D, Tuttle RM, Wartofsky L. 2015 American Thyroid Association Management Guidelines for Adult Patients with Thyroid Nodules and Differentiated Thyroid Cancer. Thyroid 2015 in press.
4. Portulano C, Paroder-Belenitsky M, Carrasco N. The Na+/I- symporter (NIS): mechanism and medical impact. Endocr Rev. 2014;35(1):106–49.
5. American Thyroid Association Taskforce on Radioiodine Safety, Sisson JC, Freitas J, et al. Radiation safety in the treatment of patients with thyroid diseases by radioiodine 131-I: Practice recommendations of the American Thyroid Association. Thyroid. 2011;21(4):335–46.
6. Stoffer SS, Hamburger JI. Inadvertent 131I therapy for hyperthyroidism in the first trimester of pregnancy. J Nucl Med. 1976;17(02):146–9.
7. Ronga G, Bruno R, Puxeddu E, et al. Radioiodine uptake in non-lactating mammary glands: evidence for a causative role of hyperprolactinemia. Thyroid. 2007;17(4):363–6.
8. Hu LH, Wang SJ, Liu RS. Hyperprolactinemia-related 131-I uptake in nonlactating breasts. Clin Nucl Med. 2012;37(3):e57–8.
9. Ryan J, Curran CE, Hennessy E, et al. The sodium iodide symporter (NIS) and potential regulators in normal, benign and malignant human breast tissue. PLoS ONE. 2011;6(1), e16023.
10. Bakheet SM, Hammami MM. Patterns of radioiodine uptake by the lactating breast. Eur J Nucl Med. 1994;21(7):604–8.
11. Sawka AM, Thabane L, Parlea L, et al. Second primary malignancy risk after radioactive iodine treatment for thyroid cancer: a systematic review and meta-analysis. Thyroid. 2009;19(5):451–7.
12. Gandhi S, Abhyankar A, Basu S. Dual malignancies in the setting of differentiated thyroid carcinoma: their synchronous or metachronous nature, impact of radioiodine treatment on occurrence of second malignancy and other associated variables. Nucl Med Commun. 2014;35(2):205–9.

13. Iyer NG, Morris LG, Tuttle RM, Shaha AR, Ganly I. Rising incidence of second cancers in patients with low-risk (T1N0) thyroid cancer who receive radioactive iodine therapy. Cancer. 2011;117(19):4439–46.
14. Van Nostrand D, Aiken M, Atkins F, et al. The utility of radioiodine scans prior to iodine 131 ablation in patients with well-differentiated thyroid cancer. Thyroid. 2009;19(8):849–55.
15. Hammami MM, Bakheet S. Radioiodine breast uptake in nonbreastfeeding women: clinical and scintigraphic characteristics. J Nucl Med. 1996;37(1):26–31.
16. Tazebay UH, Wapnir IL, Levy O, et al. The mammary gland iodide transporter is expressed during lactation and in breast cancer. Nat Med. 2000;6(8):871–8.
17. Sinha A, Bradley KM, Steatham J, Weaver A. Asymmetric breast uptake of radioiodine in a patient with thyroid malignancy: metastases or not? J R Soc Med. 2008;101(6):319–20.
18. Hsiao E, Huynh T, Mansberg R, Bautovich G, Roach P. Diagnostic I-123 scintigraphy to assess potential breast uptake of I-131 before radioiodine therapy in a postpartum woman with thyroid cancer. Clin Nucl Med. 2004;29(8):498–501.
19. Brzozowska M, Roach PJ. Timing and potential role of diagnostic I-123 scintigraphy in assessing radioiodine breast uptake before ablation in postpartum women with thyroid cancer: a case series. Clin Nucl Med. 2006;31(11):683–7.
20. Wang AT, Mullan RJ, Lane MA, et al. Treatment of hyperprolactinemia: a systematic review and meta-analysis. Syst Rev. 2012;1:33.

Part VII
High Risk Differentiated Thyroid Cancer: *The Use of Local Treatments and Novel Systemic Chemotherapies*

Chapter 30
A Case of a Patient with Radioactive Iodine Refractory Differentiated Thyroid Cancer with Progressive Neck Disease (Latero-cervical Lymph Nodes) and Stable, Small Lung Metastases

Dana M. Hartl

Case Presentation

A 69-year-old male patient was referred to our department for management of neck recurrence from papillary thyroid carcinoma.

Comorbidities included type II diabetes, hypertension, asymptomatic stenosis of one femoral artery, tobacco consumption (50 packs/year), and stable low-grade idiopathic sideroblastic anemia.

Ten years previously, the patient had undergone total thyroidectomy and therapeutic central and right lateral neck dissection, at an outside institution, followed by two therapeutic doses of radioactive iodine (RAI) after thyroid hormone withdrawal for a 3 cm, classic variety of papillary thyroid carcinoma, with minimal extrathyroidal extension and lymph node metastases in the right lateral neck (pT3N1b). No extracervical uptake was noted on the posttreatment whole-body scans. Three years later, an increase in serum thyroglobulin (Tg) led to the discovery on chest computed tomography (CT) of two small (<10 mm) lung metastases. A third therapeutic dose of RAI was delivered, but no uptake was seen in the metastases, which remained stable over serial CTs. Three years after this treatment, neck ultrasound revealed a metastatic node in neck level III on the right. A reoperative right lateral neck dissection was performed, revealing 13 metastatic nodes out of 20 resected. A fourth administration of RAI followed surgery, with no uptake on single photon emission computed tomography (SPECT). Tg after thyroid hormone withdrawal remained elevated at 37 ng/ml, however. Over the next 4 years, thyroxine-supressed

D.M. Hartl, MD, PhD (✉)
Thyroid Surgery Unit, Department of Head and Neck Oncology, Institut de Cancérologie Gustave Roussy, Paris-Sud University, 114, rue Edouard Vaillant, 94805 Villejuif Cedex, France
e-mail: dana.hartl@gustaveroussy.fr

D.S. Cooper, C. Durante (eds.), *Thyroid Cancer*,
DOI 10.1007/978-3-319-22401-5_30

Tg increased from 2 to 18 ng/ml. Ultrasound with fine-needle aspiration cytology (FNAC) revealed three previously non-identified lymph node metastases in neck levels II and VIB on the right side, measuring 15–20 mm each. All three lymph nodes were positive on 18-fluorodeoxyglucose positron emission tomography (^{18}FDG-PET) (Fig. 30.1). The lung micrometastases visible on CT were stable as compared to imaging 1 year previously and were ^{18}FDG-PET-negative. The patient was referred to our center for management.

Due to the size and progressive nature of the tumor in the neck, reoperative surgery in the neck and upper mediastinum was proposed by the multidisciplinary tumor board. Preoperative laryngoscopy was normal. Surgery was performed using intermittent recurrent nerve neuromonitoring. Intraoperative findings revealed that the level II metastasis invaded the posterior aspect of the internal jugular vein which was sacrificed. The right paratracheal node completely surrounded the inferior laryngeal (recurrent) nerve and superficially invaded the esophageal muscularis, which was resected with a shaving technique, with no perforation of the esophageal

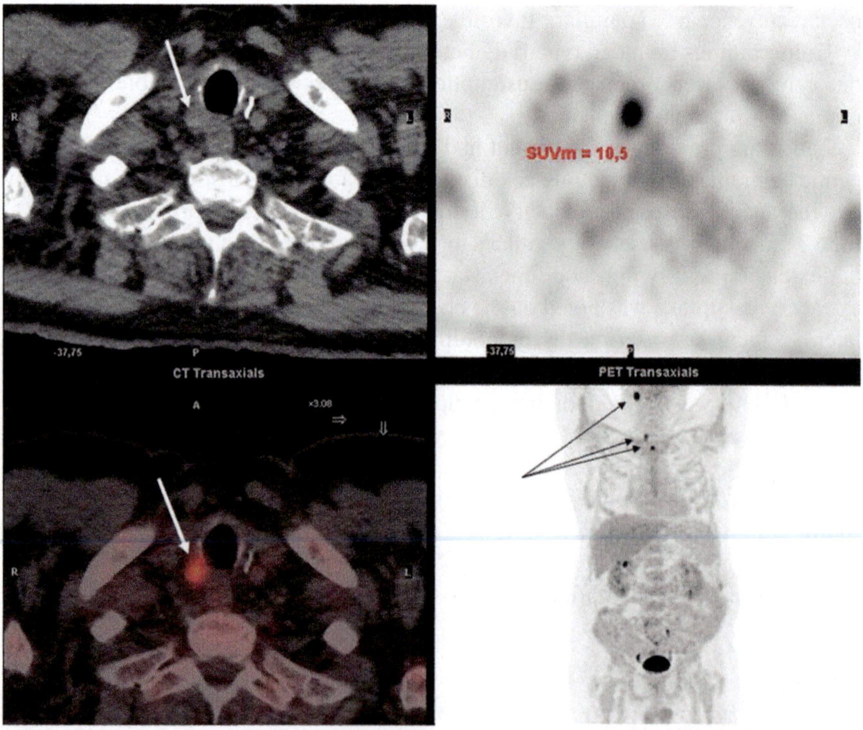

Fig. 30.1 *Upper left*: non-contrast-enhanced CT showing right paratracheal mass (*white arrow*). *Lower left*: 18FDG-PET-CT showing right paratracheal recurrent tumor (*white arrow*). *Upper right*: 18FDG uptake with a standard uptake value of 10.5. *Lower right*: 18FDG-PET showing uptake in three lesions on the *right* side of the neck—from *top* to *bottom*—level II, paratracheal and pretracheal, shown by *black arrows*

mucosa. The nerve was resected en bloc with the tumor mass. The pretracheal node was also resected en bloc with the paratracheal mass. Final pathology revealed three lymph node metastases (20–25 mm each) with the tall cell variant of papillary thyroid carcinoma and extranodal extension. The postoperative course was uneventful, with a satisfactory vocal outcome despite resection of the recurrent nerve.

Assessment and Literature Review

Evaluation and Diagnosis

How Do We Know That This Patient Has RAI-Refractory Disease?

After the fourth administration of a therapeutic dose of RAI, no uptake was seen on SPECT imaging, but the micrometastases were still visible on CT and Tg was still elevated, proof of persistent disease despite RAI [1].

Was FNAC Necessary if ^{18}FDG-PET-CT Showed Significant Uptake?

The reported specificity of ^{18}FDG-PET-CT for recurrence in the neck is 67 % [2], whereas the specificity of ultrasound is 89 %. Ultrasound-guided FNAC with Tg measured on the needle aspirate fluid has a reported specificity of 95 % [3]. Thus, FNACwith measurement of Tg in the needle washout fluid, when possible, improves diagnostic accuracy and avoids the pitfall of false-positive readings of^{18}FDG-PET-CT. FNAC also rules out other tumors, such as lung or head and neck cancer in this older patient with a history of smoking. FNAC is indicated for diagnostic purposes only when a specific treatment can be proposed. Small (<8 mm) suspicious lymph nodes may be followed safely in many cases, with little or no increase in size over time or regional complications. Surgery may be suggested for larger metastases, however, to avoid regional complications in case of tumor progression and to optimize disease-free survival.

What Does the Previous Course of the Disease Tell Us About Prognosis?

The extrathyroidal extension of the disease (pT3), the initial stage of the neck disease (N1b), the age of the patient at first diagnosis (59 years old), and his gender are risk factors for lower disease-free survival [4, 5]. The aggressive histopathological variant of differentiated thyroid carcinoma (tall cell) has also been shown to be a risk factor for recurrent/persistent disease and worse survival [6, 7]. In rare cases, tall cell carcinoma (> or =50 % tall cells) and carcinoma with tall cell features (30–49 % tall cells) have also been found to show anaplastic transformation in the recurrent tumor [6].

The lymph node ratio (the ratio of the number of metastatic nodes found to the total number of resected lymph nodes)—13/20 or 0.65 in this patient after the first reoperation—has also been shown to portend a lower rate of disease-free survival. A rate of 0.3 or above was associated with a 3.4 times higher rate of persistent or recurrent disease, in the study by Vas Nunes et al. [8]. A cutoff of 0.7 was associated with worse prognosis for Schneider et al. [9]. A number of metastatic nodes exceeding ten have also been shown to be a risk factor for persistent/recurrent disease for papillary thyroid carcinoma [10]. Extranodal spread of disease—a further risk factor [10]—was not noted on the pathological report from the first reoperation in the neck in our patient, although it was evident after the operation at our institution. Finally, the presence of macroscopic (>1 cm) metastatic nodes resected at the first operation has been shown to be a factor for persistent/recurrent neck disease [11]. Unfortunately, we were not able to verify the size of the metastatic nodes resected at the first operation in our patient, this operation having been performed at an outside institution.

What Other Imaging or Explorations Could or Should Be Performed to Determine Resectability of the Neck Disease?

In a reoperative situation with macroscopic surgical targets in proximity to the carotid artery, trachea, and esophagus, morphological imaging such as contrast-enhanced CT or MRI may improve prediction of local invasion and aid surgical planning [12]. With recurrent disease close to the esophagus, endoscopic ultrasound may also be helpful in determining the depth of any invasion of the esophageal muscle wall [13]. Finally, laryngoscopy is highly recommended in cases with recurrent disease before reoperation, to detect recurrent nerve paralysis from a previous operation or from locally invasive cancer [14, 15]. Preoperative laryngeal mobility was normal for our patient.

Management

What Are the Treatment Options?

Due to the slowly progressive nature of the disease and the relatively good prognosis over the short to medium term, surgery is generally recommended for potentially resectable lesions, unless undue morbidity is to be expected [16, 17]. External beam radiation therapy to the neck is an option for progressive but unresectable disease [17–19]. Other local therapies such as alcohol injection, radiofrequency ablation, or cryotherapy have not been widely studied in the treatment of large (>1 cm) neck recurrences. Systemic therapy with small molecule tyrosine kinase inhibitors is generally reserved for progressive distant metastases of significant volume, due to the long-term nature of this treatment and its toxicities. Confirmed invasion of the viscera or brain may be a contraindication to this type of systemic therapy with anti-angiogenic activity, however, due to the risk of perforation, fistula, or hemorrhage [20].

What Extent of Surgery Is Recommended?

For our patient, several factors favored surgery to remove the neck metastases: the good general health of the patient despite his comorbidities and age, the size of the metastases >1 cm, RAI-refractory disease, the progression of serum Tg, resectability ascertained on contrast-enhanced CT, the small volume of the lung metastases and their stability over 7 years, and the absence of other detectable lesions. The aim of surgery was to reduce tumor burden and to reduce the risk of symptoms in the neck from vascular and visceral invasion over time.

Why Was the Recurrent Nerve Resected if It Was Functional?

Dissection of the tumor off of the nerve sheath is technically feasible, but generally leaves small disease on the nerve, with resection classified as R1 (microscopic residual disease) or R2 (macroscopic residual disease) [21]. In our patient, however, the distal end of the nerve was entirely encased by the tumor, and nerve preservation would have required leaving macroscopic residual tumor near the larynx, trachea, and esophagus (R2 resection). Our aim was to optimize locoregional control in the neck and minimize the risk of invasion of the trachea and/or esophagus. With RAI-refractory tumors, this goal can be attained only with a macroscopically complete surgical resection.

Swallowing may be affected postoperatively if there is recurrent nerve damage, with aspiration of liquids, and patients should be monitored and receive swallowing rehabilitation if necessary. Voice outcomes are variable after resection of the recurrent nerve due to several factors: compensation from the contralateral side, bilateral innervation of the interarytenoid muscle, variable muscle atrophy, and some degree of reinnervation from nerve anastomoses and from the regional autonomous nerve system. Voice can be surgically improved with several methods based on volume augmentation of the paralyzed vocal fold or medialization of the vocal fold or the arytenoid cartilage, generally with excellent results [22]. Our patient did not have any postoperative dysphagia and considered his voice satisfactory; he declined any type of intervention to improve his voice.

What Outcome Can Be Expected?

A survival rate of 10 % at 10 years and 6 % at 15 years has been reported for patients harboring RAI-refractory metastatic disease [23]. In the same study, however, an intermediate group of patients aged >40 years with RAI-refractory disease but with low tumor burden and micronodular lung metastases had a survival rate of 67 % at 10 years. Our patient falls into this intermediate group with a relatively good prognosis (better than many other solid tumors). This intermediate prognosis justifies locoregional treatments when possible to maintain a low tumor burden and avoid symptoms from progressive disease. For patients with multiple recurrences in the neck, Kim et al. [24] showed a 10-year disease-specific survival rate of 83 % as compared to patients with no recurrence or only 1 recurrence whose 10-year disease-specific survival rate was 100 %.

Reoperative surgery in the neck must be preceded by a meticulous preoperative imaging and planning, in order to foresee possible complications or sequelae and inform the patient preoperatively but also to find and completely map all of the neck metastases in order to resect all of the disease at the time of the operation [25, 26]. Morbidity for reoperation is higher than for primary neck dissection, with a higher risk of unintended nerve injury (recurrent, spinal accessory, and phrenic nerves in particular), tracheal or esophageal injury, and chyle leak from thoracic duct injury [26–28]. Intentional resection of the recurrent nerve, more frequent in the reoperative setting [25], should be discussed with the patient preoperatively, with information regarding the effectiveness of a vocal rehabilitation procedure secondarily if needed.

Recurrence after reoperative surgery has been reported to occur in 40–66 % of cases [26, 27, 29–31]. When evaluated, re-recurrence may be related to inherent disease aggressiveness (particularly after an apparently disease-free interval), but insufficient preoperative workup, "missing" metastatic nodes at the first reoperation, can also be a cause of recurrent/persistent disease [26]. A persistently elevated stimulated Tg level after reoperation is a risk factor for further structural recurrence/persistence [29].

Several techniques have been developed to aid in localizing recurrences, which are often difficult to locate due to scarring from previous surgery. Intraoperative ultrasound may be performed, but requires training in ultrasonography or bringing the radiologist into the operating room. Radio-guided surgery with RAI (when uptake is present) may be helpful, particularly for metastatic nodes in the mediastinum or retropharyngeal nodes, not seen on ultrasound [32]. ^{18}FDG-PET-guided surgery has been described but is not yet widely employed due to technical constraints [33, 34]. Harpoon-guided (hooked-needle) surgery has been described, but may be hazardous for small metastases close to major vascular structures such as the carotid artery and internal jugular vein [35]. Ultrasound tattoo-guided surgery, using colloidal charcoal or methylene blue, is relatively simple to implement, with high rates of localization, but is only applicable to lesions that can be visualized on ultrasound and that are accessible with a needle [36–38]. Due to the size of the recurrences which were well visualized on CT, and their anatomic locations, we did not use localizing techniques in this patient, however.

Back to the Patient

Follow-up ^{18}FDG-PET-CT performed at 10 months revealed retrosternal uptake in the middle mediastinum, with a 1 cm lesion visualized on contrast-enhanced CT. Postoperative levothyroxine-suppressed Tg was 4 ng/ml. This new recurrence will be monitored for progression, and possibly resected via a sternotomy, if no new lesions are discovered and the lung metastases remain stable.

Clinical Pearls

- Patients with a low tumor burden and stable disease generally have a relatively long survival, and aggressive surgery may be advantageous for resectable, progressive lesions in the neck, taking into account other treatment options and quality of life.
- Recurrent lesions near the pharynx, esophagus, and trachea should be explored with morphological imaging techniques and laryngoscopy to determine resectability.
- In recurrent disease, a complete diagnostic work up is necessary, to avoid the pitfall of falsely positive lesions but also to detect the full extent and invasiveness of local disease.
- Patients should be informed of the surgical risks and be aware of the possibility of further recurrences despite apparent macroscopically complete reoperative surgery.

References

1. Schlumberger M, Brose M, Elisei R, Leboulleux S, Luster M, Pitoia F, et al. Definition and management of radioactive iodine-refractory differentiated thyroid cancer. Lancet Diabetes Endocrinol. 2014;2(5):356–8.
2. Seo YL, Yoon DY, Baek S, Ku YJ, Rho YS, Chung EJ, et al. Detection of neck recurrence in patients with differentiated thyroid cancer: comparison of ultrasound, contrast-enhanced CT and (18)F-FDG PET/CT using surgical pathology as a reference standard: (ultrasound vs. CT vs. (18)F-FDG PET/CT in recurrent thyroid cancer). Eur Radiol. 2012;22(10):2246–54.
3. Kim MJ, Kim EK, Kim BM, Kwak JY, Lee EJ, Park CS, et al. Thyroglobulin measurement in fine-needle aspirate washouts: the criteria for neck node dissection for patients with thyroid cancer. Clin Endocrinol (Oxf). 2009;70(1):145–51.
4. Mazzaferri EL. Long-term outcome of patients with differentiated thyroid carcinoma: effect of therapy. Endocr Pract. 2000;6(6):469–76.
5. Tuttle RM, Tala H, Shah J, Leboeuf R, Ghossein R, Gonen M, et al. Estimating risk of recurrence in differentiated thyroid cancer after total thyroidectomy and radioactive iodine remnant ablation: using response to therapy variables to modify the initial risk estimates predicted by the New American Thyroid Association staging system. Thyroid. 2010;20(12):1341–9.
6. Ganly I, Ibrahimpasic T, Rivera M, Nixon I, Palmer F, Patel SG, et al. Prognostic implications of papillary thyroid carcinoma with tall-cell features. Thyroid. 2014;24(4):662–70.
7. Kazaure HS, Roman SA, Sosa JA. Aggressive variants of papillary thyroid cancer: incidence, characteristics and predictors of survival among 43,738 patients. Ann Surg Oncol. 2012;19(6):1874–80.
8. Vas Nunes JH, Clark JR, Gao K, Chua E, Campbell P, Niles N, et al. Prognostic implications of lymph node yield and lymph node ratio in papillary thyroid carcinoma. Thyroid. 2013;23(7):811–6.
9. Schneider DF, Mazeh H, Chen H, Sippel RS. Lymph node ratio predicts recurrence in papillary thyroid cancer. Oncologist. 2013;18(2):157–62.
10. Leboulleux S, Rubino C, Baudin E, Caillou B, Hartl DM, Bidart JM, et al. Prognostic factors for persistent or recurrent disease of papillary thyroid carcinoma with neck lymph node

metastases and/or tumor extension beyond the thyroid capsule at initial diagnosis. J Clin Endocrinol Metab. 2005;90(10):5723–9.
11. Bardet S, Malville E, Rame JP, Babin E, Samama G, De Raucourt D, et al. Macroscopic lymph-node involvement and neck dissection predict lymph-node recurrence in papillary thyroid carcinoma. Eur J Endocrinol. 2008;158(4):551–60.
12. Urken ML. Prognosis and management of invasive well-differentiated thyroid cancer. Otolaryngol Clin N Am. 2010;43(2):301–28. viii.
13. Koike E, Yamashita H, Noguchi S, Ohshima A, Yamashita H, Watanabe S, et al. Endoscopic ultrasonography in patients with thyroid cancer: its usefulness and limitations for evaluating esophagopharyngeal invasion. Endoscopy. 2002;34(6):457–60.
14. Randolph GW, Kamani D. The importance of preoperative laryngoscopy in patients undergoing thyroidectomy: voice, vocal cord function, and the preoperative detection of invasive thyroid malignancy. Surgery. 2006;139(3):357–62.
15. Chandrasekhar SS, Randolph GW, Seidman MD, Rosenfeld RM, Angelos P, Barkmeier-Kraemer J, et al. Clinical practice guideline: improving voice outcomes after thyroid surgery. Otolaryngol Head Neck Surg. 2013;148(6 Suppl):S1–37.
16. Nixon IJ, Whitcher MM, Palmer FL, Tuttle RM, Shaha AR, Shah JP, et al. The impact of distant metastases at presentation on prognosis in patients with differentiated carcinoma of the thyroid gland. Thyroid. 2012;22(9):884–9.
17. Cooper DS, Doherty GM, Haugen BR, Kloos RT, Lee SL, Mandel SJ, et al. Revised American Thyroid Association management guidelines for patients with thyroid nodules and differentiated thyroid cancer. Thyroid. 2009;19(11):1167–214.
18. Kim JH, Kim MS, Yoo SY, Lim SM, Lee GH, Yi KH. Stereotactic body radiotherapy for refractory cervical lymph node recurrence of nonanaplastic thyroid cancer. Otolaryngol Head Neck Surg. 2010;142(3):338–43.
19. Romesser PB, Sherman EJ, Shaha AR, Lian M, Wong RJ, Sabra M, et al. External beam radiotherapy with or without concurrent chemotherapy in advanced or recurrent non-anaplastic non-medullary thyroid cancer. J Surg Oncol. 2014;110(4):375–82.
20. Leboulleux S, Bastholt L, Krause T, de la Fouchardiere C, Tennvall J, Awada A, et al. Vandetanib in locally advanced or metastatic differentiated thyroid cancer: a randomised, double-blind, phase 2 trial. Lancet Oncol. 2012;13(9):897–905.
21. Sobin LH, Gospodarowicz MK, Wittekind CW, editors. UICC International Union Against Cancer TNM classification of malignant tumors. 7th ed. West Sussex: Wiley-Blackwell; 2010.
22. Hartl DM, Travagli JP, Leboulleux S, Baudin E, Brasnu DF, Schlumberger M. Clinical review: current concepts in the management of unilateral recurrent laryngeal nerve paralysis after thyroid surgery. J Clin Endocrinol Metab. 2005;90(5):3084–8.
23. Durante C, Haddy N, Baudin E, Leboulleux S, Hartl D, Travagli JP, et al. Long-term outcome of 444 patients with distant metastases from papillary and follicular thyroid carcinoma: benefits and limits of radioiodine therapy. J Clin Endocrinol Metab. 2006;91(8):2892–9.
24. Kim KM, Park JB, Bae KS, Kang SJ. Analysis of prognostic factors in patients with multiple recurrences of papillary thyroid carcinoma. Surg Oncol. 2012;21(3):185–90.
25. Farrag TY, Agrawal N, Sheth S, Bettegowda C, Ewertz M, Kim M, et al. Algorithm for safe and effective reoperative thyroid bed surgery for recurrent/persistent papillary thyroid carcinoma. Head Neck. 2007;29(12):1069–74.
26. Onkendi EO, McKenzie TJ, Richards ML, Farley DR, Thompson GB, Kasperbauer JL, et al. Reoperative experience with papillary thyroid cancer. World J Surg. 2014;38(3):645–52.
27. Lang BH, Lee GC, Ng CP, Wong KP, Wan KY, Lo CY. Evaluating the morbidity and efficacy of reoperative surgery in the central compartment for persistent/recurrent papillary thyroid carcinoma. World J Surg. 2013;37(12):2853–9.
28. Ruggiero FP, Fedok FG. Outcomes in reoperative thyroid cancer. Otolaryngol Clin N Am. 2008;41(6):1261–8. xii.
29. Yim JH, Kim WB, Kim EY, Kim WG, Kim TY, Ryu JS, et al. The outcomes of first reoperation for locoregionally recurrent/persistent papillary thyroid carcinoma in patients who initially

underwent total thyroidectomy and remnant ablation. J Clin Endocrinol Metab. 2011;96: 2049–56.
30. Clayman GL, Shellenberger TD, Ginsberg LE, Edeiken BS, El-Naggar AK, Sellin RV, et al. Approach and safety of comprehensive central compartment dissection in patients with recurrent papillary thyroid carcinoma. Head Neck. 2009;31(9):1152–63.
31. Al-Saif O, Farrar WB, Bloomston M, Porter K, Ringel MD, Kloos RT. Long-term efficacy of lymph node reoperation for persistent papillary thyroid cancer. J Clin Endocrinol Metab. 2010;95(5):2187–94.
32. Travagli JP, Cailleux AF, Ricard M, Baudin E, Caillou B, Parmentier C, et al. Combination of radioiodine (131I) and probe-guided surgery for persistent or recurrent thyroid carcinoma. J Clin Endocrinol Metab. 1998;83(8):2675–80.
33. Kim WW, Kim JS, Hur SM, Kim SH, Lee SK, Choi JH, et al. Radioguided surgery using an intraoperative PET probe for tumor localization and verification of complete resection in differentiated thyroid cancer: a pilot study. Surgery. 2011;149(3):416–24.
34. Gulec SA. PET probe-guided surgery. J Surg Oncol. 2007;96(4):353–7.
35. Triponez F, Poder L, Zarnegar R, Goldstein R, Roayaie K, Feldstein V, et al. Hook needle-guided excision of recurrent differentiated thyroid cancer in previously operated neck compartments: a safe technique for small, nonpalpable recurrent disease. J Clin Endocrinol Metab. 2006;91(12):4943–7.
36. Hartl DM, Chami L, Al Ghuzlan A, Leboulleux S, Baudin E, Schlumberger M, et al. Charcoal suspension tattoo localization for differentiated thyroid cancer recurrence. Ann Surg Oncol. 2009;16(9):2602–8.
37. Kang TW, Shin JH, Han BK, Ko EY, Kang SS, Hahn SY, et al. Preoperative ultrasound-guided tattooing localization of recurrences after thyroidectomy: safety and effectiveness. Ann Surg Oncol. 2009;16(6):1655–9.
38. Soprani F, Bondi F, Puccetti M, Armaroli V. Charcoal tattoo localization for differentiated thyroid cancer recurrence in the central compartment of the neck. Acta Otorhinolaryngol Ital. 2012;32(2):87–92.

Chapter 31
A Case of an Elderly Patient with Advanced Disease and Non-radioiodine-avid Metastases

Fabiana Trulli, Cristina Luongo, Michele Klain, and Martin Schlumberger

Case Report

In May 2009, a 70-year-old male patient presented with a 5 cm tumor in the right thyroid lobe with ipsilateral palpable lymph node metastases. An FNAB of a palpable lymph node showed papillary thyroid cancer. A preoperative computed tomography (CT) scan with contrast confirmed the neck lesions with no apparent involvement of the aerodigestive tract but revealed multiple micronodular lung metastases <1.5 cm in diameter.

In June 2009, a total thyroidectomy with central neck and right lateral neck dissection was performed. Histology showed a 5 cm unifocal papillary thyroid cancer (PTC), classic form, with extension beyond the thyroid capsule and with six lymph node metastases in the lateral neck and four in the central neck, with extension beyond the lymph node capsule in three, and with the largest lymph node having a size of 3.5 cm; according to the TNM classification, the disease was classified as pT3-N1b-M1.

In July 2009, an activity of 3.7 GBq (100 mCi) 131-I was administered following thyroid hormone withdrawal. On the day of 131-I administration, serum TSH level was 58 mIU/L, and serum Tg level was 94 ng/mL in the absence of interfering antibodies; urinary iodine was normal. A whole body scan performed at day 3 disclosed a low thyroid bed uptake (0.5 % of the administered activity) and no detectable uptake outside the thyroid bed. A positron emission tomography (PET) scan demonstrated uptake of (18)F-fluoro-2-deoxy-D-glucose (FDG) in some lung lesions.

Thus, this patient had multiple small (<1.5 cm in diameter) lesions in the lungs that were radioactive iodine (RAI) refractory, as shown by the absence of RAI uptake, and there was no evidence of tumor progression compared to the preoperative

F. Trulli • C. Luongo • M. Klain • M. Schlumberger (✉)
Gustave Roussy and University Paris Sud, 114 rue Edouard Vaillant, 94800 Villejuif, France
e-mail: martin.schlumberger@gustaveroussy.fr

D.S. Cooper, C. Durante (eds.), *Thyroid Cancer*,
DOI 10.1007/978-3-319-22401-5_31

chest CT scan. Treatment with levothyroxine was initiated at a standard dose of 1.8 μg/kg body weight/day. Serum TSH 2 months later was 0.2 mUI/L. A repeat chest CT scan was performed in December 2009 and demonstrated an increase in the size of target lesions of 15 % and no evidence of new lesions; in the absence of significant progression, follow-up was maintained, and in May 2010, another CT scan demonstrated progression with a +44 % increase in size compared to June 2009, with the appearance of new lung, neck, and mediastinal lesions; the largest lesion now measured >2 cm. At that time, he was in good general condition (ECOG status score 0) and was being treated with amlodipine for hypertension; serum Tg level was 35 ng/mL and serum TSH <0.1 mU/L on levothyroxine therapy.

The thyroid tumor board confirmed the indication for systemic treatment, and he was included in the DECISION trial, the first randomized, double-blind, placebo-controlled phase 3 trial designed to explore the efficacy and safety of sorafenib in patients with RAI-refractory differentiated thyroid cancer (DTC). In May 2010, treatment with sorafenib 400 mg, PO twice a day, was initiated. Response to therapy was assessed with a chest CT scan every 3 months. In November 2010, a 38 % reduction in target lesion size from baseline was observed (the nadir) (Fig. 31.1a), and serum Tg level decreased by two-thirds to 13 ng/mL, TSH <0.1 mU/L. Tolerance was acceptable with hand-foot skin reaction that was controlled by local treatments, diarrhea, and fatigue (grade 2). However, he had an almost normal quality of life (ECOG 0), appetite was preserved, his weight remained stable, and the blood pressure remained well controlled with amlodipine.

In February 2011, the daily dose of sorafenib was decreased to 600 mg for painful hand-foot skin reaction (grade 3) that was no longer controlled by local treatment modalities, diarrhea (grade 2), and fatigue (grade 2).

Symptoms improved and the patient continued to receive sorafenib 600 mg a day. In April 2011, progression was observed with a 32 % increase in lesion size from the nadir (Fig. 31.1b). Treatment with sorafenib was discontinued, and the patient refused a different second-line systemic therapy.

After withdrawal of sorafenib, disease progressed at a pace similar to that observed before treatment (Fig. 31.1c). In May 2012, 12 months after discontinuation of sorafenib treatment, dyspnea occurred, indicating the need for additional treatment, but the patient refused again for personal reasons. Dyspnea progressively worsened and was accompanied by hemoptysis. In March 2013, a bronchoscopy showed a lesion in the left mainstem bronchus. Since bronchial invasion increases the risk of bleeding, enrollment in another clinical trial was not possible. Testing for BRAF and *ALK* mutations was performed because the presence of a driver mutation may lead to a specific inhibitor, but this was negative.

The tumor board decision was that second-line treatment should not be delayed, and the patient agreed to additional therapy. In May 2013, treatment with off-label sunitinib 37.5 mg/day for 3 weeks followed by 1 week off therapy was initiated. After two cycles, dyspnea improved and he had no hemoptysis. In August 2013, a CT scan demonstrated a partial tumor response (−35 %) using Response Evaluation Criteria in Solid Tumors (RECIST). He had minor adverse events, consisting in fatigue (grade 1) and intermittent diarrhea (grade 1) and enjoyed an almost normal quality of life (ECOG 0). Sunitinib treatment was maintained, and chest CT scans

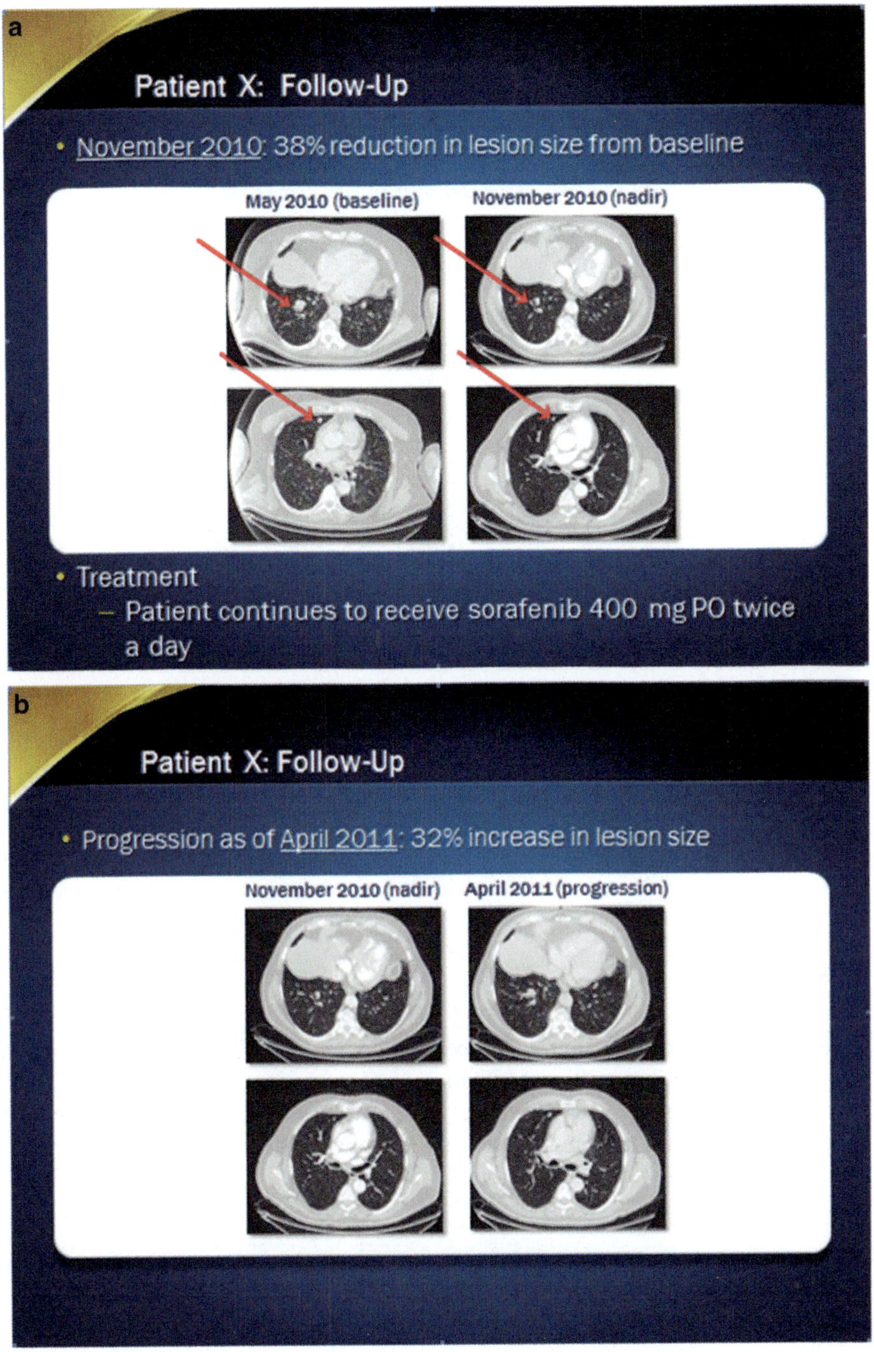

Fig. 31.1 Imaging of the patient at baseline and during sorafenib treatment. In November 2010, a partial response was observed (panel **a**), but thereafter, in April 2011, the patient progressed despite treatment (panel **b**). Less than 2 years after treatment withdrawal, in January 2013, progression was obvious (panel **c**), and the patient initiated a second-line treatment

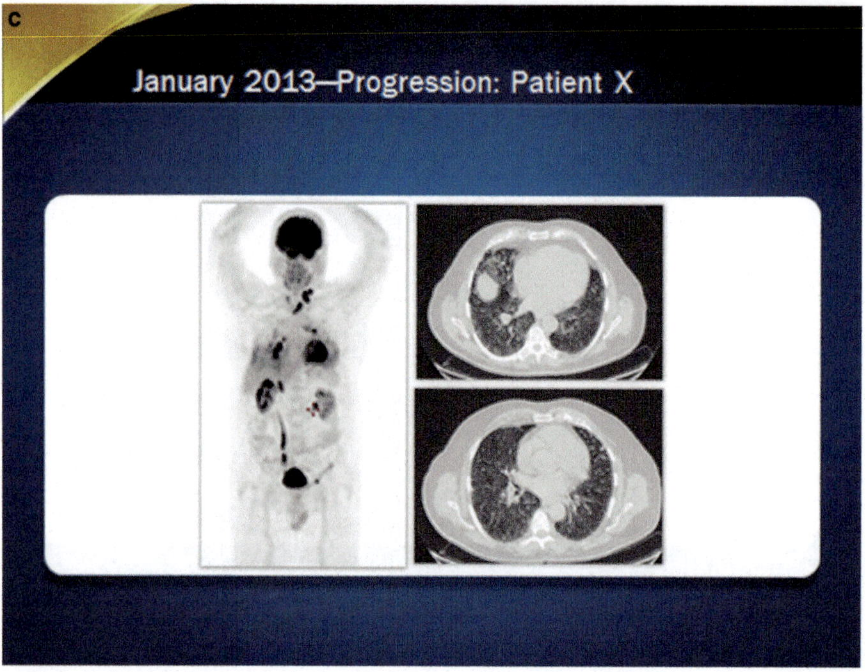

Fig. 31.1 (continued)

performed every 3 months did not show tumor progression. In December 2014, the patient was still receiving sunitinib treatment at the same dosage with no significant adverse events and a good quality of life.

Discussion

Radioiodine-refractory thyroid cancer is uncommon, with an estimated incidence of 4–5 cases per million population (5 % of patients with clinical thyroid cancer, 250 patients per year in France) [1, 2]. It occurs more frequently in older patients, in those with large metastases or with poorly differentiated thyroid cancer, and in those with high FDG uptake on PET scan [3–5].

Definition of 131I-Refractory Thyroid Cancer

Most patients with 131-I-refractory DTC fall into four categories [6]: (a) Patients with metastatic disease that does not take up 131-I at the time of the first 131-I treatment. (b) Patients whose tumors lose the ability to take up 131-I after previous evidence of uptake. This is due to the eradication by 131-I treatment of differentiated cells able to take up 131-I, but not of less differentiated cells that do not take up 131-I and that are likely to progress. (c) Patients with 131-I uptake retained in some lesions but not in others. This is frequently observed in patients with multiple large metastases. In such patients, progression is likely to occur in metastases without 131-I uptake (in particular when FDG uptake is present) [3, 5, 7]. (d) Patients with metastatic disease that progresses despite significant uptake of 131-I in all the metastases and adequate 131-I treatment. It has been shown that if progression occurs following a course of adequate radioiodine treatment, subsequent 131-I treatment will be ineffective [8].

Our patient had lung metastases with no uptake on posttherapy WBS. There was an increase in serum TSH level following thyroid hormone withdrawal, and there was no iodine contamination; therefore, technical conditions did not prevent visualization of potential uptake at distant sites. Thus, the patient was considered 131-I refractory and no further RAI was administered. This is consistent with the age of the patient (70 years) and with the presence of FDG uptake in some metastases on PET/CT.

Treatment Initiation

Patients with advanced disease who are refractory to 131-I treatment have a median survival rate of 3–6 years in the absence of effective treatment modalities and a 10-year survival rate of only 10 % [4]. However, patients with refractory thyroid cancers encompass a heterogeneous group with regard to progression rate and life expectancy. For example, more aggressive tumors occur in older patients, are poorly differentiated, and have no initial RAI uptake but a high FDG uptake, and usually large metastases are present. In contrast, young patients with non-radioiodine-avid small lung metastases from a well-differentiated thyroid carcinoma can be asymptomatically stable for long periods of time. However, there are exceptions, and the rate of progression should be documented by imaging in each patient.

Once 131-I treatment is abandoned, levothyroxine treatment is used to maintain serum TSH at a low or undetectable level, depending on other patient comorbidities, and local treatment of metastases is performed whenever needed. Surveillance includes a FDG-PET/CT scan or a CT scan of the neck, chest, abdomen, and pelvis with contrast medium, at an interval of 3–6 months. In the absence of documented progression, follow-up with anatomical imaging every 6–12 months is continued.

The decision to initiate systemic therapy in patients with 131-I-refractory thyroid cancer is based on the presence of a large tumor burden, evidence of disease progression, the presence of symptoms, a high risk of local complications, and the general condition of the patient [1]. Treatment should be initiated preferably before the occurrence of invasion of the respiratory-digestive axis or of encasement of large vessels that increases the risk of severe bleeding during treatment. Some patients may require treatment of local tumor extension with surgery or radiotherapy to permit treatment with kinase inhibitors [9].

The progression rate can also be evaluated by the doubling time of serum Tg [10] but should always be confirmed by anatomic imaging using RECIST criteria. Patients with multiple lesions >1–2 cm and with RECIST progression (i.e., at least a 20 % increase in the sum of the diameters of target lesions or the appearance of significant new metastatic lesions) within less than 12 months are considered for systemic treatment. In contrast, patients with few and/or small metastatic lesions <1 cm or those with no evidence of progression over a 12-month period are followed without treatment, and stable disease or slow progression has been observed in some patients over decades [1, 4].

Our patient had stable disease at 5 months postthyroidectomy, but disease progression was documented within 11 months, with an increase in tumor diameters by 44 % and with the appearance of new lesions. At that point, the sum of the diameters of the largest lesion was >2 cm. The thyroid tumor board concluded that he fulfilled all criteria for treatment initiation. Because of the poor efficacy of cytotoxic chemotherapy [11], the use of tyrosine kinase inhibitor was recommended as first-line treatment.

Molecular-Targeted Therapy

Gene rearrangements (*RET/PTC* and *NTRK*) or point mutations of the *RAS* and *BRAF* genes are found in two-thirds of papillary thyroid cancers, resulting in the activation of the MAP kinase pathway [2, 12]. An even greater frequency of mutations is observed using next-generation sequencing [13]. Angiogenesis is activated in thyroid cancers, with an overproduction of VEGF by cancer cells and an overexpression of VEGF receptors by cancer and endothelial cells, and is associated with a poor outcome. Furthermore, other pathways such as the fibroblast growth factor receptor (FGFR) and platelet-derived growth factor receptor (PDGFR) pathways may also be activated. Up to now, antiangiogenic drugs, some of which also target kinases in the MAP kinase pathway, have been used in refractory thyroid cancers. The relative role of the inhibition of each target or of their combined inhibition on tumor response is currently unknown.

Results of Clinical Trials with Antiangiogenic Drugs

In phase 2 trials with these agents, partial responses were observed in 0–59 % of patients and long-term stable disease in at least another third. The comparison of the outcomes among these compounds is at the present time not possible, but 50 % or even higher response rates that have been recently reported with pazopanib [14], lenvatinib [15], and cabozantinib [16] seem higher than previously reported with axitinib [9, 17], motesanib [18], sorafenib [19], sunitinib [20], and vandetanib [21]. It also appears that most drugs are more effective in treating metastases located in the lymph nodes, liver, and lungs rather than in the skeleton.

The improvement in progression-free survival (PFS) with these agents is also significant when compared with placebo. This was reported in a randomized phase 2 trial (vandetanib vs. placebo) and in two phase 3 trials (sorafenib vs. placebo and lenvatinib vs. placebo). The lack of demonstrated improvement in overall survival versus placebo in all of these trials might have been the result of the crossover design of these randomized studies.

The ZACTHYF study was a multicenter randomized phase 2 trial with vandetanib (300 mg/day) versus placebo on 145 patients with RAI-refractory, locally advanced, or metastatic DTC that had progressed within the past 14 months. Vandetanib significantly prolonged PFS compared with placebo (hazard ratio, 0.63, $p=0.008$; median, 11.1 vs. 5.9 months), but no objective response in lesion size was observed [21].

The DECISION trial was a multicenter, randomized (1:1) phase 3 trial of sorafenib (400 mg twice daily) versus placebo in 417 patients with RAI-refractory, locally advanced, or metastatic DTC that had progressed within the past 14 months [19]. Median treatment duration was 10.6 months (range, 0.07–31.1) with sorafenib and 6.5 months (range, 0.4–30.4) with placebo. The mean daily study sorafenib dose was 651 mg. Sorafenib treatment significantly improved PFS compared with placebo (hazard ratio, 0.587; 95 % CI 0.454–0.758; $p<0.0001$; median 10.8 versus 5.8 months, respectively), and the partial response rate was 12 %. The improvement in PFS was seen in all clinical and biomarker subgroups, irrespective of *BRAF* and *RAS* mutation status. Median thyroglobulin levels rose in the placebo group and decreased and then paralleled progression in the sorafenib-treated group. The safety profile of sorafenib was as expected, with most adverse events being grades 1 and 2. The most common adverse events in the sorafenib arm were hand-foot skin reaction (76 %), diarrhea (69 %), alopecia (67 %), and rash/desquamation (50 %). Toxicities led to dose reduction in 64 % of patients and to drug withdrawal in 19 %. These results led to the approval of sorafenib by the US FDA for advanced, refractory, and progressive DTC in November 2013 and by the EMA in March 2014.

The SELECT trial was a multicenter, randomized (2:1) phase 3 study of lenvatinib (24 mg/day) versus placebo in 392 patients with RAI-refractory, locally advanced, or metastatic DTC that had progressed within the past 13 months, as confirmed by independent radiological review [1]. Median treatment duration was 13.8 months (range, 0–27) with lenvatinib and 3.9 months (range, 0–24) with placebo. The mean daily study lenvatinib dose was 16.8 mg, with a median time to first dose reduction of 3 months. Lenvatinib treatment significantly improved PFS compared with placebo (hazard ratio, 0.21; 99 % CI, 0.14–0.31, $P<0.001$; median PFS, 18.3 vs. 3.6 months, respectively). At year 2, progression events occurred in 86 % of those in the placebo arm and only in 41 % of subjects in the treatment arm. The objective response rate was 65 % with complete responses in 2 %, with a median time to objective response of 2 months. Similar benefits were observed in 20 % of patients who had received prior VEGF-targeted therapy. The improvement in PFS was seen in all clinical and biomarker subgroups, irrespective of *BRAF* and *RAS* mutation status. Treatment-related adverse events were reported in all patients in the lenvatinib group. Most often, these were hypertension (68 %), fatigue (64 %), diarrhea (59 %), and decreased appetite (50 %). Proteinuria occurred in 32 % of the patients and thromboembolic events in 11 % of the patients. These adverse events were managed with dose modification and medication. Toxicities led to dose reduction in 68 % of the patients and to drug withdrawal in 14 % of patients. In the active treatment arm, there were 20 fatalities compared with six in the placebo arm. Investigators attributed six fatalities (2 %) directly to the use of lenvatinib. One person died from a pulmonary embolism, one died due to hemorrhagic stroke, and the other four patients died due to general health deterioration. In conclusion, lenvatinib seems more effective than any other kinase inhibitor with an almost 15-month improvement in median PFS compared with placebo and a response rate as high as 65 %, with few complete responses. However, efficacy and toxicity of lenvatinib have still to be evaluated in real life, outside the frame of a controlled trial.

Metabolic consequences of kinase inhibitor treatment are relevant in DTC patients. An increased need of levothyroxine is frequent, and serum TSH should be measured at each visit. An increased need for calcium and vitamin D may occur, particularly in patients with postoperative hypoparathyroidism, and ionized calcium should be measured at each visit during treatment and also when kinase inhibitor treatment is withdrawn to avoid severe hypercalcemia.

The well-described toxicities of kinase inhibitors include fatigue, diarrhea, hypertension, and skin toxicities, and there were no unexpected toxicities observed in the clinical trials mentioned above. Toxicities were significant and led to dose reduction in 11–73 % of patients and to drug withdrawal in 7–25 %. This suggests that these treatments should be initiated only in patients with a significant tumor burden and with documented progression of the disease and that such patients should be managed by experienced teams of caregivers. Aerodigestive fistula formation [22] and bleeding have been reported in patients with tumor involvement of the aerodigestive tract that may require intervention before initiating any treatment with KI. Also, prevention of adverse events whenever possible, education of patients and of care providers, assessment of adverse events using standardized guidelines, and their early management are mandatory and represent the best way to improve patient compliance.

As of now, there are no factors that are predictive of drug efficacy. In DECISION and in SELECT trials, benefits of sorafenib or lenvatinib were observed in patients with mutated or wild-type *RAS* or *BRAF* status, and thus, this status cannot be used to predict response to treatment [15, 19]. In our institution, mutational screening is performed on a routine basis in these patients, because it may lead to the use of a specific inhibitor in the presence of a driver mutation. Basal levels of some cytokine or angiogenic factors or changes in their serum level at 1–2 weeks are not reliable enough to be used in routine practice [23]. The comparison of FDG uptake on PET/CT after 1–2 weeks of therapy with baseline FDG uptake has produced inconsistent results, and the role of repeated FDG-PET/CT in the management of DTC patients during treatment with these new drugs is still unclear [20, 21].

Back to Our Patient

He was included after informed consent signature in the DECISION trial open for inclusion at that time. He experienced a typical tumor response, as observed in 12 % of responders that was partial (−38 %) and lasted for 12 months. Toxicity was observed as expected, with hand-foot skin reaction grade 2 and fatigue and diarrhea; these adverse events needed local treatment and a decrease in the sorafenib daily dosage.

Progression During Treatment with Kinase Inhibitors

The mechanism of resistance after a partial response has been obtained is unknown. It may be related to insufficient drug exposure that may be determined by pharmacokinetic studies or by the development of a resistant tumor cell population.

When a patient who responded and then slowly progresses, an unresolved question is how long should the treatment be maintained? It appears that progression rate does not change when treatment is maintained, as showed by studying secondary PFS in the DECISION trial. However, accelerated disease progression has been reported after discontinuation of treatment [24], indicating that patients with progressive disease should not remain untreated for long periods of time. This can be achieved by either maintaining treatment when there are still some clinical benefits or using another anti-angiogenic drug if this is available; indeed, PFS with a second-line antiangiogenic treatment is similar to the PFS observed with the first-line treatment [6, 25].

In our patient, in whom tumor progression occurred after a partial response, sorafenib was withdrawn because there was no persistent clinical benefit. The patient then did not want to receive a second-line treatment, and during the period of time when he was off drug therapy, the progression rate did not change. However, bronchial involvement and bleeding developed, and he was no longer a suitable candidate for clinical trials. He was still in good general condition, and we proposed treatment with sunitinib, the only commercially available drug at that time, after a thorough discussion of the risks and potential benefits of such treatment. He experienced a partial response with symptom improvement that has persisted up to his last clinic visit 18 months after the initiation of sunitinib. It is hoped that successive courses of systemic therapy will prolong his life expectancy.

The Future

In case of progression during the second line of antiangiogenic treatment, the potential benefits of further treatments with other antiangiogenic drugs are questionable, and this may lead to the combined use of two drugs with different targets. Drugs targeted at other abnormalities that are present in the tumor tissue, such as

BRAF or anaplastic lymphoma kinase (ALK) may be of benefit in future studies [25, 26]. Another potential way of treating these patients is to restore the ability of tumor cells to concentrate radioiodine and then to treat with radioiodine following preparation with rhTSH stimulation. This was reported in pilot studies after 4 weeks of treatment with a MEK inhibitor, selumetinib [27], and with a BRAF inhibitor dabrafenib [28]. Finally, immunological intervention may involve two possible strategies: One is guided by the increased number of tumor-associated macrophages (TAMs) in aggressive tumors [29, 30]. It has recently been reported in *BRAF* transgenic mice that depletion of TAM through the inhibition of the colony-stimulating factor 1 (CSF1) pathway that attracts TAMs into the tumor impairs tumor progression [31]. Another potential pathway involves tumor evasion from immunosurveillance. This can occur through a variety of mechanisms, such as tumor expression of inhibitors of T-cell function, CTLA-4, PD-1, or PD-L1. Blockade with monoclonal antibodies directed at these immune checkpoints has emerged as a successful therapeutic approach in patients with advanced melanoma and other cancer types [32]. Interestingly, *BRAF*-mutated papillary thyroid cancers have a higher expression of CTLA-4 and PD-L1 compared with *BRAF* wild-type tumors [33]. There are no available data on treatment with these antibodies in refractory DTC, but this represents a potential future avenue of research in these patients.

Conclusion

Despite the many advances achieved in recent years, there are still many questions to be answered. These include the following: (1) which drug should be used as first-line treatment, (2) what is the mechanism of resistance in case of progression, (3) how long should the treatment be maintained, (4) is combination therapy effective, and (5) what are other drugs targeting other pathways. Thus, there is a need for more clinical trials. Recent experience with trials performed in the framework of clinical oncology networks have shown that enrollment of the required number of thyroid cancer patients to reach statistically significant outcomes is possible in a limited period of time. Patients should be offered participation to trials, as this is the only way to achieve progress in this field. For patients that are not candidates for a clinical trial, a number of agents that have shown significant efficacy in delaying tumor progression are either approved or are on the horizon.

Clinical Pearls

- Radioiodine-refractory thyroid cancer is rare, and RAI treatment should be abandoned in such cases.
- Treatment with levothyroxine should maintain serum TSH to a low/undetectable level, depending on underlying comorbidities. Imaging is performed every 3–12 months.

- Treatment with a kinase inhibitor is indicated when progression occurs in a patient with a significant tumor burden.
- Kinase inhibitors induce tumor responses and significant improvement in PFS but as yet have not been shown to increase overall survival. Toxicity is significant and responses are partial and transient.
- Several different drugs may be used sequentially. Clinical trials are still warranted.

References

1. Schlumberger M, Brose M, Elisei R, Leboulleux S, Luster M, Pitoia F, Pacini F. Definition and management of radioactive iodine-refractory differentiated thyroid cancer: recommendations by an international expert panel. Lancet Diabetes Endocrinol. 2014;2:356–8.
2. Xing MM, Haugen B, Schlumberger M. Progress in molecular-based management of differentiated thyroid cancer. Lancet. 2013;381:1058–69.
3. Deandreis D, Al Ghuzlan A, Leboulleux S, Lacroix L, Garsi JP, Talbot M, Lumbroso J, Baudin E, Caillou B, Bidart JM, Schlumberger M. Do histological, immunohistochemical and metabolic (radioiodine and fluorodeoxyglucose uptake) patterns of metastatic thyroid cancer correlate with patient outcome? Endocr Relat Cancer. 2011;18:159–69.
4. Durante C, Haddy N, Baudin E, Leboulleux S, Hartl D, Travagli JP, Caillou B, Ricard M, Lumbroso JD, De Vathaire F, Schlumberger M. Long-term outcome of 444 patients with distant metastases from papillary and follicular thyroid carcinoma: benefits and limits of radioiodine therapy. J Clin Endocrinol Metab. 2006;91:2892–9.
5. Robbins RJ, Wan Q, Grewal RK, Reibke R, Gonen M, Strauss HW, Tuttle RM, Drucker W, Larson SM. Real-time prognosis for metastatic thyroid carcinoma based on 2-[18F]fluoro-2-deoxy-D-glucose-positron emission tomography scanning. J Clin Endocrinol Metab. 2006;91: 498–505.
6. Massicotte MH, Brassard M, Claude-Desroches M, Borget I, Bonichon F, Giraudet al, Docao C, Chougnet CN, Leboulleux S, Baudin E, Schlumberger M, de la Fouchardière C. Tyrosine kinase inhibitor treatments in patients with metastatic thyroid carcinomas: a retrospective study of the TUTHYREF network. Eur J Endocrinol. 2014;170:575–82.
7. Rivera M, Ghossein RA, Schoder H, Gomez D, Larson SM, Tuttle RM. Histopathologic characterization of radioactive iodine-refractory fluorodeoxyglucose-positron emission tomography-positive thyroid carcinoma. Cancer. 2008;113:48–56.
8. Vaisman F, Tala H, Grewal R, Tuttle RM. In differentiated thyroid cancer, an incomplete structural response to therapy is associated with significantly worse clinical outcomes than only an incomplete thyroglobulin response. Thyroid. 2011;21:1317–22.
9. Locati LD, Licitra L, Agate L, Ou SH, Boucher A, Jarzab B, Qin S, Kane MA, Wirth LJ, Chen C, Kim S, Ingrosso A, Pithavala YK, Bycott P, Cohen EE. Treatment of advanced thyroid cancer with axitinib: phase 2 study with pharmacokinetic/pharmacodynamic and quality-of-life assessments. Cancer. 2014;120:2694–703.
10. Miyauchi A, Kudo T, Miya A, Kobayashi K, Ito Y, Takamura Y, Higashiyama T, Fukushima M, Kihara M, Inoue H, Tomoda C, Yabuta T, Masuoka H. Prognostic impact of serum thyroglobulin doubling-time under thyrotropin suppression in patients with papillary thyroid carcinoma who underwent total thyroidectomy. Thyroid. 2011;21:707–16.
11. Sherman SI. Cytotoxic chemotherapy for differentiated thyroid carcinoma. Clin Oncol (R Coll Radiol). 2010;22:464–8.
12. Fagin JA. How thyroid tumors start and why it matters: kinase mutants as targets for solid cancer pharmacotherapy. J Endocrinol. 2004;183:249–56.
13. Cancer Genome Atlas Research Network. Integrated genomic characterization of papillary thyroid carcinoma. Cell. 2014;159:676–90. Electronic address: giordano@umich.edu.

14. Bible KC, Suman VJ, Molina JR, Smallridge RC, Maples WJ, Menefee ME, Rubin J, Sideras K, Morris 3rd JC, McIver B, Burton JK, Webster KP, Bieber C, Traynor AM, Flynn PJ, Goh BC, Tang H, Ivy SP, Erlichman C. Efficacy of pazopanib in progressive, radioiodine-refractory, metastatic differentiated thyroid cancers: results of a phase 2 consortium study. Lancet Oncol. 2010;11:962–72.
15. Schlumberger M, Tahara M, Wirth LJ, Robinson B, Brose MS, Elisei R, Habra MA, Newbold K, Shah MH, Hoff AO, Gianoukakis AG, Kiyota N, Taylor MH, Kim SB, Krzyzanowska MK, Dutcus CE, de las Heras B, Zhu J, Sherman SI. Lenvatinib versus placebo in radioiodine-refractory thyroid cancer. N Engl J Med. 2015;372:621–30.
16. Cabanillas M, Brose M, Holland J, Ferguson KC, Sherman SI. A phase I study of cabozantinib (XL184) in patients with differentiated thyroid cancer. Thyroid. 2014;24:1508–14.
17. Cohen EE, Rosen LS, Vokes EE, Kies MS, Forastiere AA, Worden FP, Kane MA, Sherman E, Kim S, Bycott P, Tortorici M, Shalinsky DR, Liau KF, Cohen RB. Axitinib is an active treatment for all histologic subtypes of advanced thyroid cancer: results from a phase II study. J Clin Oncol. 2008;26:4708–13.
18. Sherman SI, Wirth LJ, Droz JP, Hofmann M, Bastholt L, Martins RG, Licitra L, Eschenberg MJ, Sun YN, Juan T, Stepan DE, Schlumberger MJ. Motesanib diphosphate in progressive differentiated thyroid cancer. N Engl J Med. 2008;359:31–42.
19. Brose MS, Nutting CM, Jarzab B, Elisei R, Siena S, Bastholt L, de la Fouchardiere C, Pacini F, Paschke R, Shong YK, Sherman SI, Smit JWA, Chung J, Kappeler C, Pena C, Molnar I, Schlumberger M. A randomized trial of sorafenib for 131I-refractory differentiated thyroid cancer. Lancet. 2014;384:319–28.
20. Carr LL, Mankoff DA, Goulart BH, Eaton KD, Capell PT, Kell EM, Bauman JE, Martins RG. Phase II study of daily sunitinib in FDG-PET-positive, iodine-refractory differentiated thyroid cancer and metastatic medullary carcinoma of the thyroid with functional imaging correlation. Clin Cancer Res. 2010;16:5260–8.
21. Leboulleux S, Bastholt L, Krause T, de la Fouchardiere C, Tennvall J, Awada A, Gómez JM, Bonichon F, Leenhardt L, Soufflet C, Licour M, Schlumberger MJ. Vandetanib in locally advanced or metastatic differentiated thyroid cancer: a randomised, double-blind, phase 2 trial. Lancet Oncol. 2012;13:897–905.
22. Blevins DP, Dadu R, Hu M, Baik C, Balachandran D, Ross W, Gunn B, Cabanillas ME. Aerodigestive fistula formation as a rare side effect of antiangiogenic tyrosine kinase inhibitor therapy for thyroid cancer. Thyroid. 2014;24:918–22.
23. Bass MB, Sherman SI, Schlumberger MJ, Davis MT, Kivman L, Khoo HM, et al. Biomarkers as predictors of response to treatment with motesanib in patients with progressive advanced thyroid cancer. J Clin Endocrinol Metab. 2010;95:5018–27.
24. Yun KJ, Kim W, Kim EH, Kim MH, Lim DJ, Kang MI, et al. Accelerated disease progression after discontinuation of sorafenib in a patient with metastatic papillary thyroid cancer. Endocrinol Metab (Seoul). 2014;29:388–93.
25. Dadu R, Shah K, Busaidy NL, Waguespack SG, Habra MA, Ying AK, Hu MI, Bassett R, Jimenez C, Sherman SI, Cabanillas ME. Efficacy and tolerability of vemurafenib in patients with BRAFV600E-positive papillary thyroid cancer: M.D. Anderson Cancer Center off label experience. J Clin Endocrinol Metab. 2015;100:77–81.
26. Falchook GS, Millward M, Hong DS, Naing A, Piha-Paul S, Waguespack SG, Cabanillas M, Sherman SI, Ma B, Curtis M, Goodman V, Kurzrock R. BRAF inhibitor dabrafenib in patients with metastatic-BRAF-mutant thyroid cancer. Thyroid. 2015;25:71–7.
27. Ho AL, Grewal RK, Leboeuf R, Sherman EJ, Pfister DG, Deandreis D, Pentlow KS, Zanzonico PB, Haque S, Gavane S, Ghossein RA, Ricarte-Filho JC, Domínguez JM, Shen R, Tuttle RM, Larson SM, Fagin JA. Selumetinib-enhanced radioiodine uptake in advanced thyroid cancer. N Engl J Med. 2013;368:623–32.
28. Rothenberg SM, McFadden DG, Palmer EL, Daniels GH, Wirth LJ. Redifferentiation of iodine-refractory BRAF V600E-mutant metastatic papillary thyroid cancer with dabrafenib. Clin Cancer Res. 2015;21:1028–35.

29. Caillou B, Talbot M, Weyemi U, Ayache J, Pioche-Durieu C, Al Ghuzlan A, Bidart JM, Chouaib S, Schlumberger M, Dupuy C. Tumor-associated macrophages (TAMs) form an interconnected cellular supportive network in anaplastic thyroid carcinoma. PLoS ONE. 2011;6(7):e22567.
30. Ryder M, Ghossein RA, Ricarte-Filho JC, Knauf JA, Fagin JA. Increased density of tumor-associated macrophages is associated with decreased survival in advanced thyroid cancer. Endocr Relat Cancer. 2008;15:1069–74.
31. Ryder M, Gild M, Hohl TM, Pamer E, Knauf J, Ghossein R, Joyce JA, Fagin JA. Genetic and pharmacological targeting of CSF-1/CSF-1R inhibits tumor-associated macrophages and impairs BRAF-induced thyroid cancer progression. PLoS ONE. 2013;8(1):e54302.
32. Ott PA, Hodi FS, Robert C. CTLA-4 and PD-1/PD-L1 blockade: new immunotherapeutic modalities with durable clinical benefit in melanoma patients. Clin Cancer Res. 2013;19:5300–9.
33. Angell TE, Lechner MG, Jang JK, Correa AJ, LoPresti JS, Epstein AL. BRAF V600E in papillary thyroid carcinoma is associated with increased programmed death ligand 1 expression and suppressive immune cell infiltration. Thyroid. 2014;24:1385–93.
34. Dadu R, Devine C, Hernandez M, Waguespack SG, Busaidy NL, Hu MI, Jimenez C, Habra MA, Sellin RV, Ying AK, Cote GJ, Sherman SI, Cabanillas ME. Role of salvage targeted therapy in differentiated thyroid cancer patients who failed first-line sorafenib. J Clin Endocrinol Metab. 2014;99:2086–94.

Chapter 32 RAI-Refractory Differentiated Thyroid Cancer with Multiple Organ Progressive Disease

Steven I. Sherman

Case Presentation

A 55-year-old woman presented to the clinic for consideration of treatment for progressive metastases from follicular thyroid carcinoma. She had undergone a total thyroidectomy and adjuvant radioiodine at age 47 for a 3.5 cm tumor. Given persistently abnormal serum thyroglobulin levels, she received two additional radioiodine treatments for a cumulative 131I therapeutic activity of 360 mCi, but her third posttreatment scan was negative. A chest computed tomography (CT) was then performed, which demonstrated several subcentimeter lung nodules bilaterally. Subsequent growth of these nodules led to resection of two from the left lung, with pathology consistent with metastatic follicular carcinoma. One year earlier, she received a fourth treatment with radioiodine, 210 mCi, with no uptake noted in multiple lung nodules that measured between 1 and 2 cm on chest CT. Although she denied symptoms from her lung metastases such as hemoptysis or dyspnea and her physical exam yielded no evidence of her malignancy, her most recent chest CT now showed lesions that were 30–40 % larger in diameter than the previous year. Her serum thyroglobulin level was 925 ng/mL, with a concurrent TSH of 0.01 mU/L.

S.I. Sherman, MD (✉)
University of Texas MD Anderson Cancer Center,
Unit 1461, 301402, Houston, TX 77230-1402, USA
e-mail: sisherma@mdanderson.org

D.S. Cooper, C. Durante (eds.), *Thyroid Cancer*,
DOI 10.1007/978-3-319-22401-5_32

Literature Review

For patients with metastatic DTC who progress despite surgery, radioiodine, and TSH-suppressive thyroid hormone, systemic chemotherapy historically provided limited benefit and considerable morbidity. More recent efforts to apply biologically targeted therapies have emerged as promising approaches for progressive, radioiodine-refractory differentiated thyroid carcinoma (RR-DTC), although side effects remain considerable and overall patient survival has not yet been demonstrated to improve with treatment.

Given that these systemic therapies for patients with progressive RR-DTC are not curative and can have significant toxicities, careful attention must be paid to appropriate patient selection for these treatments. The first priority is to identify which patients actually have "radioiodine-refractory" and "progressive" disease [1, 2]. Various definitions have been proposed for these characteristics, both in routine clinical practice as well as for eligibility criteria for clinical trials. An evolving standard is to combine scintigraphic imaging findings with clinical outcomes, defining radioiodine-refractory disease as meeting any of the following four criteria: (1) tumors that are structurally evident on radiographic imaging that demonstrate no uptake on postthyroidectomy radioiodine imaging; (2) tumors that previously concentrated radioiodine but no longer demonstrate uptake on subsequent scanning; (3) mixed uptake, visualizing radioiodine concentration in some lesions but not others; and (4) disease that progresses radiographically despite uptake of therapeutic radioiodine. Careful review of previous radioiodine imaging and preparation regimens must be performed before declaring a patient as "radioiodine refractory," as proper dietary iodine restriction and TSH stimulation need to be assured to avoid false-negative imaging results. Finally, patients may have metastatic disease that could benefit from further treatments with radioiodine, but in whom the potential toxicity of additional radioiodine on bone marrow, pulmonary or salivary function is considered excessive and therefore radioiodine is no longer a reasonable treatment option.

"Progression" of disease also requires careful definition. For purposes of identifying patients who should be considered candidates for therapy beyond radioiodine, a combination of the extent of metastatic disease, the rate of growth of that disease, and the potential for morbidity related to further tumor growth all need to be considered [1, 2]. The extent of disease and rate of tumor growth can be assessed standardly by applying response evaluation criteria in solid tumors (RECIST) to serial CT or magnetic resonance (MR) imaging. The number and locations of "measurable" lesions at least 1 cm in diameter can be recorded, and the rate of progression can be determined by the percentage increase in the sum of the longest diameters of a representative subset of measurable lesions over a period of time. An emerging convention defines progressive disease warranting consideration of further therapy as metastatic lesions measuring at least 1–2 cm, with the sum of diameters increasing by at least 20 % over a 12 to 15-month period or the appearance of significant new metastatic lesions. The presence or absence of symptoms or complications from metastatic disease may modify the assessment. For example, a patient with a critically located vertebral metastasis may not be optimally managed by expectant observation if a minimal degree of growth threatens vertebral collapse, pain, or neurologic compromise. Similarly, a patient with extensive micrometastatic pulmonary disease that is growing very rapidly may also be considered for systemic therapy before reaching the 1–2 cm threshold.

In the setting of a limited number of progressing lesions, localized therapy can be considered. For example, palliative stereotactic radiotherapy can be administered to a patient with a painful skeletal metastasis or an enlarging pulmonary metastasis compressing a bronchus with excellent symptomatic benefit [3]. Radiofrequency and cryoablation are also useful for a variety of metastatic lesions in both soft tissue and bone.

However, the patient with multiple measurable, progressive, radioiodine-refractory metastases in one or more organs should now be considered for systemic therapy, usually with an orally administered kinase inhibitor [1]. Various kinases have emerged as potentially valuable targets for such inhibition in the treatment of cancer. In particular, proangiogenic receptors, such as the vascular endothelial growth factor receptor (VEGFR), fibroblast growth factor receptor (FGFR), and c-MET, have been demonstrated to be effective targets in the surrounding tumor microenvironment for treatment of several solid malignancies. In addition to being proangiogenic, these receptor kinases also have been identified on tumor cells themselves, thus providing a positive feedback loop by which the tumor secretes the stimulatory ligand, e.g., VEGF, that is capable of binding to the cognate receptor on the tumor cell, e.g., VEGFR, whose kinase signals upstream of multiple pro-proliferative cascades. Other oncogenic kinases, such as BRAF, are commonly mutated in papillary thyroid carcinoma and offer a second opportunity to target the tumor cell's growth pathways.

At the time of this writing, two kinase inhibitors, sorafenib and lenvatinib, have regulatory approval in the United States and Europe for treatment of RR-DTC. Sorafenib is a multikinase inhibitor, targeting VEGFR, RET/PTC, RAF, and platelet-derived growth factor receptor β. Following phase II clinical trial experience that demonstrated significant activity of sorafenib in RR-DTC, an international randomized phase III trial was performed comparing sorafenib with placebo [4]. Eligible patients had demonstrated progressive RR-DTC within 14 months of enrollment and had never been previously treated with an anti-VEGFR therapy. The starting dose of sorafenib was 400 mg by mouth, twice daily, but most patients required dose reductions and/or treatment interruptions. Median progression-free survival was significantly prolonged in the sorafenib arm compared with the placebo arm, 10.8 months versus 5.8 months (hazard ratio 0.59, 95 % confidence interval 0.45–0.76; $p<0.0001$). The most common adverse events (in decreasing frequency) due to sorafenib were hand-foot skin reaction, diarrhea, alopecia, rash or desquamation, fatigue, weight loss, and hypertension. The phase III trial is still ongoing, assessing secondary outcomes including the effect of sorafenib on overall survival; however, a preliminary analysis failed to suggest a significant impact of sorafenib on overall survival.

A second multikinase inhibitor, lenvatinib, has also been studied in an international randomized phase III trial compared with placebo [5]. Lenvatinib, in addition to targeting VEGFR and RET/PTC, also potently inhibits FGFR and therefore is likely to be a stronger antagonist of angiogenesis. In the trial, eligible patients had demonstrated progressive RR-DTC within 13 months of enrollment but were permitted to have had up to one previous anti-VEGFR therapy such as sorafenib. The starting dose of lenvatinib was 24 mg by mouth, daily, but most patients required dose reductions and/or treatment interruptions. Median progression-free survival was markedly prolonged in the lenvatinib arm compared with placebo, 18.3 months versus 3.6 months (hazard ratio 0.21, 99 % confidence interval 0.14–0.31; $p<0.0001$). The magnitude of improvement in progression-free survival was identical in the subgroup of patients previously treated with an anti-VEGFR therapy. In addition, four patients experienced prolonged complete responses on lenvatinib. The most common adverse events (in decreasing frequency) due to lenvatinib were hypertension, diarrhea, fatigue, decreased appetite, nausea or vomiting, decreased weight, and stomatitis. The phase III trial is still ongoing, assessing secondary outcomes including the effect of lenvatinib on overall survival; a preliminary analysis suggested a minimal impact of lenvatinib on overall survival.

A third multitargeted kinase inhibitor, vandetanib, is currently undergoing a randomized phase III trial, following encouraging results in a randomized phase II study performed in multiple French centers [6]. One of the earliest oral multikinase inhibitors, vandetanib, targets VEGFR, RET/PTC, and the epidermal growth factor receptor (EGFR). In the trial, eligible patients were required to have measurable, metastatic RR-DTC, but progression was not required for enrollment; prior anti-VEGFR therapy was permitted. The starting dose of vandetanib was 300 mg by mouth, daily, but 22 % of patients required dose reductions to 300 mg on alternating days, and 38 % required treatment interruptions. Median progression-free survival was significantly longer in the vandetanib arm compared with placebo, 11.1 months versus 5.9 months (hazard ratio 0.49, 95 % confidence interval 0.32–0.74; $p=0.0007$). The most common adverse events (in decreasing frequency) due to vandetanib were diarrhea, hypertension, acne, asthenia, decreased appetite, nausea, and rash. Significant QT prolongation was experienced by 14 % of vandetanib-treated patients. No impact was seen from vandetanib on overall survival.

In addition to these three drugs, several other multitargeted kinase inhibitors have been reported in phase II trials to have promising activity in treating patients with progressive RR-DTC [1]. The antiangiogenic agents axitinib, pazopanib, and sunitinib are all VEGFR inhibitors that yielded up to 50 % partial response rates in limited phase II trials. Pazopanib, which may have particular potency in treating follicular and Hurthle cell carcinomas, is under study in an ongoing randomized phase III trial in Europe.

Given the common mechanism of action among all of these multitargeted kinase inhibitors of blocking VEGFR, it might be assumed that the development of resistance to one drug would portend lack of response to another in the group. In fact, cross-resistance does not appear to occur, and patients who progress during therapy with one anti-VEGFR therapy can often be successfully treated with another [5, 7].

Given a 53 % partial response rate among all patients treated with cabozantinib (which targets VEGFR, c-MET, and RET/PTC) and a 45 % rate among patients previously treated with anti-VEGFR therapy, a phase II trial is underway studying cabozantinib specifically as second-line therapy after progression with previous anti-VEGFR agents.

In addition to the multitargeted kinase inhibitors that likely primarily affect the tumor microenvironment, more selective targeting of intracellular kinases critical to tumor proliferation is a developing approach to treatment of progressive RR-DTC. Patients whose tumors contain activating mutations in *BRAF* have been treated with selective BRAF kinase inhibitors. Using vemurafenib, which is highly selective for the V600E mutant BRAF kinase, a 35 % response rate and 15.6-month progression-free survival were reported in patients with BRAF-mutant RR-DTC [8]; similar findings were also reported using a slightly less selective BRAF inhibitor, dabrafenib. By inhibiting signaling through a second, anti-apoptotic pathway, the mTOR inhibitor everolimus has also been shown to be active in RR-DTC, particularly in Hurthle cell tumors.

A very exciting and novel application of selective kinase inhibitors has been the attempt to "redifferentiate" RR-DTC. As first suggested in preclinical models, inhibition of signaling through the mitogen-activated protein kinase (MAPK) pathway may allow restoration of sensitivity to radioiodine therapy. This hypothesis has been supported by two recent pilot trials, in which patients with RR-DTC were treated with either the MEK inhibitor selumetinib in one study and the BRAF inhibitor dabrafenib in the other. In both studies, about half of patients acquired significant radioiodine uptake in metastases previously demonstrated to lack uptake, and a subset experienced partial response after therapeutic radioiodine administration. Numerous clinical trials are now underway attempting to expand the application of this paradigm.

Cytotoxic chemotherapy has been used since the late 1960s in advanced DTC but with little enthusiasm given early reports of limited efficacy and high toxicity [9]. Monotherapy with agents such as doxorubicin, cisplatin, or bleomycin yield very few responses that are of limited durability. A randomized trial compared the combination of doxorubicin and cisplatin with doxorubicin. Of the patients with metastatic DTC, complete or partial response was seen in 16 % with combination therapy, whereas 31 % had partial response with doxorubicin monotherapy. Notably, the two complete responses seen in the combination therapy arm lasted 33 and 40 months, respectively. The combination of epirubicin and carboplatin yielded similar outcomes, though it was suggested in one study that pre-chemotherapy administration of recombinant human TSH might increase the therapeutic efficacy of the regimen.

Bone metastases often lead to considerable morbidity and increased risk for death. As first suggested with metastatic breast carcinoma, osteoclast inhibitors such as bisphosphonates may reduce the frequency of skeletal-related events (SRE) such as fracture and improve pain control from bone metastases. A retrospective study reported that monthly infusions of zoledronic acid, 4 mg, improved 3-year SRE-free rates 50–86 %, compared with no bisphosphonate treatment [10]. It remains to be reported whether thyroid cancer bone metastases respond to the anti-osteoclast monoclonal antibody denosumab, which also approved for reduction of SREs from solid tumor bone metastases.

Management of the Case

The patient had developed clear evidence of progressive RR-DTC, having had two posttreatment radioiodine scans with no uptake in growing, macronodular lung metastases that were proven to be metastatic disease. However, at that time, the only available treatments other than cytotoxic chemotherapy were investigational multitargeted kinase inhibitors. After extensive discussion about the risks and benefits of treatment in a clinical trial, she was enrolled in a phase II study of sorafenib. Her metastatic disease initially stabilized, but she eventually progressed in hilar lymph nodes and a new painful left iliac bone metastasis after 16 months. The bone lesion was treated with external beam radiotherapy, and zoledronic acid infusions were initiated, 4 mg every 3 months. Sunitinib, which had been approved for renal cell carcinoma, was then started. Considerable treatment related toxicity required frequent dose adjustment, but disease remained stable for nearly 4 years. With sudden marked elevation of her serum thyroglobulin levels, imaging revealed development of two hepatic lesions measuring 3 and 4 cm, respectively. These were treated with radiofrequency ablation, and additional radiotherapy was administered to a sacral metastasis. Her disease continued to progress despite three additional regimens in the next 2 years, particularly with multifocal bone lesions involving the calvarium, spine, and pelvis. Zoledronic acid was replaced with denosumab, and cabozantinib was initiated given initial reports of pronounced efficacy against bone metastases. Therapy was complicated by diarrhea, skin rash, fatigue, and weight loss requiring dose reduction and symptom management, but her skeletal lesions stabilized, her intrathoracic and supraclavicular nodes regressed, and she developed no new metastatic foci during 2 years of cabozantinib therapy at 100 mg by mouth daily. After 9 years of nearly continuous treatment with multitargeted kinase inhibitors and antiresorptive therapies, her performance status is excellent, and she continues to travel extensively while enjoying retirement.

Clinical Pearls

- Careful review of radioiodine imaging, clinical responses to radioiodine therapy, and serial tomographic imaging is necessary to identify patients with progressive, radioiodine-refractory DTC.
- Antiangiogenic multitargeted kinase inhibitors prolong progression-free survival and lead to frequent tumor shrinkage and partial responses, but evidence of improvement in overall survival remains lacking.

- Toxicities of multitargeted kinase inhibitors are considerable but usually can be addressed by careful symptom management and dose modification.
- As a rapidly evolving area of therapy, further results from ongoing clinical trials will likely continue to change clinical practice paradigms in the near future.

References

1. Haugen BR, Sherman SI. Evolving approaches to patients with advanced differentiated thyroid cancer. Endocr Rev. 2013;34:439–55.
2. Harris PJ, Bible KC. Emerging therapeutics for advanced thyroid malignancies: rationale and targeted approaches. Expert Opin Investig Drugs. 2011;20:1357–75.
3. Janjan N, Lutz ST, Bedwinek JM, Hartsell WF, Ng A, Pieters Jr RS, et al. Therapeutic guidelines for the treatment of bone metastasis: a report from the American college of radiology appropriateness criteria expert panel on radiation oncology. J Palliat Med. 2009;12:417–26.
4. Brose MS, Nutting CM, Jarzab B, Elisei R, Siena S, Bastholt L, et al. Sorafenib in radioactive iodine-refractory, locally advanced or metastatic differentiated thyroid cancer: a randomised, double-blind, phase 3 trial. Lancet. 2014;384:319–28.
5. Schlumberger M, Tahara M, Wirth LJ, Robinson B, Brose MS, Elisei R, et al. Lenvatinib versus placebo in radioiodine-refractory thyroid cancer. New Engl J Med. 2015;372:621–30.
6. Leboulleux S, Bastholt L, Krause T, de la Fouchardiere C, Tennvall J, Awada A, et al. Vandetanib in locally advanced or metastatic differentiated thyroid cancer: a randomised, double-blind, phase 2 trial. Lancet Oncol. 2012;13:897–905.
7. Dadu R, Devine C, Hernandez M, Waguespack SG, Busaidy NL, Hu MI, et al. Role of salvage targeted therapy in differentiated thyroid cancer patients who failed first-line sorafenib. J Clin Endocrinol Metab. 2014;99:2086–94.
8. Brose MS, Cabanillas ME, Cohen EEW, Wirth L, Sherman SI, Riehl T, et al. An open-label, multi-center phase 2 study of the BRAF inhibitor vemurafenib in patients with metastatic or unresectable papillary thyroid cancer (PTC) positive for the BRAF V600 mutation. ECCO/ESMO/ESTRO annual meeting, Amsterdam; 2013.
9. Sherman SI. Cytotoxic chemotherapy for differentiated thyroid carcinoma. Clin Oncol (R Coll Radiol). 2010;22:464–8.
10. Orita Y, Sugitani I, Toda K, Manabe J, Fujimoto Y. Zoledronic acid in the treatment of bone metastases from differentiated thyroid carcinoma. Thyroid. 2011;21:31–5.

Chapter 33
RAI-Refractory Differentiated Thyroid Cancer and Lung Lesions Causing Bleeding

Steven I. Sherman

Case Presentation

A 74-year-old woman presented for her routine follow-up noting recent development of a cough productive of blood-tinged sputum for the past 3 months, not associated with fever, shortness of breath, chest pain, or other systemic symptoms. By her report, she averaged about one to two teaspoons of bloody sputum each morning. Her past history is notable for a 3 cm, locally invasive, poorly differentiated carcinoma of the thyroid, treated with total thyroidectomy 6 years previously. Adjuvant radioiodine, 150 mCi, had been administered, with post-therapy scan uptake noted only in the thyroid bed. Two additional radioiodine treatments had been given during the next 2 years, 180 and 200 mCi, respectively, with concurrent stimulated thyroglobulin levels of about 20 ng/mL, but no pathologic uptake had been noted on post-therapy imaging. One month after her third radioiodine treatment, computed tomography (CT) scans had been performed, demonstrating extensive metastatic adenopathy in bilateral and central neck compartments and bilateral subcentimeter pulmonary nodules. Following a bilateral, central, and mediastinal neck dissection and postoperative adjuvant external beam radiotherapy, her TSH-suppressed serum thyroglobulin level had declined to 2 ng/mL. She had remained clinically and radiographically stable for the intervening 3 years until her current presentation with hemoptysis, although the serum thyroglobulin had risen to 88 ng/mL at her last evaluation 6 months ago. Examination of her upper airway including indirect laryngoscopy demonstrated no focal lesions or bleeding, there were no masses palpated in the neck, and her lungs were clear to percussion and auscultation. With an undetectable serum TSH, her thyroglobulin level was 2241 ng/mL. A CT scan demonstrated

S.I. Sherman, MD (✉)
University of Texas MD Anderson Cancer Center,
Unit 1461, 301402, Houston, TX 77230-1402, USA
e-mail: sisherma@mdanderson.org

D.S. Cooper, C. Durante (eds.), *Thyroid Cancer*,
DOI 10.1007/978-3-319-22401-5_33

an enlarging 1.6 cm pulmonary nodule in the left upper lobe and a 2.5 cm left lower paratracheal mass, along with numerous subcentimeter lung nodules that were unchanged compared with previous imaging studies.

Literature Review

Hemoptysis is commonly a distressing presenting symptom of intrathoracic disease, both benign and malignant [1]. Among patients without a known diagnosis of malignancy who present with mild hemoptysis (defined as blood-tinged or streaked sputum, blood clots, or <20 mL of blood expectorated within 24 h), most will have nonmalignant etiologies of hemoptysis including bronchitis, pneumonia, bronchiectasis, or heart failure [2]. Rarer causes of hemoptysis which also require consideration include pulmonary embolism, vascular malformations, vasculitic disorders, coagulopathies, and immunologic diseases, although many of these conditions are more likely to cause larger amounts of acute bleeding or life-threatening massive hemoptysis [1]. However, in the setting of a preexisting diagnosis of non-hematologic malignancy, fewer than 10 % will be found to have a benign cause of hemoptysis [3]. About half will have primary lung carcinoma, whereas the other half will have metastases from non-thoracic primary malignancies. When an endobronchial lesion is identified by bronchoscopy, carcinomas of the breast, colorectum, kidney, and larynx and melanoma are the most common primaries, whereas thyroid carcinoma accounts for only a few percent of reported cases [2–4]. Upper airway causes of bleeding also need to be considered, including intraluminal invasion of a malignancy of the head and neck and rarer complications of cancer therapy such as a tracheoesophageal fistula after radiation or antiangiogenic therapy.

Given this differential diagnosis, a patient with differentiated thyroid carcinoma (DTC) who develops hemoptysis requires a diagnostic evaluation before planning treatment [1]. The amount of bleeding should be assessed and the risk for hemodynamic compromise considered. Medications should be reviewed for use of anticoagulants, aspirin, and nonsteroidal anti-inflammatory drugs that increase bleeding risk. Given the amount of blood that can be lost either acutely or chronically, blood hematocrit and hemoglobin should be determined along with coagulation parameters. Computed tomography should be performed and compared with any available previous imaging studies to identify new or changing lesions, whereas chest X-ray has a very low sensitivity for identifying the etiology of hemoptysis. Combining chest CT with flexible bronchoscopy maximizes the likelihood of detecting endobronchial metastases [3, 4]. Once a suspicious lesion is visualized by bronchoscopy, a biopsy can be obtained if it is necessary to determine the histology of the tumor; alternatively, transthoracic biopsy (either CT-guided needle biopsy or an excisional procedure) can also be performed if bronchoscopic biopsy is not feasible or unsuccessful. Bronchoscopic findings may also facilitate rapid prognostication. Among patients with solid tumors and hemoptysis, bronchoscopic detection of both active bleeding and an endobronchial lesion portends a worse prognosis with a median survival of 3.5 months, compared with 66 months for those with neither active bleeding nor endobronchial lesion visualized [3]; however, whether this analysis specifically applies to DTC is unknown.

Therapeutic options for hemoptysis from metastatic DTC include bronchoscopic modalities such as argon plasma coagulation (APC) or Nd-yttrium laser resection, surgery, radiotherapy, and occasionally systemic therapy. During bronchoscopic APC, brief jets of ionized argon gas are aimed at the targeted endobronchial lesion, creating sufficient heat to coagulate and destroy the tumor tissue [5]. APC causes immediate and durable cessation of bleeding and can significantly relieve symptoms due to obstruction from endobronchial lesions. Nd-yttrium laser therapy causes photocoagulation of tumor vessels, also provides rapid relief of symptoms, and facilitates precise cutting of endotracheal and endobronchial lesions. However, the Nd-yttrium laser is considerably more expensive than the equipment required for APC [6]. Neither APC nor laser resection is appropriate for patients whose bleeding lesions are primarily intramural or peribronchial, as the risks of luminal perforation are considerable and bronchoscopic visualization of the target lesion is obviously required.

Surgical metastasectomy can be considered in patients who are inappropriate for bronchoscopic therapy but who have good performance status, sufficient pulmonary function anticipated following partial lung resection, and at least 6 months expected survival assuming local control of the cause of the hemoptysis [7]. Operative resection is usually reserved for patients in whom a complete resection of the local disease can be anticipated, and the longest survival among solid tumor patients who undergo lung metastasectomy is associated with surgery for curative intent followed by at least a 3-year disease-free interval [7]. However, palliative metastasectomy has been reported to be of symptomatic value for many patients, including those with metastatic DTC [8]. Even in the setting of residual metastatic disease following an initial surgical metastasectomy, the 5-year survival rate was more than 60 % [8].

Stereotactic radiosurgery (SRS) may also be used to control intrathoracic lesions causing hemoptysis up to 4 cm in diameter [9]. By delivering a highly targeted intense dose of high-energy radiation, SRS is capable of selectively destroying metastatic lesions that are thought to be causing hemoptysis. Synchronization of radiation delivery with the breath cycle is optimal to minimize radiation dose to surrounding uninvolved lung tissue, but this allows lesions to be safely treated in both the central as well as peripheral lung fields. Data regarding use in DTC are lacking, however. Radiofrequency ablation is another localized technique that can be employed for palliative treatment of lung metastases, although its precise application to DTC patients with hemoptysis has not been reported [10].

The systemic therapies available for use in symptomatic metastatic radioiodine-refractory DTC are primarily antiangiogenic, such as sorafenib. Bleeding complications and hemoptysis were reported in early trials of antiangiogenic therapies for intrathoracic malignancies, although they had primarily involved the anti-VEGF antibody bevacizumab in the treatment of squamous cell carcinomas in the central chest. More extensive analyses of antiangiogenic multitargeted kinase inhibitors have reduced but not completely eliminated concern for exacerbation of hemoptysis.

Alternatively, selective kinase inhibitors that have not been implicated as increasing bleeding risk, such as BRAF inhibitors, may be of benefit for patients with intrathoracic metastases causing hemoptysis.

Management of the Case

Given the possibility that the patient's hemoptysis could be arising from either her new lower paratracheal adenopathy or her enlarging left upper lobe nodule, flexible bronchoscopy was performed. The tracheal mucosa was intact, without evidence of tumor invasion or bleeding. However, fresh blood was seen within a branch off the left main stem bronchus arising from the upper lobe, suggesting a more distal source of the bleeding compatible with the enlarging mass. A median sternotomy was performed, allowing a wedge resection of the left upper lobe. In addition, metastatic adenopathy was identified encasing the recurrent laryngeal nerve but not invading the trachea, and this was successfully resected as well. Pathology confirmed metastatic poorly DTC in the metastasectomy specimens. Four months later, her TSH-suppressed serum thyroglobulin level was 5 ng/mL, and at her last follow-up 3 years after metastasectomy, she remained clinically and radiographically stable.

Clinical Pearls

- Hemoptysis is an uncommon symptom of intrathoracic metastases from radioiodine-refractory DTC.
- Careful clinical assessment is required to rule out other contributing causes of hemoptysis.
- CT scanning and flexible bronchoscopy are optimally combined to localize the cause of hemoptysis secondary to metastatic disease and to identify appropriate therapeutic options.
- Bronchoscopic treatment with argon plasma coagulation or Nd-yttrium laser is appropriate when the bleeding lesion is visualized through bronchoscopy.
- Surgical metastasectomy may be considered for palliative therapy when bronchoscopic treatment is not feasible.

References

1. Larici AR, Franchi P, Occhipinti M, Contegiacomo A, del Ciello A, Calandriello L, et al. Diagnosis and management of hemoptysis. Diagn Interv Radiol. 2014;20:299–309.
2. Hirshberg B, Biran I, Glazer M, Kramer MR. Hemoptysis: etiology, evaluation, and outcome in a tertiary referral hospital. Chest. 1997;112:440–4.

3. Grosu HB, Casal RF, Morice RC, Nogueras-Gonzalez GM, Eapen GA, Ost D, et al. Bronchoscopic findings and bleeding control predict survival in patients with solid malignancies presenting with mild hemoptysis. Ann Am Thorac Soc. 2013;10:342–9.
4. Marchioni A, Lasagni A, Busca A, Cavazza A, Agostini L, Migaldi M, et al. Endobronchial metastasis: an epidemiologic and clinicopathologic study of 174 consecutive cases. Lung Cancer. 2014;84:222–8.
5. Morice RC, Ece T, Ece F, Keus L. Endobronchial argon plasma coagulation for treatment of hemoptysis and neoplastic airway obstruction. Chest. 2001;119:781–7.
6. Freitag L. Interventional endoscopic treatment. Lung Cancer. 2004;45 Suppl 2:S235–8.
7. Pfannschmidt J, Egerer G, Bischof M, Thomas M, Dienemann H. Surgical intervention for pulmonary metastases. Dtsch Arztebl Int. 2012;109:645–51.
8. Pak H, Gourgiotis L, Chang WI, Guthrie LC, Skarulis MC, Reynolds JC, et al. Role of metastasectomy in the management of thyroid carcinoma: the NIH experience. J Surg Oncol. 2003;82:10–8.
9. Abbas G, Schuchert MJ, Pennathur A, Gilbert S, Luketich JD. Ablative treatments for lung tumors: radiofrequency ablation, stereotactic radiosurgery, and microwave ablation. Thorac Surg Clin. 2007;17:261–71.
10. Lencioni R, Crocetti L, Cioni R, Suh R, Glenn D, Regge D, et al. Response to radiofrequency ablation of pulmonary tumours: a prospective, intention-to-treat, multicentre clinical trial (the RAPTURE study). Lancet Oncol. 2008;9:621–8.

Chapter 34
A Patient with Follicular Thyroid Cancer and a Painful Bone Metastases at Risk for Pathologic Fracture

Désirée Deandreis

Case Presentation

A 56-year-old man was referred to the Gustave Roussy Institute for management of bone metastases from follicular thyroid cancer, which had been diagnosed before the primary thyroid tumor. Because of thoracic pain, a computed tomography (CT) scan had been performed and revealed a 4 cm lytic lesion of the third left rib. The CT scan showed also a 6 cm left thyroid mass and small lung nodules that were less than 1 cm in diameter. A biopsy of the rib lesion showed a metastasis from a well-differentiated follicular thyroid cancer. A 18fluorodeoxyglucose positron emission tomography (^{18}FDG PET)/CT scan showed uptake in the thyroid tumor [maximum standardized uptake value (SUVmax) of 6] and in the rib lesion (SUVmax: 3.4) and no significant uptake in multiple lung lesions (SUVmax: 1.1) (Fig. 34.1). Furthermore, a lytic lesion of the right ischium was visible on the CT scan component, but it did not disclose FDG uptake. Blood tests showed thyroglobulin (Tg) level at 7979 ng/ml with no detectable anti-Tg antibodies.

A total thyroidectomy and central neck dissection were performed. Final histology showed a polymorphic thyroid cancer measuring 10 cm with poorly differentiated areas, 6 mitoses $\times$ 2 mm^2, Ki 67 15 %, and several foci of necrosis. Due to massive extrathyroidal extension, the tumor was classified as pT4. No metastatic lymph nodes were found (N0). Two months after surgery, the patient received 100 mCi (3.7 GBq) of radioactive iodine (^{131}I) after thyroid hormone withdrawal for 4 weeks. Thyroglobulin level was 3726 ng/ml with a TSH level of 35 mIU/l. Post-therapy whole-body (WB) scan showed high ^{131}I uptake in the thyroid remnants and diffuse uptake not only in the lung and in the rib lesion but also in T8 and

D. Deandreis, MD (✉)
Nuclear Medicine and Endocrine Oncology,
Gustave Roussy, Villejuif 94805, France
e-mail: desiree.deandreis@gustaveroussy.fr

D.S. Cooper, C. Durante (eds.), *Thyroid Cancer*,
DOI 10.1007/978-3-319-22401-5_34

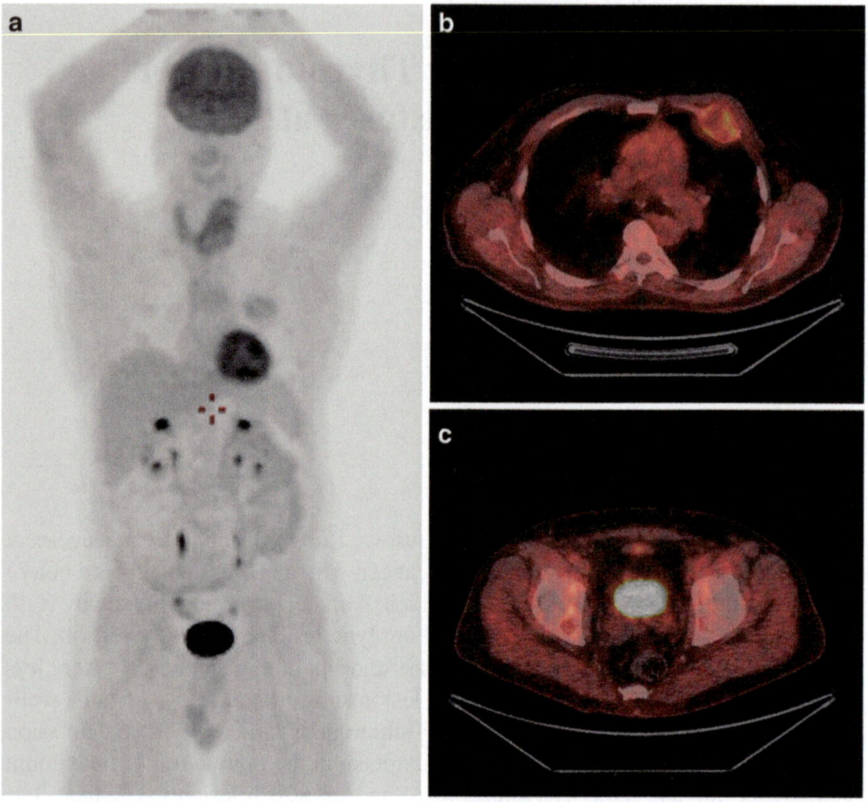

Fig. 34.1 ^{18}Fluorodeoxyglucose positron emission tomography (^{18}FDG PET)/CT scan performed at initial staging. (**a**) ^{18}FDG PET/CT whole-body maximum intensity projection (MIP) showing uptake in 6 cm left lobe thyroid cancer (SUVmax: 6) and in the third left rib (SUVmax: 3.4) corresponding to a 4 cm lytic lesion. There was no significant FDG uptake in multiple lung nodules of few millimeters diameter. (**b**) Axial fusion image showing high FDG uptake in the third left rib lesion. (**c**) Axial fusion image showing no significant FDG uptake in the right ischial lesion

right iliac bone lesions. Furthermore, ^{131}I single-photon emission tomography (SPECT)/CT scan detected three other bone lesions in the spine (C4 and L1) and in the pelvis (left iliac bone), respectively, not visible on WB scan (Fig. 34.2a, b). On the CT component, the rib and the ischial lesions both appeared as lytic lesions of 4 cm and 2.3 cm, respectively, while there was no evidence of bone lesions in the other bone ^{131}I foci. In particular, the ischial lesion showed cortical lysis with risk of fracture (Fig. 34.2c–e). Cryoablation for the rib lesion and cryoablation plus cementoplasty for the ischial lesion were performed. During local treatment, a biopsy of the ischial lesion was performed and was consistent with well-differentiated thyroid cancer.

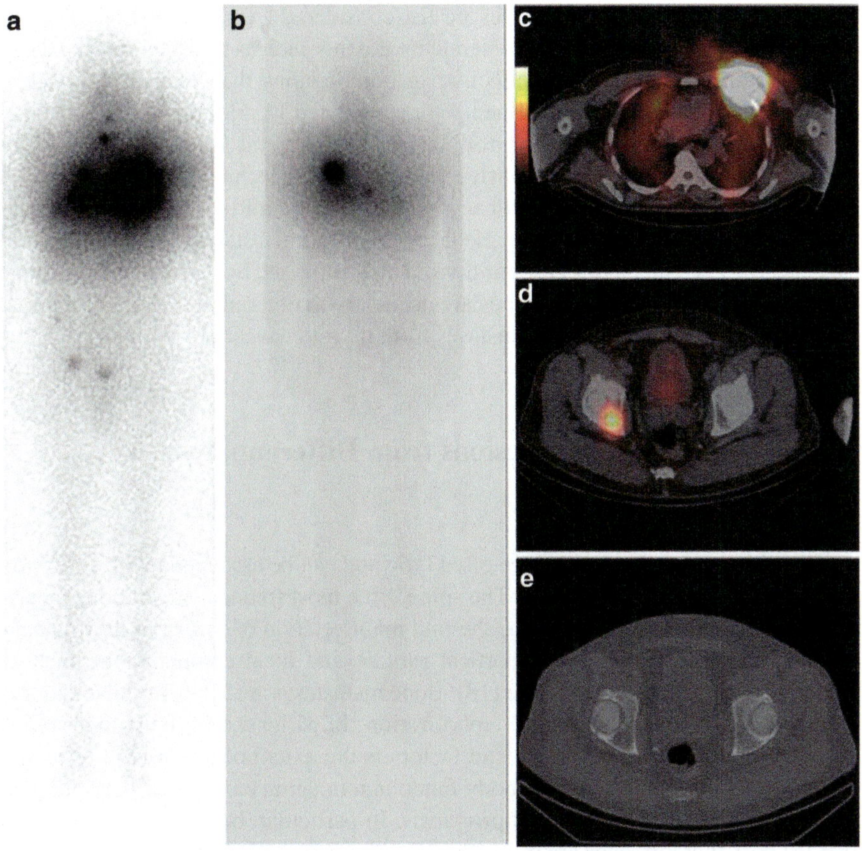

Fig. 34.2 ^{131}I post-therapy whole-body (WB) scan after administration of 100 mCi (3.7 GBq) after thyroid hormone withdrawal for 4 weeks. (**a**, **b**) Anterior and posterior view showing high 131I uptake in the third left rib lesion, in the right ischial lesion, and in the spine T8 and a diffuse uptake in the lung. (**c**) Axial fusion image (SPECT/CT) showing high ^{131}I uptake in the third left rib. (**d**) Axial fusion image (SPECT/CT) showing high ^{131}I uptake in the right ischium. (**e**) Axial image of CT component of SPECT/CT showing a 23 mm lytic lesion in the right ischium

Assessment and Literature Review

Bone metastases occur in less than 5 % of patients with thyroid cancer and are often a cause of morbidity from local pain, fracture, and neurological complications [1]. The median reported overall survival in case of bone metastases is 2–4 years after their diagnosis, but may range from 96 % at 10 years in young patients (<45 years) without radiological abnormalities to less than 10 % in older patients with multiple lesions and radiological abnormalities [1–3]. In the presence of ^{131}I uptake in the metastases, ^{131}I is used as first-line treatment [4]. Although ^{131}I may eradicate small metastases, it is poorly effective at treating large metastases, and in such cases, local treatment modalities are also considered. In patients with radioactive iodine refractory thyroid cancer, systemic treatments such as tyrosine-kinase inhibitors or chemotherapy are less effective in bone lesions than in treating visceral metastases, and again, local treatments are considered [4, 5]. Data on the management of bone metastases from thyroid cancer are rare and focused on surgery or radiotherapy [6–9]. Minimally invasive thermal ablation techniques show promising results in terms of pain control, efficacy in local tumor control, and lesion stabilization in case of fracture risk in patients with bone metastases from non-thyroid cancers [10–13]. Only a few cases of thyroid cancer treated by thermal ablation have been reported, and additional studies are necessary to determine the role of thermal ablation in patients with bone metastases from thyroid cancer [14–16].

Characteristics of Bone Lesions from Differentiated Thyroid Cancer

Thyroid cancer bone lesions are often lytic and can be associated with extension into surrounding soft tissues [17]. The spine is the most frequent site of bone metastases, and spinal metastases can be the first manifestation of follicular thyroid cancer [17, 18]. The major risk is cortical rupture and local complications such as medullary compression or fracture [18]. Bone metastases are often vascular and this pattern makes them accessible to embolization. In patients with bone metastases, one of the most important prognostic factors is the extent of the disease (size and number of lesions) [1, 2]. Whole-body functional imaging can give important information on the patient's stage and prognosis. In particular, both FDG PET/CT and WB ^{131}I post-therapy scans are recommended to stage metastatic patients at the time of diagnosis, as they will provide important information for both prognosis and therapy. Bone lesions are frequently FDG avid due to their vascularity and concomitant inflammatory bone reaction. High FDG uptake in distant metastases is a negative prognostic parameter and a negative predictive factor for response to radioactive iodine [19–22]. However in most differentiated tumors, WB ^{131}I post-therapy scan can show radioactive iodine uptake in small lesions that are not visualized on cross-sectional imaging. In addition to ^{131}I scans and FDG/PET CT, magnetic resonance imaging (MRI) is useful to evaluate the presence of local complications and medullary compression, which can help to plan radiotherapy.

Treating Bone Metastases with Radioactive Iodine

Radioactive iodine administration is recommended to explore ^{131}I avidity of distant metastases, to stage the disease, and to treat ^{131}I-avid distant metastases [4]. Two thirds of patients with distant metastases show radioactive iodine uptake, and complete response is achieved in around 40 % of these cases with initial RAI therapy, especially in case of young patients with ^{131}I-avid micrometastases without correlates on cross-sectional imaging [1]. The prognostic value of radioactive iodine uptake in patients with bone metastases has been reported [7]. Young patients with small or single bone lesions or with bone ^{131}I uptake but with no lesion visualized on CT can be treated by repeated ^{131}I administrations [2, 23]. The number of ^{131}I treatments and administered activity varies depending on institutional protocols. On the other hand, ^{131}I is not sufficient for large or multiple bone lesions and local treatment may be warranted.

In patients with distant metastases, ^{18}FDG PET/CT has to be correlated with ^{131}I treatment, especially at initial staging, to evaluate FDG uptake in distant lesions and to predict response to therapy. Patients with FDG-avid and no ^{131}I-avid distant metastases have rapidly progressive disease. In contrast, patients with ^{131}I-avid and FDG-negative lesions have a much better prognosis. Patients with both FDG and ^{131}I uptake in the same lesions or FDG and ^{131}I uptake in different lesions represent a very heterogeneous group, but their prognosis seems similar to the group with only FDG uptake.

Indications and Options of Local Treatment

In case of symptomatic lesions, fracture, local compression, or spinal neurological damage, surgery is the first therapeutic choice [8]. If complete and curative surgery can be achieved, this may improve patient survival, especially in young patients [7–9]. External beam radiation therapy has been used in association with surgery for pain palliation, but stereotactic radiotherapy is becoming a very promising technique in spinal tumors as a selective and curative treatment of bone metastases [6, 24]. Some cases of vascular embolization by polyvinyl alcohol particles have also been reported with effective and immediate pain relief after treatment [25]. Vascular embolization is routinely performed before surgery to limit bleeding. In cases of limited bone lesions without soft tissue involvement but symptomatic or at risk of fracture, local thermal ablation by radiofrequency ablation (RFA) or cryotherapy is currently used more and more frequently. These techniques are preferred to other local treatment modalities because they are well tolerated, they are minimally invasive, and they can be repeated in the same patient together with cementoplasty for lesion stabilization [13]. All local treatments can be used in association with systemic treatments, such as radioactive iodine, if the lesions are ^{131}I avid or TKIs in the case of radioactive iodine refractory cancer.

Principles and Definition of Thermal Ablation

The principle of thermal ablation action is coagulative tissue necrosis by heating a tumor with high temperature (radiofrequency ablation) or freezing it with pressurized gas (cryoablation) [26, 27]. The main effects are intracellular, vascular, and interstitial damage causing cell apoptosis. Radiofrequency ablation and cryoablation are currently the most frequently used percutaneous minimally invasive techniques, but other options such as high-intensity focused ultrasound (HIFU), irreversible electroporation, or laser ablation are evolving [28]. The selective action is achieved by inserting needles (RFA) or cryoprobes (cryoablation) under imaging guidance during the procedure. After thermal ablation of soft tissue lesions, progressive lesion shrinkage can be monitored with imaging (CT or MRI) with a fibrotic scar as final result. In some patients, ^{18}FDG PET/CT can be more sensitive in the detection of persistent disease or disease relapse earlier than anatomical imaging [29]. In contrast, the response to thermal ablation in bone lesions is more difficult to evaluate because frequently there are no changes in size or volume of treated lesions on cross-sectional imaging. In patients with bone lesions at risk for fracture due to metastases in the spine or in femoral region, percutaneous cementoplasty with cement injection can be used together with thermal ablation to stabilize the bone and for an analgesic effect [30]. Finally, screws can be also inserted percutaneously in lesions with high risk of fracture to consolidate the bone.

Thermal Ablation for Treatment of Bone Metastases

Thermal ablation has been used for several years for treating benign bone tumors and for palliation of bone metastases. The first cases examining the feasibility of percutaneous ablation and cementoplasty efficacy in treating bone metastases were reported in 1995–2000 [31–33]. In particular, these techniques have been reported as safe and effective in reducing pain and in stabilizing lesion preventing skeletal events in bone metastases [31–33]. More recently, some investigators demonstrated efficacy as curative treatment in bone metastases from solid tumors other than thyroid cancer [10, 12, 13]. In particular, Deschamps et al. evaluated the rate of complete response to thermal ablation in 89 patients with 122 bone metastases from solid tumor. The 1-year complete treatment rate was 67 %. Oligometastatic status, metachronous metastases, and small lesions without cortical bone erosion or surrounding neurological structures were all predictive factors on multivariate analysis [13]. Only a few cases with bone metastases from differentiated thyroid cancer treated with thermal ablation have been reported. All cases showed good local control with improvement of patient quality of life after the procedure. In addition to being a palliative treatment for symptomatic lesions, percutaneous ablation may also be curative in patients with localized lesions, with a favorable impact on patient survival. In three patients with bone metastases from differentiated thyroid cancer treated by RFA in association with radioactive iodine, two of three patients with lesions of 30 and 50 mm were free of disease 44 and 53 months, respectively, after ablation [14]. In one case, two repeated RF ablation treatments at 12-month intervals were necessary to achieve complete tumor regression. The third patient showed disease progression 9 months after treatment. In eight patients with symptomatic spinal metastases from thyroid cancer, treatment included a surgical approach in the case of spinal compression or percutaneous vertebroplasty associated with systemic treatment (radioactive iodine or chemotherapy). The authors confirmed that local treatment can improve patients' quality of life by reducing pain and prolonging time to skeletal events, especially spinal cord compression, and can delay initiation of systemic treatment. Finally, local treatment can improve patient survival, with a median survival reported in this paper of 50 months after treatment [16].

Further studies are needed to evaluate the efficacy and the impact of thermal ablation on prognosis. Preliminary results show that FDG PET/CT scan can be a useful tool for treatment follow-up also in bone lesions [34].

Thermal Ablation on Metastatic Sites Other Than Bone

Thermal ablation can also be performed for liver and lung metastases. Clinical trials show high efficacy of RFA on liver lesions from solid tumors, with local control equivalent to surgical resection ranging from 40 to 80 %, and a prolonged overall survival in treated patients [35, 36]. In neuroendocrine tumors, treatment of liver lesions by thermal ablation is now considered an alternative to surgery, especially when there is a small number of lesions of small diameter (< to 3 cm) [37]. A few cases of liver metastases from thyroid cancer treated by thermal ablation have been reported. In three patients with liver metastases from thyroid cancer (two medullary thyroid cancer and one follicular thyroid cancer) treated by RFA, thermal ablation reduced local symptoms due to hepatic capsular compression [38].

In a clinical trial focused on lung lesions, RFA was both effective and well tolerated, with a high complete tumor control rate (93 %) at 18 months in 100 analyzed lung lesions, including primary lung tumors and distant metastases from solid tumors [39]. Another multicenter prospective trial including 183 lung metastases showed again a high complete response rate (88 %) at 1 year and an overall survival of 92 % and 64 % at 1 year and at 2 years, respectively [40]. In all clinical trials, lesion size and lesion location are reported as the most important predictive factors of response. In particular, recurrence occurs more frequently in lesions >3 cm with soft tissue or mediastinal invasion and if the lesion is in contact with large vessels [39]. FDG PET/CT is a useful tool to evaluate response to treatment and to detect early relapse of disease when the lesions have FDG uptake on a baseline FDG PET/CT [29].

Denosumab and Bisphosphonates

To treat bone lesions, some systemic specific bone agents such as bisphosphonates and more recently the anti-RANK agent denosumab have demonstrated efficacy in reducing skeletal events in patients with bone metastases from prostate or breast cancer [41]. A beneficial effect of these agents has also been reported in patients with lytic lesions from other solid tumors such as lung, renal cell, or myeloma due to inhibition of osteoclast action. In particular, a beneficial effect of zoledronic acid treatment in terms of fewer and delayed skeletal events has been reported in some patients with bone lesions from thyroid cancer, leading to consideration of this drug as a valid therapeutic option [42]. On the other hand, no data are available on denosumab's efficacy on bone lesions from thyroid cancer, although it is a promising and potentially more effective therapy than zoledronic acid in other tumors [43]. They both may be useful in the case of disseminated and progressive bone metastases. Bisphosphonates and denosumab are administered monthly by intravenous or subcutaneous injection, respectively, with careful follow-up to monitor for jaw osteonecrosis, hypocalcemia, and renal failure that are the most common side effects. To avoid hypocalcemia, calcium and vitamin D therapy is recommended. Bisphosphonates and denosumab are not curative therapies, but they can be used in association with local treatment for symptomatic lesions or lesions at risk or with other systemic treatments such as TKI agents.

Management of the Case

This case shows that multidisciplinary treatment is frequently needed to treat bone lesions from thyroid cancer. In the case of distant metastases, there are several important prognostic factors: tumor histology, patient age, the presence or absence of radioactive iodine uptake, size of the metastases (micro or macro), and disease burden. However, therapeutic choices also may have an impact on patient quality of life and survival [2]. For bone lesions, local disease control is particularly important [15].

Radioactive Iodine Treatment

This patient presented with multiple radioiodine-avid bone lesions that were not seen on CT scan. In this situation, a favorable ^{131}I response could be expected [23, 44, 45]. Only the rib and the ischial lesions needed local treatment for their size, the pain management (for the rib lesion), and the fracture risk (ischial lesion). The use of local treatment was necessary to obtain a potential complete resolution of the lesions and to prevent skeletal events. Radioactive iodine alone would not have been efficient to treat these two larger lesions. On the other hand, the patient also had lung micrometastases with significant ^{131}I uptake. Miliary lung disease such as this typically has a good response to ^{131}I treatment [1, 46]. For these reasons, the patient received a second dose of radioactive iodine [100 mCi (3.7 GBq) after THW] 4 months after cryoablation and 6 months after the first radioactive iodine treatment. Serum thyroglobulin level decreased to 722 ng/ml with TSH level of 78 mIU/l and negative anti-Tg antibodies. The second ^{131}I post-therapy scan showed a reduction in lung uptake with a reduction in size of lung lesions on the CT component of SPECT/

CT and the disappearance of ^{131}I uptake in C4, T8, and right and left iliac bone lesions, confirming the efficacy of radioactive iodine in treating small lesions without morphological radiologic changes [23].

The post-therapy scan showed also the disappearance of rib uptake and an important reduction of ischium uptake, confirming the efficacy of local treatment of these lesions. Unfortunately, on the post-therapy scan, an increased uptake was reported in T10 and L1 with millimeter-sized lytic lesions on the CT component of the SPECT/CT. There were also two new areas of uptake in the sacrum and in the left femur without structural evidence on the CT component. Progression of disease in the bones, with appearance of new lesions, was confirmed on a third post-therapy scan after administration of 100 mCi (3.7 GBq) 6 months later, while the uptake in the lungs completely disappeared. The disease in the bones was then defined as refractory to radioactive iodine therapy due to the progression despite ^{131}I administration [4].

In our patient, FDG PET/CT was performed at initial presentation and FDG uptake was very heterogeneous. The lung metastases did not show significant FDG uptake, and several bone lesions did not show any FDG uptake and were detected only on ^{131}I WB scan. All these lesions showed a good response to ^{131}I. Only the rib lesion, the most aggressive and largest lesion, showed significant FDG uptake. The patient was reevaluated by ^{18}FDG PET scan after the third ^{131}I treatment. No FDG uptake was detected in the lung or in the lesions treated by cryoablation. This case shows that ^{18}FDG PET can be used to follow up bone lesions treated by thermal ablation as previously reported in liver and in lung lesions, but further studies are necessary to evaluate the impact of FDG uptake in this field [34]. The other new bone ^{131}I refractory lesions showed moderate FDG uptake, probably due to their small size. It was decided to evaluate disease progression with serial PET scans every 6 months, to monitor for disease progression, which might be an indication for additional local therapy or systemic treatment.

Cryoablation and Cementoplasty

This patient was a good candidate for local treatment in association with radioactive iodine. Patients who are candidates for thermal ablation are defined as follows: "*(a)* patients with limited painful metastatic disease who have failed conventional therapies or have refused conventional therapy; *(b)* patients at risk for further morbidity, with progression of a metastatic tumor that may be at risk for fracture or invasion of adjacent critical structures; and *(c)* patients with limited metastatic disease who are not surgical candidates" [28].

Our patient had limited metastatic disease without neurological compression, with at least two macrometastases (>1 cm) not treatable by ^{131}I alone: a painful lesion in the rib and a cortical lytic lesion with fracture risk in the ischium. Surgery was not indicated because of the absence of local compression. Lesion size and location were favorable for needle access and for good efficacy of thermal ablation [13].

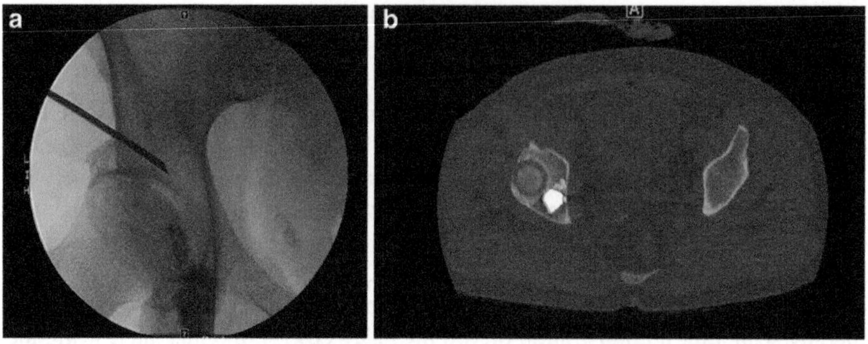

Fig. 34.3 Interventional radiology images during cementoplasty procedure in the right ischium lesion. (**a**) Fluoroscopy image showing cement injection in the right ischium lesion. (**b**) Axial CT image showing cement in the right ischium lesion

The goal was reducing the local pain and the fracture risk, but also to obtain a local control of these lesions. Thermal ablation was performed on the two macrometastases that were visible on morphological imaging in association with cementoplasty in the ischial lesion. Cryoablation was chosen over RFA and was performed under conscious sedation using special probes (IceRod®, Galil Medical, Yokneam, Israel) inserted into the tumor under imaging (CT) guidance. The passage of pressurized gas (argon) through the probes rapidly freezes the lesion with no damage to surrounding tissues. The effect of ablation by "cold temperature" is the formation of the so-called iceball that can be seen and followed up by imaging during the procedure. Cryotherapy is frequently preferred to RFA because it is less painful during and after the procedure, due to a more selective action on the target lesion and also because the "iceball" can be seen by unenhanced CT during the procedure to monitor the completeness of treatment of the target lesion [13].

Cementoplasty was performed after thermal ablation to consolidate the bone lytic lesion. The cement injection is normally performed in the same manner used to insert the cryoprobe in the bone lesion. Also, the cement is a dense material that can be easily visualized at imaging (Fig. 34.3). During the procedure, potential collateral effects such as pain or neurological symptoms are evaluated by the operator. The risk of collateral effects is higher in case of lesions in the spine.

Clinical Pearls/Pitfalls

- In case of bone lesion at risk for fracture or invasion of adjacent critical structures, a multidisciplinary approach is necessary.
- The goal of local treatments is to reduce pain, to treat and possibly eliminate the lesion, and to avoid local complications such as pathological fracture or medullary compression.
- Local treatments can also prolong patient survival and delay systemic treatment such as TKI.

References

1. Schlumberger M, Challeton C, De Vathaire F, et al. Radioactive iodine treatment and external radiotherapy for lung and bone metastases from thyroid carcinoma. J Nucl Med. 1996; 37(4):598–605.
2. Durante C, Haddy N, Baudin E, et al. Long-term outcome of 444 patients with distant metastases from papillary and follicular thyroid carcinoma: benefits and limits of radioiodine therapy. J Clin Endocrinol Metab. 2006;91(8):2892–9.
3. Schlumberger M, French TUTHYREF Network. Targeted therapy in refractory thyroid cancer. Eur J Cancer. 2011;47 Suppl 3:S328–9.
4. Cooper DS, Doherty GM, Hauguen BR, et al. Revised American thyroid association management guidelines for patients with thyroid nodules and differentiated thyroid cancer. Thyroid. 2009;19:1167–214.
5. Haissaguerre M, Leboulleux S, Bonichon F, et al. Impact of molecular targeted therapies in patients with bone metastases of differentiated thyroid carcinoma. Poster, 54th American Thryoid Association meeting; 24–27 Oct 2012.
6. Tubiana M, Haddad E, Schlumberger MJ, et al. External radiotherapy in thyroid cancers. Cancer. 1985;55:2062–71.
7. Bernier MO, Leenhardt L, Hoang C, et al. Survival and therapeutic modalities in patients with bone metastases of differentiated thyroid carcinomas. J Clin Endocrinol Metab. 2001;86(4): 1568–73.
8. Zettining G, Fueger BJ, Passler C, et al. Long-term follow-up of patients with bone metastases from differentiated thyroid carcinoma—surgery or conventional therapy? Clin Endocrinol. 2002;56:377–82.
9. Kushchayeva YS, Kushchayev SV, Wexler JA, et al. Current treatment modalities for spinal metastases secondary to thyroid carcinoma. Thyroid. 2014;24:1443–55.
10. Goetz MP, Callstrom MR, Charboneau JW, et al. Percutaneous image-guided radiofrequency ablation of painful metastases involving bone: a multicenter study. J Clin Oncol. 2004;22: 300–6.
11. Thanos L, Mylona S, Galani P, et al. Radiofrequency ablation of osseous metastases for the palliation of pain. Skelet Radiol. 2008;37(3):189–94.
12. Dupuy DE, Liu D, Hartfeil D, et al. Percutaneous radiofrequency ablation of painful osseous metastases: a multicenter American College of Radiology Imaging Network trial. Cancer. 2010;116:989–97.
13. Deschamps F, Farouil G, Ternes N, et al. Thermal ablation techniques: a curative treatment of bone metastases in selected patients? Eur Radiol. 2014;8:1971–80.
14. Monchik JM, Donatini G, Iannuccilli J, Dupuy DE. Radiofrequency ablation and percutaneous ethanol injection treatment for recurrent local and distant well-differentiated thyroid carcinoma. Ann Surg. 2006;244:296–304.
15. Sugitani I, Fujimoto Y, Yamamoto N. Papillary thyroid carcinoma with distant metastases: survival predictors and the importance of local control. Surgery. 2008;143:35–42.
16. Quan GM, Pointillart V, Palussière J, Bonichon F. Multidisciplinary treatment and survival of patients with vertebral metastases from thyroid carcinoma. Thyroid. 2012;22:125–30.
17. Pittas AG, Adler M, Fazzari M, Tickoo S, Rosai S, Larson SM, Robbins RJ. Bone metastases from thyroid carcinoma: clinical characteristics and prognostic variables in one hundred forty-six patients. Thyroid. 2000;10(3):261–8.
18. Kushchayeva YS, Kushchayev SV, Carroll NM, et al. Spinal metastases due to thyroid carcinoma: an analysis of 202 patients. Thyroid. 2014;24:1488–500.
19. Wang W, Larson SM, Fazzari M, et al. Prognostic value of [18F] fluorodeoxyglucose positron emission tomographic scanning in patients with thyroid cancer. J Clin Endocrinol Metab. 2000;85:1107–13.
20. Wang W, Larson SM, Tuttle RM, et al. Resistance of [18f]-fluorodeoxyglucose-avid metastatic thyroid cancer lesions to treatment with high-dose radioactive iodine. Thyroid. 2001;11: 1169–75.

21. Robbins RJ, Wan Q, Grewal RK, et al. Real-time prognosis for metastatic thyroid carcinoma based on 2-[18F]fluoro-2-deoxy-D-glucose-positron emission tomography scanning. J Clin Endocrinol Metab. 2006;91:498–505.
22. Deandreis D, Al Ghuzlan A, Leboulleux S, et al. Histological, immunohistochemical and metabolic (radioiodine and FDG uptake) patterns of metastatic thyroid cancer: do they correlate with patients outcome? Endocr Relat Cancer. 2011;18:159–69.
23. Robenshtok E, Farooki A, Grewal RK, Tuttle RM. Natural history of small radioiodine-avid bone metastases that have no structural correlate on imaging studies. Endocrine. 2014;47(1): 266–72.
24. Lo SS, Fakiris AJ, Chang EL, et al. Stereotactic body radiation therapy: a novel treatment modality. Nat Rev Clin Oncol. 2010;7:44–54.
25. Smit JW, Vielvoye GJ, Goslings BM. Embolization for vertebral metastases of follicular thyroid carcinoma. J Clin Endocrinol Metab. 2000;85:989–94.
26. Erinjeri JP, Clark TW. Cryoablation: mechanism of action and devices. J Vasc Interv Radiol. 2010;21 Suppl 8:S187–91.
27. Hong K, Georgiades C. Radiofrequency ablation: mechanism of action and devices. J Vasc Interv Radiol. 2010;21(8 Suppl):S179–86.
28. Rosenthal D, Callstrom MR. Critical review and state of the art in interventional oncology: benign and metastatic disease involving bone. Radiology. 2012;262(3):765–80.
29. Deandreis D, Leboulleux S, Dromain C, et al. Role of FDG-PET/CT in the follow up of lung lesions treated with radiofrequency ablation. Radiology. 2011;258:270–6.
30. Proschek D, Kurth A, Proschek P, et al. Prospective pilot-study of combined bipolar radiofrequency ablation and application of bone cement in bone metastases. Anticancer Res. 2009; 29(7):2787–92.
31. Chiras J, Sola-Martinez MT, Weill A, et al. Percutaneous vertebroplasty. Rev Med Intern. 1995;16:854–9.
32. Cotten A, Dewatre F, Cortet B, et al. Percutaneous vertebroplasty for osteolytic metastases and myeloma: effects of the percentage of lesion filling and the leakage of methyl methacrylate at clinical follow-up. Radiology. 1996;20:525–30.
33. Fourney DR, Schomer DF, Nader R, et al. Percutaneous vertebroplasty and kyphoplasty for painful vertebral body fractures in cancer patients. J Neurosurg. 2003;98:21–30.
34. Deandreis D, Dechamps F, Nascimento C, et al. Role of FDG-PET/CT in the follow up of bone lesions treated with thermal ablation. Abstract CL-NMS-MO3B. Radiological Society of North America (RSNA), Chicago, Dec 2013.
35. de Baere T, Elias D, Dromain C, et al. Radiofrequency ablation of 100 hepatic metastases with a mean follow-up of more than 1 year. AJR Am J Roentgenol. 2000;175:1619–25.
36. Solbiati L, Livraghi T, Goldberg SN, et al. Percutaneous radio-frequency ablation of hepatic metastases from colorectal cancer: long-term results in 117 patients. Radiology. 2001;221: 159–66.
37. de Baere T, Deschamps F, Tselikas L, et al. GEP-NETS update: interventional radiology: role in the treatment of liver metastases from GEP-NET tumors. Eur J Endocrinol. 2014;172(4):R151–66. pii: EJE-14-0630.
38. Wertenbroek MW, Links TP, Prins TR, et al. Radiofrequency ablation of hepatic metastases from thyroid carcinoma. Thyroid. 2008;18:1105–10.
39. de Baère T, Palussière J, Aupérin A, et al. Midterm local efficacy and survival after radiofrequency ablation of lung tumors with minimum follow-up of 1 year: prospective evaluation. Radiology. 2006;240:587–96.
40. Lencioni R, Crocetti L, Cioni R, et al. Response to radiofrequency ablation of pulmonary tumours: a prospective, intention-to-treat, multicentre clinical trial (the RAPTURE study). Lancet Oncol. 2008;9:621–8.
41. Coleman R, Body JJ, Aapro M, Hadji P, Herrstedt J, ESMO Guidelines Working Group. Bone health in cancer patients: ESMO Clinical Practice Guidelines. Ann Oncol. 2014;25 Suppl 3:iii124–37.

42. Orita Y, Sugitani I, Toda K, Manabe J, Fujimoto Y. Zoledronic acid in the treatment of bone metastases from differentiated thyroid carcinoma. Thyroid. 2011;21(1):31–5.
43. Fizazi K, Carducci M, Smith M, et al. Denosumab versus zoledronic acid for treatment of bone metastases in men with castration-resistant prostate cancer: a randomised, double-blind study. Lancet. 2011;377(9768):813–22.
44. Proye CA, Dromer DH, Carnaille BM, et al. Is it still worthwhile to treat bone metastasis from differentiated thyroid carcinoma with radioactive iodine? World J Surg. 1992;16:640–6.
45. Petrich T, Widjaia A, Musholt TJ, et al. Outcome after radioiodine therapy in 107 patients with differentiated thyroid carcinoma and initial bone metastases: side effects and influence of age. Eur J Nucl Med Mol Imaging. 2001;28:203–8.
46. Ilgan S, Karacalioglu AO, Pabuscu Y, et al. Iodine-131 treatment and high-resolution CT: results in patients with lung metastases from differentiated thyroid carcinoma. Eur J Nucl Med Mol Imaging. 2004;3:825–30.

Chapter 35
Differentiated Thyroid Cancer and Brain Metastases

Steven I. Sherman

Case Presentation

A 68-year-old woman presented to the emergency room having awoken with the "worst headache of her life," followed by several episodes of emesis. The pain was most severe behind the right orbit, radiating to the occiput and associated with photophobia and phonophobia. Her past history was notable for papillary thyroid carcinoma diagnosed 27 years previously, initially treated with thyroidectomy and adjuvant radioiodine. She had undergone four additional neck operations in the succeeding 15 years for radioiodine refractory recurrences, the last surgery having been followed by external beam radiotherapy to the neck. Eleven years before her emergency room (ER) visit, wedge biopsy of her right lung revealed metastatic thyroid carcinoma, and her bilateral pulmonary nodules remained radiographically stable throughout the intervening years on TSH-suppressive levothyroxine therapy. With a rising thyroglobulin level, extensive imaging including magnetic resonance imaging (MRI) of the brain had failed to identify other sites of metastases when performed 6 months previously. On presentation to the ER, her blood pressure was 185/80 mmHg, without papilledema or neurologic abnormalities on exam. An emergent head computed tomography (CT) revealed a 3.4 cm hemorrhagic lesion extending into the right lateral ventricle with a low-density solid component felt most consistent with a hemorrhagic metastasis. MR angiogram showed no evidence of aneurysm, vasculitis, or spasm, but patchy contrast enhancement was interpreted as consistent with a hemorrhagic metastasis. Dexamethasone, 4 mg twice daily, was initiated, along with aggressive blood pressure and pain control; a fluid restriction was transiently required to manage hyponatremia due to syndrome of inappropriate

S.I. Sherman, MD (✉)
University of Texas MD Anderson Cancer Center,
Unit 1461, 301402, Houston, TX 77230-1402, USA
e-mail: sisherma@mdanderson.org

D.S. Cooper, C. Durante (eds.), *Thyroid Cancer*,
DOI 10.1007/978-3-319-22401-5_35

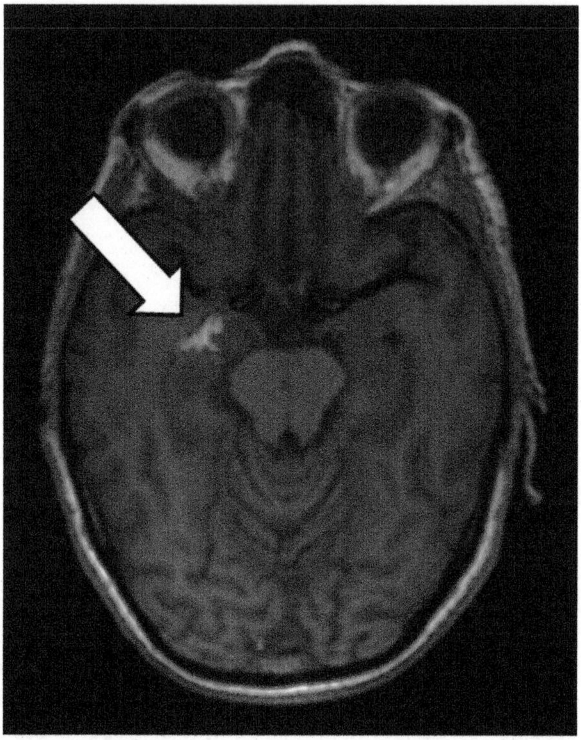

Fig. 35.1 Computed tomography (CT) of the head. Arrow indicates a 3.4 cm hemorrhagic lesion extending into the right lateral ventricle with a low-density solid component, consistent with a hemorrhagic metastasis from DTC

antidiuretic hormone. As the hemorrhage reabsorbed, a 1.5 cm solid lesion was seen enhancing brightly on T1-weighted MRI consistent with a solitary metastatic focus (Fig. 35.1). Stereotactic radiosurgery was performed, using a gamma knife machine to deliver 16 Gy at the 50 % isodense line with 22 shots. She experienced an uncomplicated full recovery from the hemorrhage and treatment and survived another 2 years before dying due to cardiac failure associated with a right ventricular metastasis.

Literature Review

Brain metastases from differentiated thyroid carcinoma are uncommon, reported in only 1–2 % of all patients [1–3]. They are typically identified in older patients, with the median age of detection of brain metastases in these recent reports ranging from 61 to 63 years, and the median time interval between initial cancer diagnosis and brain metastasis ranges from 4 to 10 years. Although most cases have been reported arising from papillary carcinomas, there may be a particular predisposition for the oxyphilic or Hürthle cell variant [1]. Usually, patients have had evidence of distant metastatic disease detected previously, such as in the lungs or bones [4], though some patients may present with symptomatic brain metastasis at their initial diagnosis. A majority of patients are initially identified with oligometastatic brain disease, with three or fewer lesions detected by imaging [1, 3]. Historically, imaging to detect these lesions was triggered by symptoms; however, with the introduction of systemic therapy options and more comprehensive staging examinations for patients with progressive distant metastatic disease, patients are now also being identified with brain metastases at an earlier, presymptomatic phase [3].

Compared with most patients with differentiated thyroid carcinoma, the prognosis of patients with brain metastases is poor. Median overall survival after the diagnosis of brain metastases has been reported as between 7 and 21 months [2, 3], with almost all patients dying of complications of disease and/or treatment. Prognostic factors for prolonged survival include disease amenable to localized intervention such as surgical excision or stereotactic radiosurgery (which is likely to be oligometastatic) and good performance status [1–3]. Median survival for patients with Karnofsky performance status at least 70 was 31 months in one series and for patients with WHO performance status of zero or one was 27 months in another [2, 3].

Treatment options for patients with brain metastases include surgical resection and various modalities of radiotherapy including radioactive iodine, TSH-suppressive thyroid hormone therapy, and systemic therapy. Supportive care must also be considered, particularly for patients with poor performance status and/or widespread intracranial disease [5]. Of note, there have been no randomized clinical trials specifically devoted to treatment of brain metastases from differentiated thyroid carcinoma, and thus recommendations rely primarily upon trials that included patients with various solid tumors or retrospective case series of thyroid patients (with their inherent risk for bias in selection of treatments).

Surgical excision is the traditional approach to treatment for solitary or oligometastatic brain lesions and has been associated with improved survival. In one series, median overall survival was nearly five times longer (16.7 versus 3.4 months) for patients who underwent surgical excision of one or more intracranial lesions compared with those who did not [1]. Resection may be preferred for patients whose metastatic tumors are greater than 3 cm in diameter [6]. Surgical excision can provide diagnostic information when there is uncertainty about the histologic diagnosis (e.g., patients with another primary malignancy as well as thyroid) and can be beneficial for relief of acute intracranial swelling if high-dose glucocorticoids are insufficiently effective. On the other hand, surgery requires time for recovery both before and after hospital discharge, carries a degree of risk, and may not be appropriate for patients with an expected short survival time due to rapidly progressive systemic metastases or poor performance status. Whether surgery should be followed by adjuvant whole-brain radiotherapy (WBRT) is controversial, as randomized studies in patients with metastatic solid tumors have failed to demonstrate an improvement in overall survival or performance status with combination treatment despite improvements in intracerebral recurrence-free survival [7].

The development of stereotactic radiosurgery (SRS) provided an attractive new option for patients with multiple small intracerebral metastases by allowing the delivery of a highly focused radiation dose to the tumors while minimizing radiation damage to surrounding uninvolved brain tissue [6]. In one series of thyroid cancer patients, median overall survival was 37.4 months after SRS [2], and in a second series, median overall survival was prolonged more than threefold after SRS [3]. Multiple lesions can be treated simultaneously with a limited number of outpatient treatment sessions, and recovery can be rapid. SRS is most appropriate for patients with tumors up to 3 cm in diameter, minimal intracerebral shift as evidence of mass effect, and good performance status [6]. Due to the highly focused radiation dosimetry of SRS, necrosis of surrounding brain tissue is uncommon and usually asymptomatic. Like surgery, there is no evidence to support an overall survival advantage by adding WBRT after SRS for metastases from solid tumors, although intracerebral recurrence-free survival may be enhanced by the combination [6].

WBRT can be of benefit in the local control of multifocal brain metastases [5, 8]. A standard treatment approach to deliver 3000 cGy in ten fractions is commonly employed. Studies in other solid tumors have failed to demonstrate a significant advantage to the use of altered dosing strategies or concomitant radiosensitizers [5]. Combining WBRT with subsequent SRS or using WBRT following either surgery or SRS has been associated with improved intracerebral recurrence-free survival, but overall survival has not been improved in multiple trials for either oligometastatic or widely metastatic disease [5, 8]. Unfortunately, eventual development of broad cognitive decline has been associated with WBRT, limiting the attractiveness of this intervention in patients anticipated to have longer survival.

Radioiodine has a potential role unique to treating metastases from differentiated thyroid carcinoma. In one report, only 17 % of patients scanned with radioiodine had visible uptake concentrated in a brain metastasis, which may be expected given the older age of these patients and their advanced disease [1]. In those cases, surgical resection combined with high administered activities of radioiodine was employed successfully for intracerebral disease control. The use of exogenous recombinant human TSH to stimulate radioiodine uptake instead of endogenous TSH elevation following thyroid hormone withdrawal may be theoretically preferable to minimize the period of excessive thyrotropin stimulation to tumor growth [1]. Dexamethasone should also be given prophylactically to minimize risk for peritumoral edema or hemorrhage following recombinant human TSH or therapy with radioiodine [1].

Recent publications suggest that systemic therapy with kinase inhibitors might play a role in treating solid tumor brain metastases [9]. In one report, a partial response was described in a patient with follicular thyroid carcinoma treated with sorafenib following failure of stereotactic radiosurgery. A clinical trial for *BRAF*-mutated solid tumors noted that patients with brain metastases from melanoma often experienced marked reduction in tumor size with therapy with the BRAF kinase inhibitor dabrafenib, despite intentional design of the drug to minimize penetration of the blood-brain barrier; given the high frequency of *BRAF* mutations in aggressive papillary thyroid carcinoma, treatment with a BRAF kinase inhibitor can also be considered.

High-dose glucocorticoids may be helpful in the control of cerebral edema that often accompanies brain metastases from solid malignancies. In the presence of neurologic symptoms but without impending herniation, a randomized trial suggested that a starting dose of dexamethasone of 4 or 8 mg daily followed by rapid tapering appears to provide optimal symptomatic relief while minimizing cushingoid toxicities associated with higher doses [10]. Conversely, in the setting of severe neurologic compromise or risk for herniation, higher daily doses of dexamethasone may be warranted. It is reasonable to use thyroid hormone to suppress TSH levels, given the stimulatory effect reported from high levels of TSH on tumor growth, but data are lacking regarding actual efficacy of this approach. For supportive care, antiseizure medications are warranted in the presence of seizure activity but have not been shown to be of value when given prophylactically.

Management of the Case

The patient unfortunately presented with significant morbidity from an undiagnosed brain metastasis despite extensive efforts to identify such a lesion 6 months before her symptomatic presentation. Initially, it was somewhat unclear whether she had experienced intracerebral hemorrhage from a vascular lesion or from a metastasis, and confirmation of metastatic disease was somewhat delayed. Symptomatically, she responded very well to supportive treatments with dexamethasone and pain relief. SRS provided long-term control of her intracerebral disease, without the addition of adjuvant WBRT. She was offered systemic therapy with either sorafenib or vemurafenib for her $BRAF^{V600E}$-mutant papillary carcinoma, which she refused, and she died from extracerebral metastases subsequently.

Clinical Pearls

- Brain metastases are an uncommon, late event in differentiated thyroid carcinoma.
- Prognosis is poor, similar to other solid tumors that metastasize to the brain.
- Selected patients with oligometastatic disease and good performance status may benefit from either surgical excision or SRS.
- Radioiodine uptake occasionally permits additional intervention with this modality.
- Supportive care with judiciously administered dexamethasone can help provide symptomatic relief while minimizing symptoms of glucocorticoid excess.
- Future studies are required to evaluate the role of new systemic therapy options for brain metastases from thyroid carcinoma.

References

1. Chiu AC, Delpassand ES, Sherman SI. Prognosis and treatment of brain metastases in thyroid carcinoma. J Clin Endocrinol Metab. 1997;82:3637–42.
2. Bernad DM, Sperduto PW, Souhami L, Jensen AW, Roberge D. Stereotactic radiosurgery in the management of brain metastases from primary thyroid cancers. J Neurooncol. 2010;98:249–52.
3. Henriques de Figueiredo B, Godbert Y, Soubeyran I, Carrat X, Lagarde P, Cazeau AL, et al. Brain metastases from thyroid carcinoma: a retrospective study of 21 patients. Thyroid. 2014;24:270–6.
4. Dinneen SF, Valimaki MJ, Bergstralh EJ, Goellner JR, Gorman CA, Hay ID. Distant metastases in papillary thyroid carcinoma: 100 cases observed at one institution during 5 decades. J Clin Endocrinol Metab. 1995;80:2041–5.
5. Tsao MN, Lloyd N, Wong R, Chow E, Rakovitch E. Laperriere N whole brain radiotherapy for the treatment of multiple brain metastases. Cochrane Database Syst Rev. 2006;3, CD003869.
6. Linskey M, Andrews D, Asher A, Burri S, Kondziolka D, Robinson P, et al. The role of stereotactic radiosurgery in the management of patients with newly diagnosed brain metastases: a systematic review and evidence-based clinical practice guideline. J Neurooncol. 2010;96:45–68.
7. Kalkanis S, Kondziolka D, Gaspar L, Burri S, Asher A, Cobbs C, et al. The role of surgical resection in the management of newly diagnosed brain metastases: a systematic review and evidence-based clinical practice guideline. J Neurooncol. 2010;96:33–43.
8. Gaspar L, Mehta M, Patchell R, Burri S, Robinson P, Morris R, et al. The role of whole brain radiation therapy in the management of newly diagnosed brain metastases: a systematic review and evidence-based clinical practice guideline. J Neurooncol. 2010;96:17–32.
9. Soffietti R, Trevisan E, Ruda R. Targeted therapy in brain metastasis. Curr Opin Oncol. 2012;24:679–86.
10. Vecht CJ, Hovestadt A, Verbiest HB, van Vliet JJ, van Putten WL. Dose-effect relationship of dexamethasone on Karnofsky performance in metastatic brain tumors: a randomized study of doses of 4, 8, and 16 mg per day. Neurology. 1994;44:675–80.

Part VIII
High Risk Differentiated Thyroid Cancer: *Novel Chemotherapy and Toxicity*

Chapter 36
RAI-Refractory, Advanced Differentiated Thyroid Cancer Receiving Tyrosine Kinase Inhibitor Treatment: Checking for Drug-Drug Interactions

Steven I. Sherman

Case Presentation

A 67-year-old man presented to his local emergency room with complaints of light-headedness and an intermittently irregular heart rhythm, without chest pain or shortness of breath. His past medical history was notable for diagnosis of papillary thyroid carcinoma 5 years previously, treated initially with total thyroidectomy, bilateral modified neck dissection, and adjuvant radioiodine. His post-therapy scan showed minimal uptake in the neck, but a TSH-stimulated thyroglobulin level of 524 ng/mL had subsequently prompted tomographic imaging that revealed bilateral lung lesions compatible with metastatic thyroid carcinoma. With progressive radiographic enlargement over the succeeding 12 months and repeat radioiodine imaging that was negative, he was started on oral therapy with sorafenib for radioiodine-refractory progressive metastases. He initially responded well, but with subsequent progression, his therapy was switched 14 months prior to this emergency room visit to sunitinib. Treatment was complicated by adverse events, including hypertension, diarrhea, and hypomagnesemia. Two weeks before his emergency room visit, he presented to his local primary care physician with acute bronchitis, and antibiotic therapy with clarithromycin was initiated. He returned to his physician 4 days later complaining of worsening diarrhea and was found to have a blood pressure of 170/100 mmHg and a pulse of 96 beats per minute. Verapamil was added to his chronic valsartan therapy, along with an increase in his dosing of diphenoxylate/atropine for his diarrhea. On examination in the emergency room, his pulse was 52 beats per minute and blood pressure 126/62 mmHg. An electrocardiogram revealed sinus bradycardia, with a prolonged QT_c of 520 msec. His serum magnesium level

S.I. Sherman, MD (✉)
University of Texas M.D. Anderson Cancer Center,
Unit 1461, 301402, Houston, TX 77230-1402, USA
e-mail: sisherma@mdanderson.org

D.S. Cooper, C. Durante (eds.), *Thyroid Cancer*,
DOI 10.1007/978-3-319-22401-5_36

was low, 0.9 mg/dL. While preparing an intravenous magnesium infusion, his heart rate was noted to increase acutely to 140 beats per minute, and a transient episode of torsades de pointes was identified on his cardiac monitoring. An infusion of magnesium, 16 mEq, was initiated, and subsequent monitoring demonstrated improvement in the QT_c to 470 msec and resolution of his tachyarrhythmia to baseline sinus bradycardia.

Literature Review

With the introduction of multitargeted tyrosine kinase inhibitors (TKIs) for the treatment of individuals with radioiodine-refractory differentiated thyroid carcinoma, new patient safety risks have appeared that require extreme caution on the part of all physicians involved in these patients [1, 2]. These adverse events range from common toxicities, such as diarrhea and skin rashes, to uncommon events that can occasionally be life threatening, such as prolongation of QT intervals that can trigger arrhythmias. Those adverse events that are directly related to the concentration of the drug in circulation can be potentiated by concomitant use of other drugs that alter the metabolic clearance or pharmacokinetics of the TKI itself. Thus, knowledge of the potential for drug-drug interactions is critical whenever medications are prescribed for a thyroid cancer patient being treated for metastatic disease with a TKI. Patient education is also critical, so that the patient is able to alert whoever is prescribing a medication for them to check for possible drug-drug interactions that either increase risk or decrease the effectiveness of the TKI. Most available TKIs used for treating thyroid carcinoma are dosed once or twice per day, with long half-lives that facilitate such dosing schedules. With slow metabolic clearance and often active metabolites, the blood concentration of TKIs can be significantly altered by other agents that interact with the enzymes metabolizing their clearance, thus potentially contributing to concentration-related toxicities. Most TKIs, e.g., sunitinib, are primarily metabolized through hepatic cytochrome P450s such as CYP3A4 [3]. Thus, drugs that activate CYP3A4 might reduce the therapeutic effectiveness of sunitinib by enhancing its metabolic clearance, whereas drugs that inhibit the cytochrome might be anticipated to increase susceptibility to toxic side effects. Further, some TKIs carry the potential to inhibit other drug-metabolizing enzymes, thus introducing the potential for the TKI to interfere with metabolism of other therapies.

The potential to prolong the QT interval and increase risk for torsades de pointes has been a key focus for studies of drug-drug interactions for multitargeted TKIs relevant to thyroid carcinoma [4]. The interval, defined as the time between the beginning of the QRS complex and the end of the T wave, is highly sensitive to inhibition of the myocyte potassium channel associated with human ether-a-go-go-related gene (hERG) that mediates ventricular repolarization during phase 2–3 of the action potential [5]. No single mechanism has emerged to explain the ability of multitargeted TKIs to inhibit the hERG, and it appears to vary among the different

TKIs themselves. However, alterations in the function of numerous intracellular protein kinases including PI3K, AKT, and protein kinase A that function downstream from the tyrosine kinases affected by TKIs have all been implicated to contribute [5]. Electrolyte abnormalities, such as hypokalemia and hypomagnesemia which can commonly result from TKI-induced diarrhea, may also independently contribute to a risk of QT prolongation and torsades de pointes.

The magnitude of the effect of TKIs on significant QT prolongation was evaluated in a trial-level meta-analysis of placebo-controlled studies that included EKG monitoring while on therapy with any of the following drugs: sunitinib, sorafenib, pazopanib, axitinib, vandetanib, cabozantinib, ponatinib, and regorafenib; note that all of the first six drugs have been formally studied in phase II or phase III trials in radioiodine-refractory differentiated thyroid cancer [4]. More than 4 % of patients experienced any grade of prolongation of the QT interval during therapy with a multitargeted TKI, in contrast with 0.25 % for those untreated, and high-grade prolongation was 2.7-fold more likely in the TKI-treated patients. The risks were highest for patients treated with sunitinib or vandetanib, and importantly a significant correlation was noted between drug dosing and frequency of QT prolongation.

The dose-response effect on QT intervals suggests that the risk for proarrhythmic adverse effect from the TKI can be enhanced by concomitant drugs that increase TKI levels by inhibiting TKI metabolism though CYP3A4. Unfortunately, many drugs that might be used during supportive care of oncology patients have the potential to inhibit CYP3A4, including macrolide and azole antibiotics and calcium channel blockers. Ketoconazole, for example, increases plasma levels of sunitinib and its active metabolite SU12662 by 51 % which could be expected to have a major effect on the QT interval [6].

An alternative concern results from concomitant use of drugs that stimulate CYP3A4 activity, thereby accelerating the clearance of TKIs and potentially reducing their effectiveness. For example, rifampin, a potent inducer of CYP3A4, reduces sunitinib and SU12662 plasma levels by nearly 50 % and also increases sorafenib levels [1, 7]. Complementary and alternative medicines may also interact. Both St. John's wort (*Hypericum perforatum*) and *Echinacea*, which are available as over-the-counter medicinal herbs, induce CYP3A4 and have been implicated in altering TKI pharmacokinetics [6]. With evidence that declining plasma sorafenib concentrations over time may permit progression of metastatic thyroid carcinoma, careful attention must be paid to the contribution of concomitant medications if a patient begins to progress while on TKI therapy [8].

Less commonly, TKIs themselves create drug-drug interactions that alter the effectiveness of other medications. Most relevant to patients with thyroid carcinoma is the common effect of all TKIs to contribute to rising TSH levels [1]. Although some TKIs, most notably sunitinib, cause hypothyroidism when used to treat other malignancies in patients with baseline normal thyroid function, the mechanism of this effect likely differs in postthyroidectomy patients. Whereas induction of autoimmune thyroiditis and/or regression of intrathyroidal capillaries may be causes of primary hypothyroidism secondary to sunitinib, inadequate thyroid hormone absorption or accelerated thyroid hormone metabolism is more likely to contribute to loss of TSH suppression in thyroid carcinoma patients, necessitating careful monitoring of TSH levels and frequent increases in hormone dosing [2]. A similar effect of TKIs is postulated to contribute to a need for increased vitamin D dosing in postthyroidectomy patients with decreased parathyroid function or frank hypoparathyroidism [2]. Non-cytochrome-mediated pathways of drug clearance can secondarily be affected by TKIs, altering drug exposure of other medications and predisposing to drug toxicity. For example, sorafenib partially inhibits several UDP-glucuronosyltransferases (such as UGT1A9 and UGT1A1), which can lead to slower clearance of acetaminophen and increased risk for hepatotoxicity [6].

The frequency of co-administration of medications that could lead to drug-drug interactions is surprisingly high. In one study of patients treated with TKIs at the Mayo Clinic, the rate of co-administration of medications that could increase TKI-induced toxicity ranged from 25 % for sunitinib to 75 % for pazopanib [9]. In a second study in renal cell carcinoma, 47 % of sunitinib-treated patients were co-administered medications that would inhibit CYP3A4 and potentiate sunitinib concentration-dependent toxicities [10].

With the plethora of possible drug-drug interactions that could increase TKI drug levels and risk for TKI-induced toxicities or otherwise alter the effectiveness or tolerance of TKI therapy for metastatic thyroid carcinoma, it is imperative that a patient's medications be reviewed at multiple key points in their clinical care to identify potential problems that could emerge [2]. At baseline, before a patient is initiated on TKI therapy, the clinician should review and reconcile the medication list including all over-the-counter nonprescription drugs as well as complementary or alternative medications that the patient may be obtaining from other sources. If potential drug-drug interactions are identified, the clinician can proactively change one of the offending medications or alter drug dosing so as to minimize the impact of the anticipated interaction. Similarly, such medication reconciliation should take place whenever a new concomitant drug is added to the patient's therapies. The difficulty, as demonstrated in this case, is that multiple providers may all be involved in the patient's care, introducing greater risk from polypharmacy and the potential for drug-drug interactions. Thus, there is also a need for thorough communication among all providers for the patient, such that awareness of all medications being prescribed is universal. Perhaps most critical, the patient must be educated and reminded by the provider team prescribing the TKI of the risk for drug-drug interactions and of the importance of medication review by each prescribing provider to minimize that risk. This should certainly be a component of the initial informed consent process prior to starting a TKI, as well as a part of each subsequent follow-up visit [2].

Several tools are available online that simplify the ability to screen for significant drug-drug interactions, in addition to those that exist within electronic health record and medication-prescribing software. The risk for life-threatening arrhythmia due to QT interval prolongation has led to creation of a specific website, www.qtdrugs.org, which provides the most up-to-date and well-annotated summary of information. For more general information and to search for other types of interactions, websites such as www.lexi.com, www.webmd.com/interaction-checker/, and www.druginteractioninfo.org (maintained by the University of Washington School of Pharmacy) are reputable sources.

Management of the Case

The patient experienced a combination of events that led to heightened risk for cardiac arrhythmia. In addition to the potential for QT prolongation by sunitinib, the patient developed significant electrolyte loss due to drug-induced diarrhea. With the onset of bronchitis, he was given clarithromycin, a recognized inhibitor of CYP3A4, which likely led to increased sunitinib concentrations. Regardless of whether the worsening diarrhea was secondary to higher sunitinib levels or was antibiotic induced, his electrolyte loss worsened, and he developed even greater risk for QT prolongation due to severe hypomagnesemia. Exacerbation of hypertension led to addition of a calcium channel antagonist that likely altered the QT interval even further, eventually leading to a typical acquired torsades de pointes that fortunately was self-limited and did not degenerate into ventricular tachycardia or fibrillation. By treating the hypomagnesemia, the acute risk was averted, and gradual clearance of the interacting medications allowed eventual restoration of sunitinib therapy.

Clinical Pearls

- Drug-drug interactions are common with the use of TKI therapy.
- Interactions can markedly increase risk for drug toxicity, particularly life-threatening complications such as torsades de pointes and other cardiac arrhythmias.
- Loss of TKI efficacy and alteration in the effectiveness and toxicities of other concomitant medications can also result from unanticipated drug-drug interactions, including effect on levothyroxine and vitamin D therapy.
- All involved providers and most critically the patient must be made aware of the risk for drug-drug interactions throughout the course of TKI therapy.

References

1. Cabanillas ME, Hu MI, Durand J, Busaidy NL. Challenges associated with tyrosine kinase inhibitor therapy for metastatic thyroid cancer. J Thyroid Res. 2011;2011:985780.
2. Carhill AA, Cabanillas ME, Jimenez C, Waguespack SG, Habra MA, Hu M, et al. The noninvestigational use of tyrosine kinase inhibitors in thyroid cancer: establishing a standard for patient safety and monitoring. J Clin Endocrinol Metab. 2013;98:31–42.

3. Duckett DR, Cameron MD. Metabolism considerations for kinase inhibitors in cancer treatment. Expert Opin Drug Metab Toxicol. 2010;6:1175–93.
4. Ghatalia P, Je Y, Kaymakcalan MD, Sonpavde G, Choueiri TK. QTc interval prolongation with vascular endothelial growth factor receptor tyrosine kinase inhibitors. Br J Cancer. 2014;112:296–305.
5. Shah RR, Morganroth J, Shah DR. Cardiovascular safety of tyrosine kinase inhibitors: with a special focus on cardiac repolarisation (QT interval). Drug Saf. 2013;36:295–316.
6. Thomas-Schoemann A, Blanchet B, Bardin C, Noe G, Boudou-Rouquette P, Vidal M, et al. Drug interactions with solid tumour-targeted therapies. Crit Rev Oncol Hematol. 2014;89:179–96.
7. van Erp NP, Gelderblom H, Guchelaar HJ. Clinical pharmacokinetics of tyrosine kinase inhibitors. Cancer Treat Rev. 2009;35:692–706.
8. Bellesoeur A, Carton E, Mir O, Groussin L, Blanchet B, Billemont B, et al. Critical role of sorafenib exposure over time for its antitumor activity in thyroid cancer. Invest New Drugs. 2014;32:569–72.
9. Bowlin SJ, Xia F, Wang W, Robinson KD, Stanek EJ. Twelve-month frequency of drug-metabolizing enzyme and transporter-based drug-drug interaction potential in patients receiving oral enzyme-targeted kinase inhibitor antineoplastic agents. Mayo Clin Proc. 2013;88:139–48.
10. Kruse V, Somers A, Van Bortel L, De Both A, Van Belle S, Rottey S. Sunitinib for metastatic renal cell cancer patients: observational study highlighting the risk of important drug-drug interactions. J Clin Pharm Ther. 2014;39:259–65.

Chapter 37
A Patient with Advanced Differentiated Radioactive Iodine-Refractory Thyroid Cancer Receiving Tyrosine Kinase Inhibitor Treatment: Managing Hypertension, QTc Prolongation, Dermatologic and Gastrointestinal Adverse Events

Roberta Granata, Laura Locati, and Lisa Licitra

Case Presentation

In June 2012, a 67-year-old woman was diagnosed with thyroid cancer. She had a history of an enlarging nodular goiter, and for this reason, she underwent total thyroidectomy and neck dissection. Pathologic examination revealed the presence of a 9 cm widely invasive follicular thyroid carcinoma, staged pT3pN0. Later she received radioactive iodine (RAI) treatment for three cycles receiving a cumulative activity of 18.55 GBq (500 mCi), until March 2013. RAI administration was prompted by the detection of inappropriately high serum thyroglobulin values, in the absence of structurally identifiable disease. In May 2013, an ^{18}F-fluorodeoxyglucose positron emission tomography (^{18}FDG)/computed tomography (CT) scan showed disease progression according to RECIST criteria because of the appearance of ^{18}FDG-avid lung and liver metastases. These lesions were RAI refractory as they did not concentrate iodium on radioiodine scintigraphy.

Management of the Case

In February 2014, a CT scan showed further progression of liver and lung metastases. At the end of February, she began systemic therapy in a clinical trial with vandetanib 300 mg daily, an oral multitarget tyrosine kinase inhibitor (TKI) that targets the activities of rearranged during transfection (RET), the vascular endothelial growth

R. Granata (✉) • L. Locati • L. Licitra
Head and Neck Cancer Medical Oncology Unit, Fondazione IRCCS Istituto Nazionale dei Tumori, via Venezian 1, Milan, Italy
e-mail: roberta.granata@istitutotumori.mi.it; laura.locati@istitutotumori.mi.it; lisa.licitra@istitutotumori.mi.it

D.S. Cooper, C. Durante (eds.), *Thyroid Cancer*,
DOI 10.1007/978-3-319-22401-5_37

factor receptor (VEGFR), and the epidermal growth factor receptor (EGFR) [1, 2]. The patient was enrolled into a clinical trial [3], because at that time, there were no approved drugs for treatment of advanced differentiated thyroid carcinoma.

In her past medical history, the patient had mild hypertension and was receiving atenolol 50 mg once daily. The patient measured and reported her arterial pressure daily using a home monitoring diary, and her hypertension was managed with the assistance of her cardiologist. After 2 weeks on vandetanib, the patient developed grade 2 hypertension (according to common terminology criteria for adverse events [CTCAE] version 4, systolic blood pressure 140–159 mmHg or diastolic blood pressure 90–99 mmHg) and the cardiologist added amlodipine to the atenolol. After 1 week, the hypertension was still grade 2 and irbesartan and hydrochlorothiazide were started while atenolol was stopped, resulting in better blood pressure control. The following week, the patient developed a QT prolongation [QT corrected by Bazett's formula (QTcB): 524 msec], grade 2 diarrhea, and grade 1 skin rash (Figs. 37.1 and 37.2). Because of QTcB prolongation, vandetanib was temporarily discontinued and the patient was monitored over the next week with electrocardiogram (ECG) and serum electrolytes. When the QTcB was 471 msec, vandetanib 200 mg was restarted. The diarrhea was controlled with loperamide. One week later, the patient developed a worsening skin rash to grade 2 (papules and/or pustules covering 10–30 % body surface area, which may or may not be associated with symptoms of pruritus or tenderness or associated with psychosocial impact, limiting instrumental ADL). The patient started oral antibiotics (doxycycline 100 mg once a day) and oral steroids (methylprednisolone 16 mg once a day) that improved the skin condition.

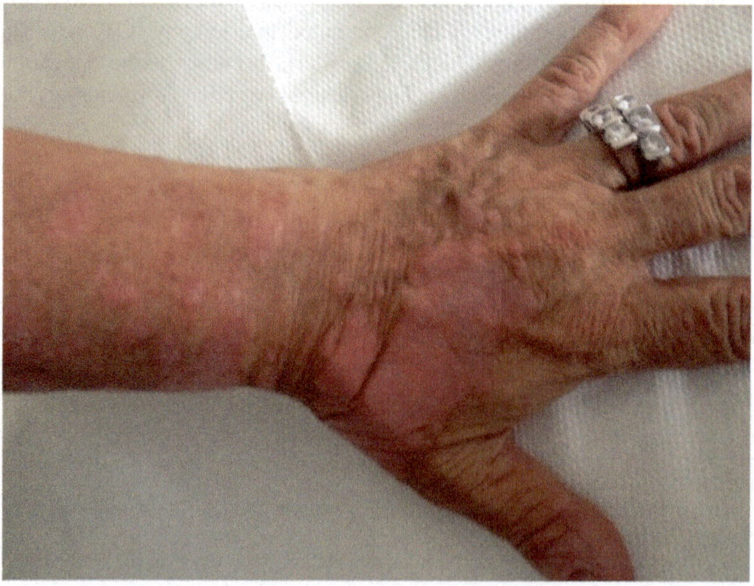

Fig. 37.1 Skin rash of the hand of the patient

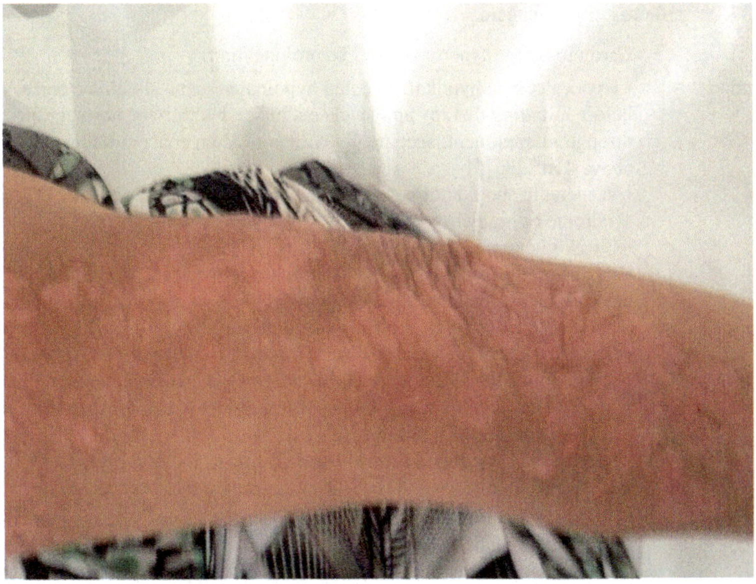

Fig. 37.2 Skin rash of the arm of the patient

In summary, this patient developed a complex combination of well-known TKI toxicities: hypertension, QTc prolongation, diarrhea, and skin rash. The recommendations on the management of these toxicities are reported in Tables 37.1, 37.2, and 37.3.

The effective management of TKI toxicity starts with comprehensive patient education regarding anticipated side effects, patient compliance, and medical recommendations, together with complete screening with laboratory tests (blood count and thyroid, renal, and liver function) and ECG before initiation of therapy. As drug interactions are potentially important in patients treated with TKI, it is essential to know all the drugs that the patient is taking.

The management of toxicities also requires a multidisciplinary approach [4].

Outcome

As of this writing, the patient has had two CT scans that showed stable disease. Currently, the patient has had to stop vandetanib for a new worsening of her skin rash after two courses of antibiotics (doxycycline and amoxicillin), topical and oral steroids, and oral antihistamines. Another dermatological consultation is planned.

Table 37.1 Cardiotoxicity management

	Cardiotoxicity (hypertension, QTc prolongation)
Prevention	• Hypocalcemia, hypokalemia, and hypomagnesemia should be corrected before initiating therapy and levels maintained within the normal range throughout treatment, specifically with potassium concentrations maintained above 4 mEq/L [5] • Vandetanib should not be used in patients with a history of long QT syndrome or bradyarrhythmias [5] • Check interactions with drugs [5][a] • Assess pretreatment risk with a minimum of two standardized blood pressure measurements, a thorough patient history, physical examination, and laboratory evaluation to determine specific cardiovascular risk factors [6] • Set a goal blood pressure at 140/90 mmHg for most patients, in accordance with recommendations for all adults. Higher-risk patients, including those with diabetes and/or chronic kidney disease, should achieve a lower blood pressure goal (e.g., 130/80 mmHg) [6] • Actively monitor blood pressure weekly during the first cycle of TKI therapy and then at least every 2–3 weeks for the duration of treatment [6]
Management	• Electrocardiogram as well as serum levels of calcium, potassium, and magnesium should be obtained at baseline and during weeks 2 to 4, weeks 8 to 12, and every 3 months thereafter during therapy • Ensure that patients for whom antihypertensive therapy has already been prescribed are adherent and that therapy has been titrated to effective doses. For newly diagnosed patients with hypertension, therapy should be initiated and titrated to effective doses, ideally, before initiating TKI therapy [6] • Aggressively manage blood pressure to avoid the development of complications associated with excessive or prolonged blood pressure increases [6] • Dose reduction or discontinuation of TKI therapy may be considered if blood pressure cannot be controlled; once the desired blood pressure is achieved, TKI therapy should be reinstituted at the same or lower dose to achieve maximum efficacy on the tumor growth [6]

[a]Some of the common drug interactions that can be associated with QT prolongation include the use of the following medications: alfuzosin, amiodarone, amitriptyline, azithromycin, ciprofloxacin, citalopram, clarithromycin, erythromycin, fluconazole, furosemide, granisetron, ondansetron, hydrochlorothiazide, levofloxacin, paroxetine, sertraline, and others (see: http://www.qtdrugs.org)

Table 37.2 Gastrointestinal management

	Gastrointestinal (diarrhea, nausea, vomiting)
Prevention	• Discuss the potential development of diarrhea with the patient. Obtain medication and dietary profile to identify potential diarrhea-causing agents [4] • Give the patient some dietary recommendations [4]
Management	• Loperamide and codeine • Hydration

Table 37.3 Dermatologic management

	Skin rash
Prevention	• Discuss the potential development of skin reactions with patients, initiate preventive measures, and provide reassurance that these can usually be managed effectively [4] • Skin care guidelines
Management	• Strict photoprotection (e.g., use of a broad-spectrum UVA/UVB sunscreen with a sun protection factor of 30 or higher, avoidance of any sun exposure by cloth protection) [4] • Avoidance of products that dry the skin (e.g., soaps, alcohol-based or perfumed products) [4] • Steroids, antibiotic, antihistamine creams • Oral glucocorticoids, antibiotics, antihistamines [4]

Clinical Pearls/Pitfalls

- There are no evidence-based guidelines for the management of TKI toxicities.
- The management of TKI toxicities always requires a multidisciplinary approach.
- Even low-grade side effects can significantly impair the patients' quality of life, as they are expected to require lifelong TKI therapy.

References

1. Carlomagno F, Vitagliano D, Guida T, Ciardiello F, Tortora G, Vecchio G, Ryan AJ, Fontanini G, Fusco A, Santoro M. ZD6474, an orally available inhibitor of KDR tyrosine kinase activity, efficiently blocks oncogenic RET kinases. Cancer Res. 2002;62:7284–90.
2. Wedge SR, Ogilvie DJ, Dukes M, Kendrew J, Chester R, Jackson JA, Boffey SJ, Valentine PJ, Curwen JO, Musgrove HL, Graham GA, Hughes GD, Thomas AP, Stokes ES, Curry B, Richmond GH, Wadsworth PF, Bigley AL, Hennequin LF. ZD6474 inhibits vascular endothelial growth factor signaling, angiogenesis, and tumor growth following oral administration. Cancer Res. 2002;62:4645–55.
3. https://clinicaltrials.gov/ct2/show/NCT01876784?term=vandetanib&rank=6
4. Grande E, Kreissl MC, Filetti S, et al. Vandetanib in advanced medullary thyroid cancer: review of adverse event management strategies. Adv Ther. 2013;30:945–66.
5. Cooper MR, Yi SY, Alghamdi W, Shaheen DJ, Steinberg M. Vandetanib for the treatment of medullary thyroid carcinoma. Ann Pharmacother. 2014;48(3):387–94.
6. Lenihan DJ, Kowey PR. Overview and management of cardiac adverse events associated with tyrosine kinase inhibitors. Oncologist. 2013;18(8):900–8.

Part IX
Medullary Thyroid Cancer: *Postoperative Management*

Chapter 38
Management of Postoperative Hypercalcitoninemia in MTC

Farouk Drissi and Eric Mirallié

Case Presentation

A 62-year-old man, without any significant medical history, presented to a gastroenterologist with chronic diarrhea of 1-year duration. He did not take any medications except for occasional anti-inflammatory drugs. In general, he felt well. The diarrhea was sometimes associated with hematochezia. The patient's physical examination was normal. The endoscopic work-up (upper endoscopy and colonoscopy) and abdominal ultrasound (US) were normal. Laboratory testing revealed a serum calcitonin (Ct) level of 1000 pg/mL and CEA level was 86.7 ng/mL. Thyroid and neck US showed a posterior right 13 × 10 × 10 mm hypoechoic, irregular thyroid nodule. Furthermore, a right jugular (8 × 3 mm) and a left subclavicular lymph node (47 × 19 mm) were identified. Chest and abdominal computed tomography (CT) scans showed another left jugular lymph node (23 × 20 mm), small mediastinal lymph nodes, and two left adrenal nodules (12 and 18 mm). These findings were highly suggestive of the diagnosis of medullary thyroid carcinoma (MTC). Biologic measurements excluded associated pheochromocytoma and primary hyperparathyroidism (PHPT).

Total thyroidectomy with bilateral central and jugular lymph node dissection was performed. Histological examination confirmed the diagnosis of MTC on the right (primary tumor: 2 cm in diameter), with mild C-cell hyperplasia in the left thyroid lobe and major lymph node invasion (36 out of 52 bilateral lymph nodes were involved: 15 involved nodes out 21 in the central compartment, 17/23 in ipsilateral lateral compartments, and 4/8 in the contralateral lateral compartment).

F. Drissi • E. Mirallié (✉)
Clinique de Chirurgie Digestive et Endocrinienne (CCDE), Institut des Maladies de l'Appareil Digestif (IMAD), Hôtel Dieu, CHU Nantes,
Place Ricordeau, 44093 Nantes cedex 1, France
e-mail: eric.mirallie@chu-nantes.fr

D.S. Cooper, C. Durante (eds.), *Thyroid Cancer*,
DOI 10.1007/978-3-319-22401-5_38

The primary tumor had minimal extrathyroid extension (pT3) and the resection margins were positive (R1). Tumor was finally classified pT3 N1b Mx R1. The postoperative serum Ct level was 71 pg/mL.

Assessment and Literature Review

MTC accounts for 5–10 % of thyroid cancers. It is histologically defined as a tumor arising from the calcitonin-secreting parafollicular C cells of the thyroid gland. MTC is known as an indolent disease despite early lymph node and distant metastatic spread. Cervical lymph node metastases are identified in 25–82 % of MTC cases [1–3]. Distant metastases at presentation are found in 7–23 % of patients [4–8]. The main distant metastatic sites are the bone, liver, and lung [9]. In general, when MTC has spread out of the neck, there are no established therapies that can offer the possibility of a cure, and the 10-year survival rate drops below 40 % [10].

Postoperative Staging of MTC Patients

Postoperative biologic monitoring mainly relies on serum Ct, a sensitive and specific indicator of residual tumor. For practical purposes, persistently elevated serum Ct levels mean that disease still exists [4]. A serum Ct level >150 pg/mL should lead to an extensive work-up to detect and localize residual disease [4]. Giraudet et al. [11] proposed a standard optimal imaging work-up to detect MTC metastases, consisting of neck US, chest CT, liver magnetic resonance imaging (MRI), bone scintigraphy, and axial skeletal MRI. Using that protocol, the authors were able to detect 98 % of neck recurrences, 100 % of mediastinal lymph nodes, lung and liver metastases, and 94 % of bone metastases.

Bone involvement in advanced medullary thyroid cancer is frequent; in one French series, 74 % of patients developed skeletal metastases. Bone MRI and post-radioimmunotherapy (RIT) immunoscintigraphy appeared to have a higher sensitivity to detect bone involvement compared with bone scintigraphy, with a 100 %, 100 %, and 72.7 % sensitivity, respectively, in a population treated by RIT [12].

Prognosis of Postoperative Patients

The TNM classification is presented in the box. Global 10-year disease survival of MTC is about 75 % [13]. Specific 10-year survival rate decreases from 100 % to 93 %, 71 %, and 21 %, respectively, for stage I, II, III, and IV [14]. For patients with distant metastasis at diagnosis, the 10-year survival rate is 40 % [10].

Box: TNM Classification (American Joint Committee on Cancer)

Primary tumor (T)

T0—No evidence of primary tumor
T1—Tumor 2 cm or less in greatest dimension limited to the thyroid (T1a: tumor 1 cm or less; T1b: tumor more than 1 cm but not more than 2 cm)
T2—Tumor more than 2 cm, but not more than 4 cm, in greatest dimension limited to the thyroid.
T3—Tumor more than 4 cm in greatest dimension limited to the thyroid or any tumor with minimal extrathyroidal extension (e.g., extension to sternothyroid muscle or perithyroid soft tissues)
T4a—Tumor of any size extending beyond the thyroid capsule to invade subcutaneous soft tissues, larynx, trachea, esophagus, or recurrent laryngeal nerve
T4b—Tumor invades prevertebral fascia or encases carotid artery or mediastinal vessels

*Regional lymph nodes (N)**

NX—Regional lymph nodes cannot be assessed
N0—No regional lymph node metastases
N1—Regional lymph node metastases

N1a—Metastasis to level VI (pretracheal, paratracheal, and prelaryngeal/delphian lymph nodes)
N1b—Metastasis to unilateral, bilateral, or contralateral cervical or superior mediastinal lymph nodes

*Central compartment, lateral cervical and upper mediastinal lymph nodes

Distant metastases (M)

MX—Distant metastasis cannot be assessed
M0—No distant metastasis
M1—Distant metastasis

Stage

Stage I: T1, N0, M0
Stage II: T2, N0, M0
Stage III: T3, N0, M0 T1, N1a, M0T2, N1a, M0T3, N1a, M0
Stage IVA: T4a, N0, M0T4a, N1a, M0T1, N1b, M0T2, N1b, M0T3, N1b, M0T4a, N1b, M0
Stage IVB: T4b, any N, M0
Stage IVC: Any T, any N, M1

The strongest prognostic factors are an advanced age at diagnosis and the stage of disease based on the tumor size, the lymph node status, and the presence of distant metastases. Quality of initial surgical treatment is also important. Subtotal thyroidectomy versus total thyroidectomy has been associated with decreased survival [10].

Barbet et al. described serum Ct doubling time (DT) as a powerful prognostic indicator in MTC, probably superior to initial pathological staging (TNM) [15]. A cohort of 65 patients was followed for 6 months to 29.5 years after surgery. Patients with Ct DT<6 months had the worst prognosis; 5- and 10-year survival rates were, respectively, 25 and 8 %. When Ct DT was between 6 months and 2 years, those rates increased respectively to 92 and 37 %. All patients with Ct DT>2 years were still alive at the end of the study [15]. Ct DT is more accurate to predict outcome than CEA DT.

Another French study evaluated relationships between progression status of MTC according to the Response Evaluation Criteria in Solid Tumors (RECIST) and calcitonin/CEA DT. Ninety-four percent of patients with Ct/CEA DT<25 months had progressive disease and 86 % with DT>24 months had stable disease [16]. These results confirm that CEA and Ct DT are strongly related to disease progression, and thus, they represent useful biologic markers in the assessment of MTC progression.

Practically speaking, measurement of Ct and CEA DT postoperatively allows the detection of high-risk patients (DT<6 months) who are then followed and potentially be treated more aggressively. For low-risk patients (DT>2 years), monitoring can be done with reduced frequency and aggressive treatment would not be required.

Treatment

This section will discuss the benefit of both prophylactic and therapeutic neck dissection toward achieving postoperative biochemical remission and the surgical approach to patients with persistent or recurrent MTC.

Initial Surgical Approach to Patients with Clinically Apparent MTC

Before looking ahead to surgical treatment, it is mandatory to exclude a potential associated pheochromocytoma with measurement of plasma-free metanephrines or normetanephrines or 24-h urine metanephrines or normetanephrines. A positive result should lead to adrenal imaging for a pheochromocytoma (CT scan or MRI). Patients with associated pheochromocytoma must undergo adrenalectomy prior to surgical treatment of the MTC.

Optimal surgical treatment of MTC consists of a total thyroidectomy associated with a variable degree of lymph node dissection [4]. Bilateral central neck dissection is recommended for all patients, but the rationale for lateral nodal dissection is controversial. The debate is fueled by the early and frequent ipsilateral lateral cervical lymph node involvement in MTC. Indeed, ipsilateral lateral cervical lymph node spread appears to be approximatively as frequent as central nodal involvement [3]. Furthermore, contralateral lateral nodal invasion is present in about 44 % of patients with a unilateral MTC and 25 % of patients with a tumor size <1 cm.

An appropriate lymph node dissection is associated with a higher biochemical cure rate at the time of the initial procedure. The recommendation of Scollo et al. is to perform a central and complete bilateral neck dissection irrespective of the sporadic/hereditary feature or the tumor size [17]. However, the authors of the present article, in accordance with the "Groupe d'Etude des Tumeurs Endocrines" (French Neuroendocrine Tumor Group), recommend that the initial surgical treatment should include bilateral central and at least ipsilateral lateral lymph node dissection. When lymph nodes are diagnosed preoperatively with imaging, bilateral central and lateral lymph node dissections should be performed. These considerations are weighed against surgical complications of such a procedure (hypoparathyroidism, recurrent laryngeal nerve palsy).

Surgical Approach to Patients with Persistent or Recurrent MTC

For patients with local recurrent or persistent disease, a second surgery can be justified if the initial surgery was incomplete (subtotal thyroidectomy or incomplete lymph node dissection). However, only a minority of patients are cured after a second surgery. For example, Moley et al. reported a 38 % of biochemical cure after reoperation. Those patients undergoing reoperation must be restricted to selected patients with disease confined to the neck [18]. Most often, a second surgery is not associated with long-term biochemical cure, but may be associated with a decreased rate of disease progression [19].

The place of external beam radiation therapy in the treatment of locoregional disease is not clearly defined. It seems to improve locoregional disease control in patients with high risk of locoregional relapse without evidence of improvement in survival rates [20].

In patients with distant metastatic disease, less aggressive neck surgery must be considered in order to preserve speech, swallowing, and parathyroid functions [4]. However, in select cases, single organ invasion can be managed with surgical resection or specific local treatment.

Management of the Case

Postoperative serum Ct level was 71 pg/mL (2 days after surgery) and increased to 163 pg/mL 1 month later and remained stable at 5 months (152 pg/mL). At 6 months, CEA level was 17.1 ng/mL. Therefore, the patient was included in a research protocol using radiolabelled anti-CEA monoclonal antibodies to detect residue of the MTC. The imaging displayed a right supraclavicular and left paratracheal uptake. Similar findings were observed following a fluorine-18-dihydroxyphenylalanine (F-DOPA) positron emission tomography. He also had liver and axial skeletal MRI, which were normal.

Based on these findings, it was decided to check periodically serum Ct level in order to evaluate its doubling time and to perform periodic imaging studies to estimate the disease progression and the need of a re-intervention.

Because of the detection of a C-cell hyperplasia in the context of the thyroid tissue, a genetic analysis was performed. RET testing was negative.

Clinical Pearls

- MTC prognosis depends on age, TNM staging, quality of initial surgery, and Ct/CEA DT.
- CEA and Ct DT are strongly related to disease progression, and thus, they can be exploited in the assessment of MTC progression.
- Ct and CEA doubling time may guide the timing of diagnostic imaging procedures and therapeutic interventions.

References

1. Raue F, Kotzerke J, Reinwein D, et al. Prognostic factors in medullary thyroid carcinoma: evaluation of 741 patients from the German medullary thyroid carcinoma register. Clin Investig. 1993;71:7–12.
2. Rossi RL, Cady B, Meissner WA, et al. Non familial medullary thyroid carcinoma. Am J Surg. 1980;139:554–60.
3. Moley JF, De Benedetti MK. Patterns of nodal metastases in palpable medullary thyroid carcinoma: recommendations for extent of node dissection. Ann Surg. 1999;229:880–7.
4. Kloos RT, Eng C, Evans DB, et al. Medullary thyroid cancer: management guidelines of the American Thyroid Association. Thyroid. 2009;19:565–612.
5. Atkins D, Eccles M, Flottorp S, et al. GRADE Working Group: grading quality of evidence and strength of recommendations. BMC Health Serv Res. 2004;4:38.
6. Swiglo BA, Murad MH, Schünemann HJ, et al. A case for clarity, consistency, and helpfulness: state-of-the-art clinical practice guidelines in endocrinology using the grading of recommendations, assessment, development, and evaluation system. J Clin Endocrinol Metab. 2008;93:666–73.
7. Guyatt G, Gutterman D, Baumann MH, et al. Grading strength of recommendations and quality of evidence in clinical guidelines: report from an American college of chest physicians task force. Chest. 2006;129:174–81.
8. Schlumberger M, Carlomagno F, Baudin E, et al. New therapeutic approaches to treat medullary thyroid carcinoma. Nat Clin Pract Endocrinol Metab. 2008;4:22–32.
9. Kraeber-Bodéré F, Salaun PY, Oudoux A, et al. Pretargeted radioimmunotherapy in rapidly progressing, metastatic, medullary thyroid cancer. Cancer. 2010;116(4 Suppl):1118–25.

10. Roman S, Lin R, Sosa JA. Prognosis of medullary thyroid carcinoma: demographic, clinical and pathologic predictors of survival in 1252 cases. Cancer. 2006;107:2134–42.
11. Giraudet al, Vanel D, Leboulleux S, et al. Imaging medullary thyroid carcinoma with persistent elevated calcitonin levels. J Clin Endocrinol Metab. 2007;92:4185–90.
12. Mirallié E, Vuillez JP, Bardet S, et al. High frequency of bone/bone marrow involvement in advanced medullary thyroid cancer. J Clin Endocrinol Metab. 2005;90:779–88.
13. Hundahl SA, Fleming ID, Fremgen AM, et al. A national cancer data base report on 53,856 cases of thyroid carcinoma treated in the US 1985-1995. Cancer. 1998;83:2638–48.
14. Modigliani E, Cohen R, Campos JM, et al. Prognostic factors for survival and for biochemical cure in medullary thyroid carcinoma: results in 899 patients. The GETC Study Group. Clin Endocrinol. 1998;48:265–73.
15. Barbet J, Campion L, Kraeber-Bodere F, et al. Prognostic impact of serum calcitonin and carcinoembryonic antigen doubling-times in patients with medullary thyroid carcinoma. J Clin Endocrinol Metab. 2005;90:6077–84.
16. Giraudet al, Al Ghulzan A, Aupérin A, et al. Progression of medullary thyroid carcinoma: assessment with calcitonin and carcinoembryonic antigen doubling times. Eur J Endocrinol. 2008;158:239–46.
17. Scollo C, Baudin E, Travagli JP, et al. Rationale for central and bilateral lymph node dissection in sporadic and hereditary medullary thyroid cancer. J Clin Endocrinol Metab. 2003;88:2070–5.
18. Moley JF, Dilley WG, DeBenedetti MK. Improved results of cervical reoperation for medullary thyroid carcinoma. Ann Surg. 1997;225:734–40.
19. Kebebew E, Kikuchi S, Duh QY, et al. Long-term results of reoperation and localizing studies in patients studies in patients with persistent or recurrent medullary thyroid cancer. Arch Surg. 2000;135:895–901.
20. Brierley J, Tsang R, Simpson WJ, et al. Medullary thyroid cancer: analyses of survival and prognostic factors and the role of radiation therapy in local control. Thyroid. 1996;6:305–10.

Chapter 39
A Patient with Metastatic Medullary Thyroid Carcinoma (MTC) and Tumor-Related Diarrhea

Patricia Cortez, Teresa Alonso-Gordoa, and Enrique Grande

Case Presentation

A 46-year-old male patient, with no relevant previous medical or family history, presented to the emergency department with a 2-month history of dysphonia, found to be due to left vocal cord paralysis and progressively enlarging bilateral cervical lymphadenopathy. A cervical computed tomography (CT) scan showed an intrathoracic goiter. With this finding, the patient was referred to the endocrinology department. Thyroid ultrasound showed an enlarged thyroid gland with multiple nodules, the largest measuring 29 × 19 × 13 mm in the left lobe, and multiple sonographically suspicious homolateral lymph nodes. Fine needle aspiration (FNA) cytology of a thyroid nodule was interpreted as thyroid carcinoma (Bethesda class V), suggesting a medullary thyroid carcinoma (MTC). FNA performed on one of the left-sided cervical lymph nodes confirmed the presence of metastatic disease. The patient underwent a total thyroidectomy with central and left lateral neck dissection with resection of the recurrent laryngeal nerve by tumor infiltration. The pathology revealed a 64 × 31 × 30 mm MTC with lymphatic and vascular invasion and extrathyroidal extension in the left lobe. In addition, microscopic tumor foci were reported in the right lobe, and metastases were found in 24 of 34 lymph nodes, some of them with extranodal extension (Fig. 39.1). Final pathology staging after surgery was pT4a N1b Mx, stage IVA. The level of serum calcitonin before surgery was 875 pg/ml (upper limit of normal 7.40 pg/ml), and serum carcinoembryonic antigen (CEA) was 53.9 ng/ml (upper limit of normal 3.4 ng/dl), both dropping to 795 pg/ml and 36.4 ng/ml, respectively, after surgery. Postsurgical body CT scan identified three space-occupying lesions in the liver that were confirmed as metastases from

P. Cortez • T. Alonso-Gordoa • E. Grande (✉)
Medical Oncology Department, Hospital Ramón y Cajal,
Carretera de Colmenar km 9, 1, 28034 Madrid, Spain
e-mail: egrande@oncologiahrc.com

D.S. Cooper, C. Durante (eds.), *Thyroid Cancer*,
DOI 10.1007/978-3-319-22401-5_39

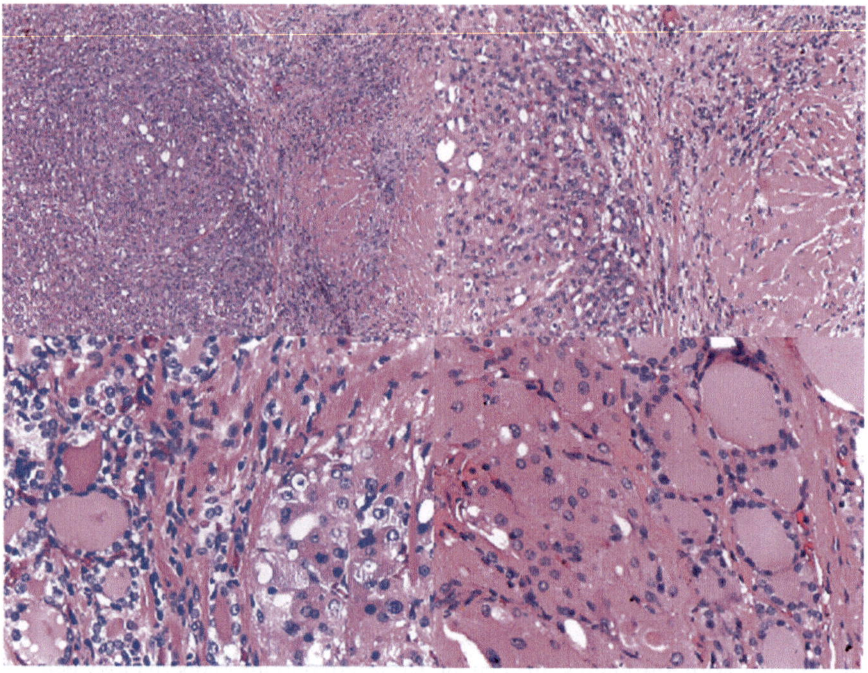

Fig. 39.1 *Microscopic high power of the medullary thyroid cancer*. Tumor is composed of solid nests of variable size, separated by the presence of areas with collagen connective tracts and foci of amyloid deposits from calcitonin. The cells are usually round and fusiform, with poorly defined and finely granular eosinophilic cytoplasm, uniform nuclei, and punctate chromatin

MTC in a subsequent CT-guided FNA. The multidisciplinary endocrine tumors team met and decided to initiate systemic tyrosine-kinase inhibitor treatment for metastatic MTC. At that time, our institution was participating in a named compassionate use program with sunitinib for advanced thyroid cancer. Sunitinib was started at a dose of 50 mg/day (with a 4 weeks "on" and 2 weeks "off" schedule). After three cycles, the patient developed grade 1 diarrhea (Table 39.1) that was attributed to drug toxicity. Progression of the liver metastases was documented on CT scan, and second-line "off-label" treatment with sorafenib was begun at a dose of 400 mg twice daily under a compassionate use protocol. Unfortunately, the patient experienced grade 3 hand-foot syndrome (severe skin changes, e.g., peeling, blisters, bleeding, edema, or hyperkeratosis with pain limiting self-care activities of daily living) and grade 2 diarrhea (Table 39.1) within the first month; therefore, dose was reduced to 200 mg twice daily. With that change in the dose, the drug was well tolerated and biochemical and partial radiological response was achieved. The patient experienced clinical relief of the diarrhea coinciding with a serum calcitonin reduction down to 163 pg/ml after 3 months of treatment with sorafenib. However, during the following 13 months, there was a continuous and slow increase in serum calcitonin levels, reaching values above 1000 pg/ml, associated with a worsening of the asthenia and diarrhea without observation of tumor progression on the CT scan

Table 39.1 Classification and treatment of the drug-related diarrhea according to common terminology criteria for adverse events (CTCAE) v4.0

	Diarrhea	Treatment
Grade 1	Increased of <4 stools per day over baseline, mild increase in ostomy output compared with baseline	No change in treatment Medical intervention not indicated
Grade 2	Increased of 4–6 stools per day over baseline, moderate increase in ostomy output compared with baseline	No change in treatment Initiating supportive care
Grade 3	Increased of ≥7 stools per day over baseline, incontinence, hospitalization indicated, severe increase in ostomy output compared with baseline. Limiting self-care ADL	Discontinue treatment until recover to grade ≤2 Hospitalization is required for intensive supportive care
Grade 4	Life-threatening consequence	Discontinue treatment until recovery to grade ≤2 and reintroduce with dose reduction Hospitalization is required for urgent treatment
Grade 5	Death	

performed at this time. Sixteen months after starting sorafenib, lung metastases were identified and hepatic tumor progression was observed. At that point, the patient began treatment with vandetanib 300 mg daily under the authorization treatment use (ATU) program available at the Spanish Agency for Medicines and Sanitary Products (AEMPS). Vandetanib was given for 12 months with stable disease as the best objective response from a radiologic point of view (Fig. 39.2). In addition, a biochemical response and subjective clinical benefit were obtained. Tolerability of vandetanib was acceptable with grade 1 skin rash (papules and/or pustules covering <10 % body surface area, which may or may not be associated with symptoms of pruritus or tenderness) and asthenia (fatigue relieved by rest). During vandetanib treatment, diarrhea control was obtained by using loperamide occasionally. After 12 months of treatment with vandetanib, radiologic and biochemical progression was observed with an increase in liver and nodal lesions and in calcitonin levels reaching 4100 pg/ml. At that time, a treatment with axitinib 5 mg twice daily was started on a compassionate use basis. With axitinib, a rapid decrease in calcitonin levels was observed (1150 pg/ml), with clinical benefit in the first 2 months of treatment, but 6 months later, the patient complained of weight loss and growth of laterocervical lymph nodes. Locoregional palliative radiotherapy was administered for pain relief and sunitinib was rechallenged. A minor disease response was obtained, but significantly worsening diarrhea required the administration of a long-acting somatostatin analog (lanreotide 60 mg subcutaneously every 28 days) to control the diarrhea after 3 months of treatment. Sorafenib was reintroduced after clinical progression on sunitinib. Unfortunately, neither clinical nor radiological benefit was seen with sorafenib thus far. After six courses of treatment with four different chemotherapeutic agents for advanced disease, the multidisciplinary team decided to initiate supportive care, and patient died few weeks after sorafenib withdrawal, 38 months after the diagnosis of metastatic MTC.

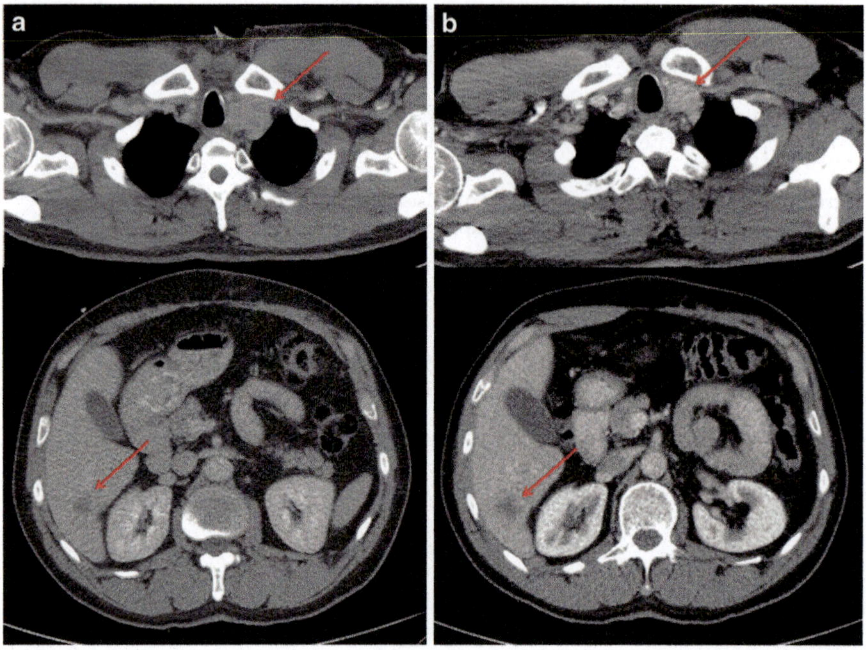

Fig. 39.2 Radiographic assessment conducted in February 2012 (**a**) and September 2012 (**b**) during treatment with vandetanib. Stable disease was achieved on the *left* supraclavicular lymph node (*arrow*) and the *right* liver lobe lesion (segment VI) according to RECIST criteria v1.1

Literature Review

The appearance of diarrhea has been described in approximately 30 % of patients with MTC and has been suggested to precede the identification of the thyroid mass in some cases [3]. Calcitonin plays a key role in this disturbance and it seems to be related to an alteration in water and electrolyte movement from absorption to secretion in the intestinal tract [4]. However, intestinal motor dysfunction has been suggested as the main mechanism for diarrhea related to hypercalcitoninemia [5]. Adequate symptomatic control will improve the quality of life of these patients.

Definition

MTC derives from the thyroid parafollicular C cells that are able to produce and secrete calcitonin. This thyroid cancer subtype occurs as a sporadic tumor or as part of a hereditary syndrome (multiple endocrine neoplasia (MEN), 2A and 2B, or familial MTC). Sporadic MTC accounts for 75 % of all cases (Table 39.2). Median age at diagnosis occurs during fifth or sixth decade of life and remains slightly more

Table 39.2 Mutation profile of hereditary and sporadic medullary thyroid cancer (MTC) [1, 2]

	Hereditary MTC (25 %)	Sporadic MTC (75 %)
RET	≈100 %	40–65 %
HRAS	–	12.1 %
KRAS	–	3.7 %
NRAS	–	1.8 %
Unknown	–	40 %

frequent in women [6]. In 35–50 % of patients, lymph node metastases are observed at diagnosis. When MTC metastasizes, the most common distant sites are the liver, lung, bones, and, with less frequency, brain and skin [7].

Their neural crest origin is responsible for the ability of C cells to take up amine precursors as well as the secretion of neuroactive peptides that include calcitonin, CEA, serotonin, ACTH, chromogranin A, somatostatin, neurotensin, pro-opiomelanocortin, prostaglandins, kinins, histaminase, and vasoactive intestinal peptide (VIP) [8]. Serum calcitonin or CEA elevations are almost universal and are key in MTC diagnosis, monitoring the clinical course of disease, and evaluating the response to therapy.

Symptoms Related to MTC

Typically, patients present with a palpable asymptomatic neck mass. However, with the appearance of a thyroid nodule, clinicians should be aware of the presence of an MTC if patients suffer from symptoms such as diarrhea, flushes, weight loss, and, more rarely, Cushing's syndrome or if it is associated with a familial history of MTC, pheochromocytoma, and hyperparathyroidism. The systemic symptoms may occur due to hormonal excess or to distant metastatic disease.

In case of a large palpable thyroid nodule, local compressive symptoms, such as dysphagia or a choking sensation, may occur. Rarely, the mass can infiltrate the recurrent nerve and cause hoarseness [9].

Diarrhea in MTC

When faced with a patient with chronic diarrhea, neuroendocrine tumors should always be considered in the differential diagnosis. Clues should be sought in the clinical history, physical examination, complementary studies, and laboratory tests. They can help rule out more common causes of chronic diarrhea such as infections, drug use, chronic inflammatory diseases, cathartic agent use, and diabetic diarrhea.

Diarrhea in MTC is caused by two main pathophysiological mechanisms: the most important one suggests a motor dysfunction diarrhea leading to decreased transit time due to hyperactivity of small intestinal and colonic tone, leading to insufficient absorption. It has been reported in 28–39 % of cases [10]. The second possible mechanism is a secretory impairment as the origin of the diarrhea caused by substances other than calcitonin. This postulated mechanism is based on an increase in fluid and electrolyte secretion induced by prostaglandins (E_2 or $F_2\alpha$), serotonin, or substance P that worsens the absorptive dysfunction in the intestinal tract caused by increased colonic tone and decreased transit time [11]. Circulating agents enter the intestinal epithelial cells (located in the jejunum and ileum) and reverse the absorption of water and electrolytes into a secretory process. The rapid emptying of the proximal colon may contribute to the increase stool weight in these patients. While sodium plays a key role in the absorption of water and electrolytes, chloride is the most important electrolyte involved in the secretion of ions. Several intracellular pathways result in the output of chloride ions from the intestinal epithelial cells via a specific chloride channel in the luminal membrane. The process can start on the luminal side, as occurs in infections, or on the serosal side, for example, when related to circulating agents such as serotonin or VIP. Thus, elevated circulating concentrations of hormones such as gastrin, somatostatin, and VIP can alter both gastrointestinal motor function and intestinal secretion and contribute to the diarrhea associated with MTC [12].

This phenomenon usually occurs in advanced disease, so patients can suffer from a syndrome similar to the carcinoid syndrome with flushing and/or diarrhea. Because the increased levels of circulating calcitonin or other peptides stimulate secretion by the small intestine mucosa, the diarrhea can be severe with a large volume of watery stools, often exceeding 1 L per day, without any specific treatment [11].

Management of Diarrhea in MTC

The optimal management of the diarrhea in advanced MTC represents a key therapeutic goal to improve the quality of life of these patients (Table 39.3). The initial treatment approach is based on antimotility agents such as loperamide, diphenoxylate with atropine, and tincture of deodorized opium. The treatment should begin with loperamide, because of its low potential for abuse and dependence. Deodorized tincture of opium is very powerful and is useful in severe cases but can induce drug dependence.

Table 39.3 Supportive treatment for the management of diarrhea in patients with medullary thyroid cancer (MTC)

Hydration	Electrolyte replacement
Antidiarrheal drugs	Loperamide 4 mg followed by 2 mg/4 h (dose max. 16 mg/day)
Somatostatin analogs	Lanreotide (60–120 mg/28 days sc) Octreotide (2–3 × 50–500 μg sc/day) Octreotide LAR (10–30 mg/28 days im)
Antibiotics	Metronidazole, quinolones
Analgesia	Spasmolytic drugs

Concomitant with dietary measures (fasting, solid food eating, and hydration), patients should avoid drinks that contain caffeine, as well as sugar-rich beverages that can worsen the diarrheal syndrome due to a hyperosmolar effect.

On the whole, it is important to maintain adequate hydration with electrolyte replacement and antispasmodic and analgesic treatment to control cramps and, if infection is suspected, administer appropriate antibiotics (Table 39.3).

In refractory cases, patients may obtain relief of symptoms with therapy directed at the tumor, such as tumor ablation or debulking. Unfortunately, symptoms reappear with disease recurrence or progression [13]. There is a clinical benefit of using somatostatin analogs but the mechanism is uncertain, since a reduction in calcitonin concentrations has not been demonstrated with those agents [14]. Somatostatin analogs are generally well tolerated but have some side effects such as nausea, abdominal discomfort, bloating, diarrhea, and fat malabsorption within the first weeks of treatment. The most important is the reduction of gallbladder contractility and delay in postprandial gallbladder emptying; up to 25 % of patients develop asymptomatic cholesterol gallstones during the first 18 months of treatment.

Diarrhea as an Adverse Event of Novel Targeted Agents in MTC

Although some tyrosine-kinase inhibitors (TKIs) may be effective in treating advanced MTC, these systemic therapies also cause diarrhea as a side effect.

In the phase II trial of vandetanib that included 30 patients with hereditary MTC, the most common adverse events were diarrhea, which was observed in 21 patients (three patients with grade >3), fatigue, rash, and nausea. Interruption or dose reduction was required in 24 patients due to adverse events, most commonly due to diarrhea ($N=7$) [15]. In patients receiving vandetanib, skin rash and diarrhea were suggested to be associated with the anti-EGFR effects of this therapy. In the phase III ZETA trial, all grades of diarrhea were observed in 56 % of patients ($N=130$) in the vandetanib arm and 26 % of patients ($N=26$) in the placebo arm [16]. Final recommendations for the use of vandetanib in patients with MTC require close monitoring of diarrhea that can be related either to the disease or to an adverse drug reaction. In case of diarrhea, the presence of dehydration, electrolyte imbalance, and/or impaired renal function may increase the risk of prolonging the QTc interval and predispose to malignant cardiac arrhythmias, so close ECG monitoring is mandatory. It is also important to maintain normal serum potassium, magnesium, and calcium levels as well as renal function during treatment with vandetanib.

Cabozantinib was the second drug approved for the treatment of MTC. In the phase I dose escalation study of oral cabozantinib, 37 patients with MTC were included [17]. Grade 1–2 diarrhea was observed in 50 % of patients ($N=43$) and grade 3–4 diarrhea was described in 7 % of patients ($N=6$). In the EXAM phase III trial, all grades of diarrhea were described in 63.1 % of patients ($N=135$) treated with cabozantinib vs. 33.0 % of patients ($N=36$) treated with placebo [18].

In the phase II trial of sorafenib that included 21 patients with MTC, grade 1–2 diarrhea was reported in 71 % ($N=15$) of patients and grade ≥ 3 in 10 % ($N=2$) of patients [19]. The occurrence of drug-related diarrhea was well managed with symptomatic treatment and dose reduction when required.

In an open-label phase II trial of sunitinib, 35 patients with progressive refractory thyroid cancer ($N=7$ with MTC) were included. Dose reduction related to grade 3 diarrhea was described in 17 % ($N=6$) of patients [20].

As we attempted to achieve in our patient, optimal management of TKIs is required to obtain the maximum therapeutic effect with an acceptable tolerability profile. In clinical trials, diarrhea-related adverse event was manageable with antidiarrheal medications, dose interruption, and/or dose reduction. If severe diarrhea is identified (grade 3 according to the common terminology criteria for adverse events), the TKI should be discontinued until the patient recovers with intensive supportive hydration and electrolyte replacement. Once the diarrhea has been fully treated, vandetanib or cabozantinib can be reintroduced at the same or a reduced dose, according to the adverse event severity (see Table 39.1).

Back to the Patient

Symptomatic Management of the Case

Our patient had advanced sporadic MTC that metastasized early, requiring a multidisciplinary approach and multiple courses of systemic TKI-based treatment and achieving a prolonged progression-free survival, with proper management of symptoms.

In the case presented above, diarrhea was a symptom that worsened with biochemical and radiological disease progression and ameliorated with response to systemic treatment. The occurrence of drug-related diarrhea was well managed with symptomatic treatment and dose reduction when required. After adjusting the daily dose of sorafenib, our patient was able to receive the drug continuously and achieved a good tumor response and symptom relief.

Diarrhea was initially treated with hydration and diet and antiperistaltic drugs like loperamide (maximum dose of 16 mg/day). This approach was not adequate when the disease progressed with an increase in tumor burden, requiring somatostatin analog therapy for symptomatic relief.

Clinical Pearls/Pitfalls

- Patients with MTC may suffer from chronic diarrhea that has been attributed to intestinal motor dysfunction due to hypercalcitoninemia and can be worsened with a disturbance in water and electrolyte secretion mediated by other substances released by tumor cells.

- The treatment of diarrhea in a patient with MTC begins with replacement of fluid and electrolyte. Antidiarrheal drugs that act by slowing intestinal motility can be effectively used as first-line therapies. In more severe cases, somatostatin analogs may be useful. In refractory patients, surgical and ablation techniques represent a more aggressive but effective alternative.
- It is important to differentiate between the diarrhea from targeted agents and the diarrhea caused by the MCT or by other complications (infections) in order to offer the most specific and effective treatment.
- Control of disease-related symptoms and side effects in patients with MTC is essential to provide an optimal quality of life to our patients.

References

1. Mulligan LM. RET revisited: expanding the oncogenic portfolio. Nat Rev. 2014;14:173–86.
2. Ciampi R, Mian C, Fugazzola L, Cosci B, Romei C, Barollo S, et al. Evidence of a low prevalence of RAS mutations in a large medullary thyroid cancer series. Thyroid. 2013;23:50–7.
3. Kebebew E, Ituarte PH, Siperstein AE, et al. Medullary thyroid carcinoma: clinical characteristics, treatment, prognostic factors, and a comparison of staging systems. Cancer. 2000;88:1139.
4. Gray IK, Brannan P, Juan D, et al. Ion transport changes during calcitonin-induced intestinal secretion in man. Gastroenterology. 1976;71:392–8.
5. Rambaud JC, Hautefeuille M, Ruskone A, et al. Diarrhea due to circulating agents. Clin Gastroenterol. 1986;15:603–29.
6. Jin J, Phitayakorn R, Wilhelm SM, et al. Advances in management of thyroid cancer. Curr Probl Surg. 2013;50:241–89.
7. American Cancer Society. Cancer facts & figures 2013. Atlanta, GA: American Cancer Society; 2013.
8. Machens A, Hauptmann S, Dralle H. Increased risk of lymph node metastasis in multifocal hereditary and sporadic medullary thyroid cancer. World J Surg. 2007;31:1960.
9. Pacini F, Castagna MG, Cipri C, Schlumberger M. Medullary thyroid carcinoma. Clin Oncol (R Coll Radiol). 2010;22:475.
10. Bergholm U, Bergström R, Ekbom A. Long-term follow-up of patients with medullary carcinoma of the thyroid. Cancer. 1997;79(1):132–8.
11. Rambaud JC, Jian R, Flourie B, et al. Pathophysiological study of diarrhoea in a patient with medullary thyroid carcinoma. Evidence against a secretory mechanism and for the role of shortened colonic transit time. Gut. 1988;29:537–43. PubMed: 3371722.
12. Rambaid J-C, Hautefeuille M, Ruskone A, Jacquenod P. Diarrhea due to circulating agents. Clin Gastroenterol. 1986;15:603–29.
13. Kloos RT, Eng C, Evans DB, et al. Medullary thyroid cancer: management guidelines of the American Thyroid Association. Thyroid. 2009;19:565–612.
14. Díez JJ, Iglesias P. Somatostatin analogs in the treatment of medullary thyroid carcinoma. J Endocrinol Invest. 2002;25(9):773–8.
15. Wells SA, Gosnell JE, Gagel RF, et al. Vandetanib for the treatment of patients with locally advanced or metastatic hereditary medullary thyroid cancer. J Clin Oncol. 2010;28:767.
16. Wells Jr SA, Robinson BG, Gagel RF, et al. Vandetanib in patients with locally advanced or metastatic medullary thyroid cancer: a randomized, double-blind phase III trial. J Clin Oncol. 2012;30:134.
17. Kurzrock R, Sherman SI, Ball DW, et al. Activity of XL184 (Cabozantinib), an oral tyrosine kinase inhibitor, in patients with medullary thyroid cancer. J Clin Oncol. 2011;29:2660.

18. Schoffski P, Elisei R, Muller S, et al. An international, double-blind, randomized, placebo-controlled phase III trial (EXAM) of cabozantinib (XL184) in medullary thyroid carcinoma (MTC) patients (pts) with documented RECIST progression at baseline. J Clin Oncol. 2012;30(suppl):5508.
19. Lam ET, Ringel MD, Kloos RT, et al. Phase II clinical trial of sorafenib in metastatic medullary thyroid cancer. J Clin Oncol. 2010;28:2323.
20. Carr LL, Mankoff DA, Goulart BH, et al. Phase II study of daily sunitinib in FDG-PET-positive, iodine-refractory differentiated thyroid cancer and metastatic medullary carcinoma of the thyroid with functional imaging correlation. Clin Cancer Res. 2010;16:5260.

Chapter 40
Clinical Management of a Patient with a Locally Recurrent Medullary Thyroid Cancer and Asymptomatic Slowly Progressing Distant Metastases

Virginia Cappagli, Valeria Bottici, and Rossella Elisei

Case Presentation

On May 1994, a 21-year-old woman with a 3.5 cm left thyroid nodule underwent total thyroidectomy mainly for aesthetic reasons. Paratracheal lymph nodes were also removed because they were found to be enlarged and suspicious by the surgeon. The histology identified a 3.2 cm medullary thyroid cancer (MTC) with three metastases out of six paratracheal lymph nodes (T2N1aM0). No information about presurgical functional thyroid status or serum calcitonin (Ct) levels were available. Fine needle aspiration cytology (FNAC) was indeterminate showing a microfollicular cell pattern that could be nowadays included in the category III of Bethesda cytological classification.

In October 1994, the patient arrived at our center for consultation: serum Ct was 118 pg/ml (normal <14 pg/ml), and neck ultrasound showed the presence of a post-surgical remnant thyroid tissue in the thyroid bed with no evidence of suspicious lymph nodes in the neck. The screening for germline *RET* mutations was negative.

In the subsequent 2 years, serum Ct progressively, but slowly, increased with no evidence of structural disease on neck ultrasound or computerized tomography (CT). In November 1996, a suspicious left laterocervical lymph node measuring 1.2 cm was found on neck ultrasound; at that time, serum Ct was 736 pg/ml; the cytology of the lymph node and the high values of Ct in the washout of the needle used for the aspiration (1648 pg/ml) confirmed an MTC lymph node metastasis. In February 1997 [serum Ct, 1360 pg/ml, and carcinogenic embryonic antigen (CEA), 46.3 ng/ml], the patient underwent bilateral and central compartment nodal dissections. However, out of 32 lymph nodes that were removed, only the

V. Cappagli • V. Bottici • R. Elisei, M.D. (✉)
Endocrine Unit, Department of Clinical and Experimental Medicine, University Hospital of Pisa, Via Paradisa, 2, 56124 Pisa, Italy
e-mail: rossella.elisei@med.unipi.it

D.S. Cooper, C. Durante (eds.), *Thyroid Cancer*,
DOI 10.1007/978-3-319-22401-5_40

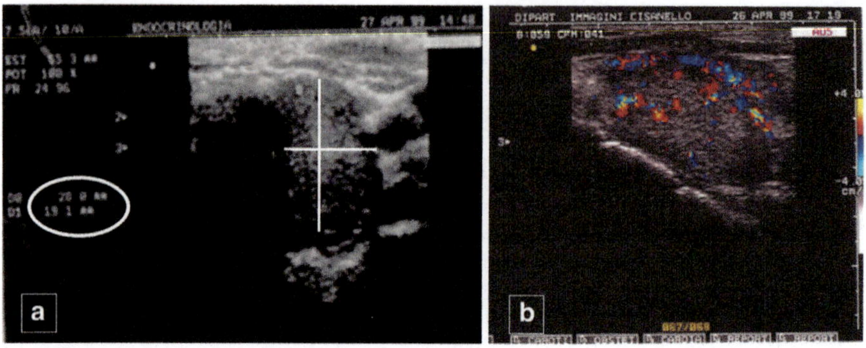

Fig. 40.1 Neck ultrasound of the *left* paratracheal lesion in April 1999, before the surgical excision, the histology of which demonstrated a medullary thyroid cancer local recurrence. (Panel **a**) Standard neck ultrasound transverse section with the anteroposterior (28.0 mm) and latero-lateral (19.1 mm) diameters of the paratracheal lesion. (Panel **b**) Color-Doppler imaging of the paratracheal lesion showing the intralesion irregular hypervascularity (sagittal section, 32 mm)

left laterocervical lymph node, corresponding to the one observed on neck ultrasound, was metastatic.

Two months after surgery, serum Ct was still elevated (1048 pg/ml) and increasing up to 2240 pg/ml in July 1997; a neck CT scan performed in September 1997 showed a left paratracheal/mediastinal nodule of 19 × 23 × 32 mm, with a suspicious cytology and Ct in the needle washout >2400 pg/ml. Because a total body (TB) CT scan did not show any other lesion in extracervical sites, we decided to proceed with local therapy. In November 1997, the patient underwent a diathermy ablation of the lesion with a 40 % reduction in its volume. Eighteen months later, at the end of April 1999, the lesion measured at neck ultrasound was even bigger than before (19 × 28 × 32 mm) (Fig. 40.1); total body CT scans confirmed that this was the only lesion, and we performed a surgical paratracheal dissection. The histology showed that the removed tissue was a recurrence of the primary tumor, since only medullary cancer cells and no lymphoid elements were present. The tissue analysis for somatic *RET* mutation showed the presence of a somatic M918T mutation. The postsurgical serum Ct progressively dropped and become <14 pg/ml (Fig. 40.2). Neck ultrasound and CT scan were negative in follow-up.

In 2001, basal Ct was still <14 pg/ml but a pentagastrin stimulation test showed a peak Ct of 88 pg/ml. At this time, both neck ultrasound and total body CT scan were still negative.

From 2001 to 2005, the patient, by her choice, did not undergo any biochemical or radiological assessment. In February 2005, she returned to our center, and at that time, serum Ct was 21 pg/ml; neck ultrasound and neck CT scan showed subcentimeter lymph nodes that were not clearly metastatic. No distant metastases were present, and a total body bone scan was negative. We continued to follow our patient with clinical, biochemical, and imaging assessment every 12 months, and from 2005 to 2009, the disease was stable.

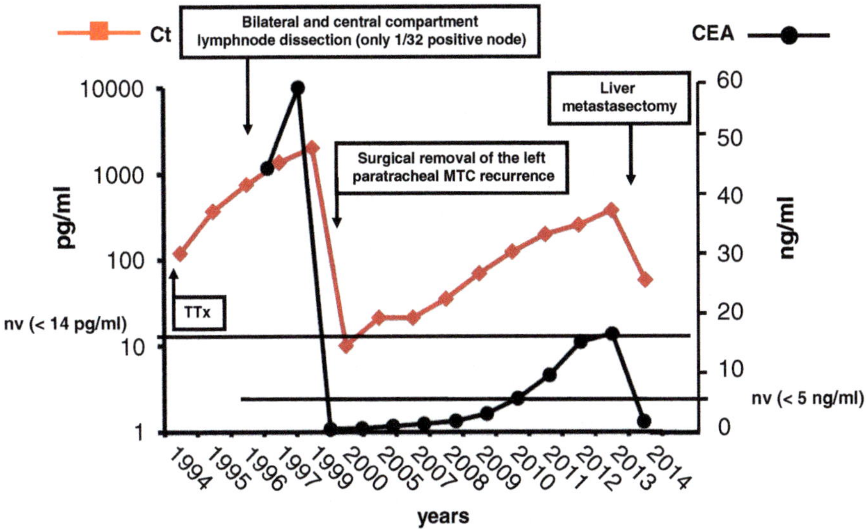

Fig. 40.2 Serum Ct and CEA variations during the follow-up of the patient: a correlation between the two markers is evident as well as a correlation with therapeutic interventions

In June 2009, the total body CT scan showed the persistence of small lymph nodes in the neck, the appearance of micronodules in the lung, and three new hepatic lesions (largest was 12 mm) with radiographic characteristics suspicious for metastatic lesions. Serum Ct levels had slowly increased up to 69 pg/ml while serum CEA was in the normal range (<5 ng/ml). We decided to not recommend active therapies but to follow the strategy of "wait and see."

During the following 3 years, radiological assessments showed the progression of the hepatic metastases; in particular, the one that had been 12 mm in 2009 grew to 14 mm in 2010, 15 mm in 2011, and 17 mm in September 2012 (Fig. 40.3, Panel a) with a mean size increase of 20% per year. In parallel, serum Ct increased from 69 pg/ml on June 2009 to 314 pg/ml on September 2012 and CEA levels from 3.12 ng/ml on June 2009 to 15.6 ng/ml on September 2012 (Fig. 40.2). At this moment, the doubling time of both Ct and CEA was 1.5 years.

In January 2013, the total body CT scan confirmed that the only growing lesion was the hepatic one which was now 19 mm. At this point, we explored the possibility of performing locoregional percutaneous thermoablation, but because of its close relationship with the gallbladder and the risk for unsuccessful treatment, we agreed on a surgical approach and the patient underwent hepatic metastasectomy.

One year later, at the last visit in February 2014, serum Ct was greatly reduced (25 pg/ml, normal range <11.5 pg/ml) as well as the CEA (1.7 ng/ml, normal range <5 ng/ml), and radiological assessments confirmed the stability of small cervical lymph nodes, small lung nodules, and the other two subcentimeter hepatic lesions, in the absence of new metastatic or suspicious lesions (Fig. 40.3, Panel b). The patient is now 42 years old; her general health is good as is her quality of life.

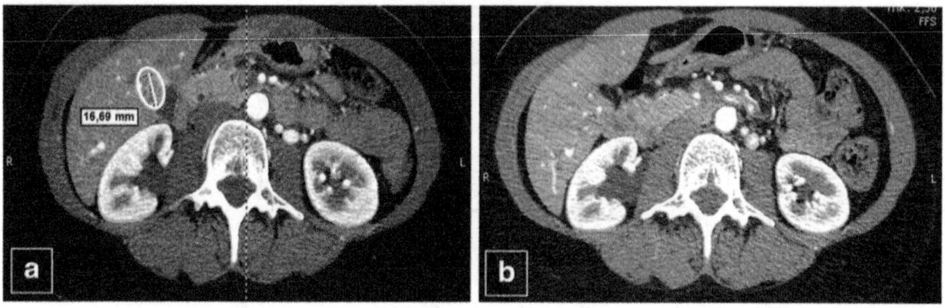

Fig. 40.3 (Panel **a**) CT scan of the hepatic metastases, with the largest one located very close to the gallbladder and measuring 17 mm in September 2012. (Panel **b**) Patient's liver CT scan 12 months after metastasectomy in 2014: no recurrence of the largest lesion was visible

Diagnosis/Assessment

This case offers the opportunity to discuss several still controversial issues related to the diagnosis and the assessment of metastatic disease in MTC patients.

MTC is a rare thyroid tumor representing only 5–7 % of all thyroid malignancies. It can be sporadic (80%) or familial (20%). Its pathogenesis is related to a molecular alteration of *RET* oncogene that can be present at the germline level in familial cases or at somatic level in sporadic cases [1]. MTC prognosis is strongly related to the presence of metastatic disease outside the neck, with a survival rate of about 30–35 % at 10 years when distant metastases are present at the time of diagnosis [2]. Also the presence of a somatic *RET* mutation has been demonstrated to be correlated to an advanced stage and a lower survival [3–5]. The detection of a somatic *RET* mutation in the paratracheal tissue of the patient is suggestive of a more aggressive phenotype, with a higher risk of disease-related mortality even though the absence of distant metastases at the time of diagnosis likely reduces this risk [3].

This is a typical case in which the presurgical diagnosis of MTC was missed since the serum Ct was not measured and the cytological diagnosis of the nodule was indeterminate, as it can sometimes happen in MTC. An international and multicenter study recently demonstrated that the FNAC was able to identify only 46 % of 245 sporadic MTCs evaluated in 12 centers across 7 nations in 4 continents [6]. In this case, the measurement of serum Ct could have helped to avoid this mistake and allowed the appropriate surgical procedure to have been performed, which would possibly have changed the long-term outcome.

The measurement of Ct in the washout of the needle used for aspiration is of great help in the diagnosis of both primary MTC and lymph node metastases [7]. This procedure is particularly useful when the cytology is unclear or undefined and the serum Ct is borderline. Sometimes, if the serum Ct levels are very high, blood contamination can lead to a false-positive result, but the identification of a cutoff above which metastatic disease is likely can solve this problem [8].

At a certain point during the follow-up of this patient, she could have been considered to be "cured" since the serum Ct was undetectable (<14 pg/ml) from 1999 to 2001. However, the pentagastrin stimulation test demonstrated a peak Ct of 88 pg/ml suggesting that residual disease was still present. It is still a matter of discussion if postsurgical Ct stimulation testing is worthwhile when the postsurgical basal serum Ct is undetectable or in the normal range. There are studies showing that MTC patients with a basal Ct lower than the upper limit of the reference range have a risk of recurrence of 10 %, and therefore they can be considered to be cured, and their follow-up can be less intensive [9]. However, this percentage is reduced to 3 % in patients with negative Ct stimulation test [10], and thus, we believe that at least one stimulation Ct test after surgery can be useful to better identify patients who have a higher probability of being free of disease [11].

Management

Newly diagnosed patients with MTC are usually 45–50 years old at the time of the diagnosis, and thus our patient was rather young. However, age at presentation is not a risk factor neither for the progression of the disease nor survival. However, younger age can impact on the choice of therapy. For example, after the third surgery, external radiotherapy (ERT) might have been considered, but the patient was only 25 years old, and her young age was a relative contraindication to ERT [12]. Nevertheless, no further recurrence in the neck has been observed thus far, after 15 years from the last surgery.

The choice to repeat surgery in the neck was made because of the evidence that the disease was locally metastatic without distant metastases. There is a general agreement among experts [13] that when MTC is characterized by a single metastatic lesion or several but subcentimeter lesions and not progressive, a local treatment is preferred, thus delaying systemic therapy, especially in young patients. The rationale underlying this concept is related to two major factors: the slow growth that characterizes the biological behavior of many MTCs and the multiplicity of adverse effects of systemic therapy. As far as the degree of progression is concerned, only a progression rate of the target lesion(s) greater than 20 % in at least 12–14 months is considered sufficiently worrisome to consider initiation of systemic therapy [14]. If the growth rate is slower, it is better to wait and see with periodical imaging controls. The doubling times of both serum Ct and CEA are good indicators of progression [15–17] and are very helpful in planning the follow-up schedule: if the doubling time is shorter than 6–12 months, the patient must be revaluated at shorter time intervals, and it is likely that at one of these assessments cross-sectional imaging will demonstrate a significant increase of one or more lesions. In contrast, if the doubling time is greater than 12–24 months, the patient can be monitored less frequently, e.g., every 12–18 months, because of a lower risk of significant progression on imaging. Our patient had a Ct and CEA doubling time of 1.5 years, and for this reason, we monitored her once a year. However, since one of her several distant micrometastases was growing and because it was very close to the gallbladder, we decided to treat the patient surgically rather than with systemic therapy.

Outcome

This is a very typical intermediate risk MTC patient with a long survival from the time of the diagnosis (i.e., 20 years, at present), with a good quality of life and a low relative risk of death from the disease. All together she has had four surgical treatments in 20 years, with many years of good health between procedures. If, during her follow-up, we had decided to initiate systemic therapy, only standard chemotherapy would have been available until 2005. Several regimens have been proposed over the years, but none of them has been demonstrated to be clinically effective despite having high levels of toxicity [18]. After 2005, several clinical trials with new targeted therapies were initiated, based on the ability of some of these drugs to inhibit tyrosine kinase receptors (TKIs) which are frequently involved in tumor transformation and progression. One of these receptors is coded by *RET* oncogene that is frequently altered in MTC, which is the rationale for such therapy in this condition. Unfortunately, these therapies have a host of adverse reactions, including life-threatening events that, if not controlled or limited, can greatly affect the quality of life of treated patients and potentially even cause mortality [19, 20]. This was the reason we postponed for as long as possible the initiation of systemic therapy in our young patient, especially considering the slow rate of growth of her disease.

In accord with the natural history of MTC and the fact that a somatic *RET* mutation was present in the tumor tissue, we can anticipate progression of the metastatic lesions that have already been detected or the appearance of new lesions within a few years. At that time, together with the patient, we will decide if it will be the right time to start systemic therapy or if there will still be a role for local treatment. In the meantime, she will continue to have a good quality of life.

Conclusions

This case represents a typical MTC case in which the combination of local treatments and "wait-and-see" strategy allowed the patient to have a relatively normal life with no other medication other than levothyroxine therapy.

Clinical Pearls/Pitfalls

- Serum Ct measurement may be a useful test in the initial evaluation of thyroid nodules, especially in those cases who are scheduled for surgery.
- The serum Ct and CEA doubling time can predict the growth rate of metastatic lesions, thus being a valuable tool for planning the schedule of follow-up controls and imaging and biochemical testing.
- Single metastatic lesions should be treated, if necessary, with local therapies.

- Systemic therapy should be reserved for MTC patients with multiple distant metastases or unresectable local disease with a clear evidence of progression on imaging.
- MTC patients with somatic *RET* mutations typically have more aggressive disease.

References

1. Elisei R, Romei C, Cosci B, Molinaro E, Agate L, Bottici V, Pinchera A. RET point mutations in thyroid carcinoma. Atlas Genet Cytogenet Oncol Haematol. 2009;13:325–32.
2. Gharib H, et al. Medullary thyroid carcinoma: clinicopathologic features and long-term follow-up of 65 patients treated during 1946 through 1970. Mayo Clin Proc. 1992;67(10): 934–40.
3. Elisei R, et al. Prognostic significance of somatic RET oncogene mutations in sporadic medullary thyroid cancer: a 10-year follow-up study. J Clin Endocrinol Metab. 2008;93(3):682–7.
4. Mian C, et al. Combined RET and Ki-67 assessment in sporadic medullary thyroid carcinoma: a useful tool for patient risk stratification. Eur J Endocrinol. 2011;164(6):971–6.
5. Moura MM, et al. Correlation of RET somatic mutations with clinicopathological features in sporadic medullary thyroid carcinomas. Br J Cancer. 2009;100(11):1777–83.
6. Essig Jr GF, et al. Fine needle aspiration and medullary thyroid carcinoma: the risk of inadequate preoperative evaluation and initial surgery when relying upon FNAB cytology alone. Endocr Pract. 2013;19(6):920–7.
7. Boi F, et al. Calcitonin measurement in wash-out fluid from fine needle aspiration of neck masses in patients with primary and metastatic medullary thyroid carcinoma. J Clin Endocrinol Metab. 2007;92(6):2115–8.
8. Trimboli P, et al. Calcitonin measurement in aspiration needle washout fluids has higher sensitivity than cytology in detecting medullary thyroid cancer: a retrospective multicentre study. Clin Endocrinol (Oxf). 2014;80(1):135–40.
9. Pellegriti G, et al. Long-term outcome of medullary thyroid carcinoma in patients with normal postoperative medical imaging. Br J Cancer. 2003;88(10):1537–42.
10. Franc S, et al. Complete surgical lymph node resection does not prevent authentic recurrences of medullary thyroid carcinoma. Clin Endocrinol (Oxf). 2001;55(3):403–9.
11. Elisei R, et al. 2012 European thyroid association guidelines for genetic testing and its clinical consequences in medullary thyroid cancer. Eur Thyroid J. 2013;1(4):216–31.
12. Sun XS, et al. Indications of external beam radiation therapy in non-anaplastic thyroid cancer and impact of innovative radiation techniques. Crit Rev Oncol Hematol. 2013;86(1):52–68.
13. Schlumberger M, et al. 2012 European thyroid association guidelines for metastatic medullary thyroid cancer. Eur Thyroid J. 2012;1(1):5–14.
14. Eisenhauer EA, et al. New response evaluation criteria in solid tumours: revised RECIST guideline (version 1.1). Eur J Cancer. 2009;45(2):228–47.
15. Barbet J, et al. Prognostic impact of serum calcitonin and carcinoembryonic antigen doubling-times in patients with medullary thyroid carcinoma. J Clin Endocrinol Metab. 2005;90(11): 6077–84.
16. Meijer JA, et al. Calcitonin and carcinoembryonic antigen doubling times as prognostic factors in medullary thyroid carcinoma: a structured meta-analysis. Clin Endocrinol (Oxf). 2010;72(4):534–42.
17. Laure Giraudet A, et al. Progression of medullary thyroid carcinoma: assessment with calcitonin and carcinoembryonic antigen doubling times. Eur J Endocrinol. 2008;158(2):239–46.

18. Orlandi F, et al. Treatment of medullary thyroid carcinoma: an update. Endocr Relat Cancer. 2001;8(2):135–47.
19. Elisei R, et al. Cabozantinib in progressive medullary thyroid cancer. J Clin Oncol. 2013;31(29):3639–46.
20. Wells Jr SA, et al. Vandetanib in patients with locally advanced or metastatic medullary thyroid cancer: a randomized, double-blind phase III trial. J Clin Oncol. 2012;30(2):134–41.

Chapter 41
A Patient with an Advanced Medullary Thyroid Cancer and Progressive, Symptomatic Distant Metastases: When to Start Systemic Therapy

Carlotta Giani, Antonio Matrone, and Rossella Elisei

Case Presentation

A 39-year-old man was diagnosed with a multinodular goiter after a neck ultrasound was performed because of familial thyroid disease. Neck ultrasound (US) showed the presence of a solid hypoechoic nodule measuring 3.8 cm in the left lobe and an anechoic nodule measuring 1.2 cm in the right lobe. Laboratory findings showed a TSH of 1.2 mU/l, negative TgAb and TPOAb, and normal values of both FT3 and FT4. A fine needle aspiration cytology (FNAC) of the biggest nodule revealed a microfollicular lesion (Bethesda class III) and surgical treatment was suggested.

In April 2003, the patient was referred to our institution for a second opinion. A neck US performed in our center confirmed the presence of the two thyroid nodules but also showed three right hypoechoic laterocervical nodules with microcalcifications that were highly suspicious for lymph node metastases. Serum calcitonin (Ct) was markedly elevated at 3654 pg/ml (normal <10 pg/ml). Fine needle aspiration cytology of the 3.8 cm thyroid nodule was positive for medullary thyroid cancer (MTC), and cytology of a 1.4 cm right laterocervical lymph node was positive for MTC as well. We performed germline *RET* mutational testing and a Ser891Ala mutation was found, thus converting the case from apparently sporadic to a hereditary form of MTC. Thereafter, the screening of his first-degree relatives (parents and siblings) was started and several of them were found to be positive. A program of clinical and biochemical (i.e., basal and stimulated Ct) screening was initiated. The patient was submitted to clinical and biochemical evaluations to verify the presence of other endocrine neoplasia such as multiple adenomatosis of parathyroid glands and pheochromocytoma, but he was negative for both of them.

C. Giani • A. Matrone • R. Elisei, MD (✉)
Endocrine Unit, Department of Clinical and Experimental Medicine, University Hospital of Pisa, Via Paradisa 2, 56124 Pisa, Italy
e-mail: rossella.elisei@med.unipi.it

D.S. Cooper, C. Durante (eds.), *Thyroid Cancer*,
DOI 10.1007/978-3-319-22401-5_41

In May 2003, the patient underwent a total thyroidectomy with central and right laterocervical compartmental lymph node dissections. The histological examination showed an MTC of 2.9 cm with metastatic lymph nodes of the central (5/8) and right laterocervical (4/10) compartments (pT2N1bMx). Four months after surgery (September 2003), a neck ultrasound was performed that showed the presence of 4 new suspicious left laterocervical lymph nodes. The largest, measuring 1.2 cm, was biopsied and its metastatic nature was confirmed with Ct on the needle washout fluid >10,000 pg/ml; at this time, serum Ct was 1000 pg/ml and carcinoembryonic antigen (CEA) was 20 ng/ml (normal <5.0 ng/ml). Computerized tomography (CT) scan of the neck, mediastinum, and thorax confirmed the presence of metastatic lymph nodes in the neck and also revealed the presence of 2 suspicious metastatic lymph nodes in the mediastinum and some subcentimeter lung lesions which were too small to be better characterized; there were no other suspicious lesions.

At this point, we decided to perform a left laterocervical lymph node dissection with the simultaneous removal of the lymph nodes in the mediastinum. Histological examination confirmed the metastatic nature of the laterocervical (4/5) and mediastinal (2/2) MTC lymph nodes.

The first clinical follow-up visit after this second neck surgery was performed 6 months later (April 2004). Serum Ct was 650 pg/ml, CT scan confirmed the presence of unchanged lung micronodules, and neck US was negative for suspicious lymph nodes.

During the following annual visits and biochemical assessments, serum Ct slightly but progressively increased over the years (Fig. 41.1) but the chest CT scan showed a stable disease. After 2 years of stable disease, the patient started to complain about diarrhea. The diarrhea was well controlled with medication (loperamide 2 mg, until eight tablets daily), but because of the progressive increase in serum Ct and the symptomatic disease (diarrhea), the patient was enrolled in the first experimental clinical trial with the tyrosine kinase inhibitor AMG 706 (i.e., motesanib) in February 2006. After 3 weeks of treatment, his diarrhea was completely controlled with no more need for loperamide, and his Ct levels remained substantially stable, with no evidence of progressive disease on the chest CT scan. In January 2007, despite the stable disease, motesanib was discontinued due to the development of hydrops of the gallbladder, one of the most common side effects of this drug. In February 2007, serum Ct was 824 pg/ml, CEA was 24 ng/ml, neck US was negative for lymph node metastases, and CT scan showed the stability of the microlesions of the lung.

From January 2007 to April 2010, no clinical, biochemical, and radiological findings of progression of MTC were observed; the diarrhea was under control with loperamide, and our patient had an acceptable quality of life. In October 2010, we found a slight increase of serum Ct and CEA with a relatively short and concerning doubling time (i.e., 1.4 year); the total body (TB) CT scan showed the presence of at least 4 mediastinal suspicious but subcentimeter lymph nodes and confirmed the stable lung microlesions. At this time, we decided upon a *wait-and-see* strategy, because of no evidence of significant radiological progression of the disease. The patient's clinical status remained stable until November 2013, when a rising serum

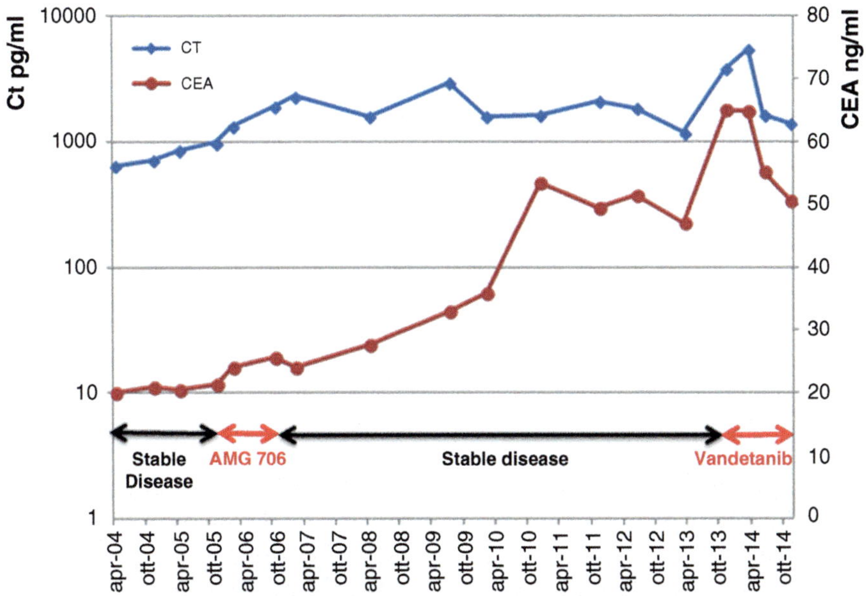

Fig. 41.1 Serum calcitonin (Ct) and carcinoembryonic antigen (CEA) during the years of follow-up of the patient: a more significant increase of both markers was observed just before the starting point of the TKI therapies just anticipating the imaging evidence of a significant increase of the size of the metastatic lesions

Ct value was observed, with a doubling time <0.5 years (i.e., 3797 pg/ml vs. 1180 pg/ml of March 2013); similarly, an increase in CEA was found with a doubling time of 1.4 years (65 ng/ml vs. 47 ng/ml of March 2013). The neck US revealed the presence of a new 11 mm lymph node in the right paratracheal area. The CT scan showed a new metastatic lymph node in the right hilum measuring 24 mm and a 116 % increase of the largest diameter of a mediastinal lymph node (from 12 mm to 26 mm in 6 months). In this period, the diarrhea was no longer well controlled despite regular therapy with loperamide.

Because of clear progression of the disease, in July 2014, we decided to initiate therapy with the TKI vandetanib (which became available for prescription in our country in June 2014 with the commercial name Caprelsa) with a starting dose of 300 mg daily. The severity of diarrhea immediately improved, but 6 weeks after the initiation of vandetanib, the patient developed a severe and extensive papular rash on the face, hands, and head (Fig. 41.2). This adverse event (AE) was considered to be grade 3 (i.e., very severe) and required the suspension of the TKI therapy until its complete resolution. In the meantime, topical and oral glucocorticoids, antihistamines, and antibiotics to prevent microbial superinfection were administered. After the resolution of this AE, we restarted vandetanib but at a reduced daily dose (100 mg daily).

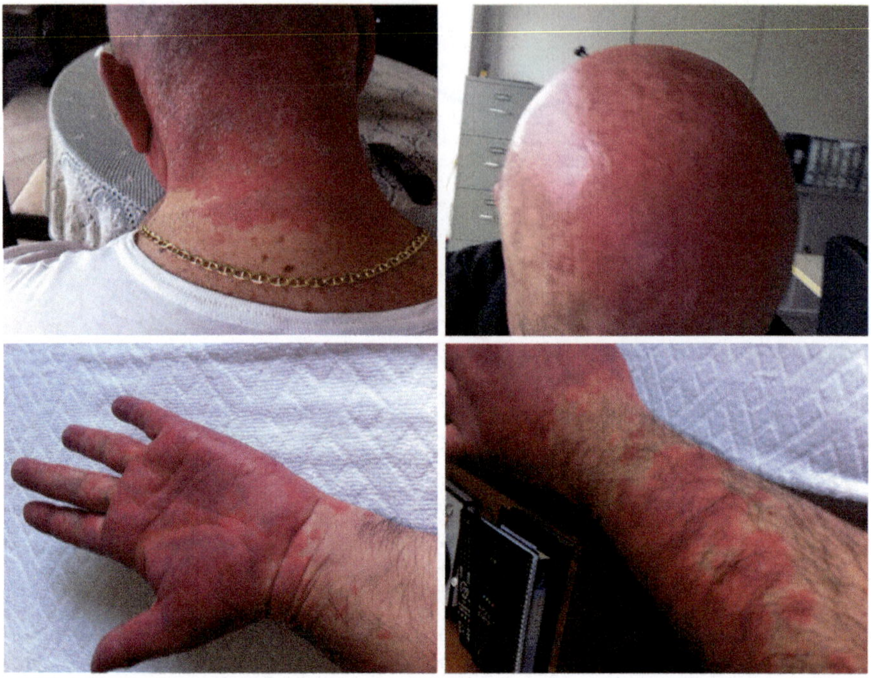

Fig. 41.2 The patient developed a severe erythroderma a few weeks after the start of the vandetanib therapy, mainly involving the sunlight-exposed areas of the body

At the last evaluation on November 2014 (after 3 months of vandetanib therapy at 100 mg daily), the patient presented for follow-up in good clinical condition, without diarrhea or the need for antidiarrheal medication. His ECG showed a normal QTc interval, and serum electrolytes were in the normal range as were thyroid function tests after a levothyroxine dose adjustment performed in September 2014 because of an elevated serum TSH. TB CT scan showed a slight reduction of the right paratracheal lymph node (10 mm vs. 11 mm) and a significant reduction of the lesions in the mediastinum (20 mm vs. 26 mm) and in the hilum (10 mm vs. 24 mm) (Fig. 41.3); the microlesions in the lung remained stable. He will continue vandetanib until there is no longer evidence of clinical benefit or if there is the development of another severe AE.

Diagnosis/Assessment

This case offers the opportunity to discuss some issues related to the diagnosis and treatment of advanced and metastatic disease in MTC patients. It is known that MTC can be sporadic (80 %) or familial (20 %), and the latter condition can be isolated (i.e., familial medullary thyroid cancer, FMTC) or associated with other

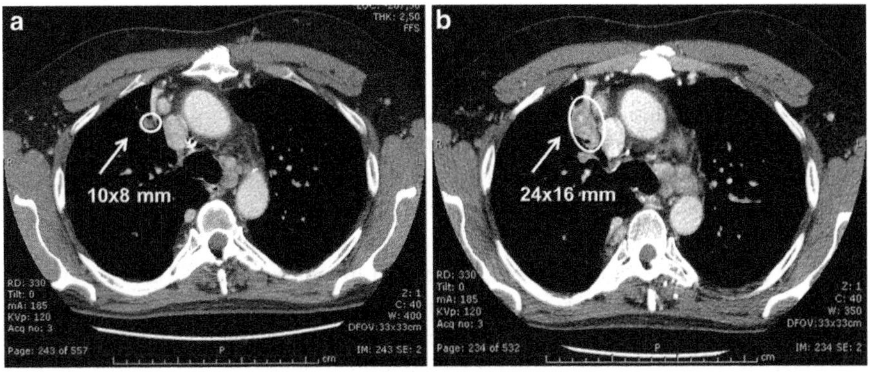

Fig. 41.3 CT scan of the lung performed 6 months after the vandetanib treatment (Panel **a**) showed a significant reduction of the metastatic lesions and in particular of the lymph node of the hilum with respect to the CT scan performed before starting vandetanib (10 mm vs. 24 mm: –58 %) (Panel **b**)

endocrine neoplasia (i.e., multiple endocrine neoplasia type 2, MEN 2) [1]. In both cases, sporadic or familial, the pathogenesis of MTC is associated with the presence of a somatic or germline *RET* oncogene mutation, respectively [2]. This case had an apparently sporadic MTC without any familial history of MTC or any other associated endocrine neoplasia. However, *RET* mutational screening revealed a germline *RET* Ser891Ala mutation consistent with familial MTC. This finding is not unexpected since 6–7 % of apparently sporadic MTCs are positive for a *RET* germline mutation when the genetic screening is performed [3]. The case illustrates the importance of performing *RET* genetic screening in all MTC cases, regardless of the clinical presentation. The finding of a germline *RET* mutation does not have any impact on the clinical management of the MTC of index case, but at variance, it is of great relevance for the first-degree relatives, who gain the knowledge of either having or not having the inherited *RET* mutation. The *RET*-positive cases (i.e., gene carriers) require further investigation because they are at high risk of developing the MEN 2 syndrome. A prophylactic thyroidectomy potentially allows a definitive cure of these individuals, who probably would have had the diagnosis made too late if the *RET* screening was not performed. The timing of thyroidectomy and the modalities of follow-up should be personalized according to the specific *RET* mutation and the levels of serum Ct [4, 5].

Management

As previously stated, the finding of a germline *RET* mutation does not change the therapeutic strategy of MTC for this patient, who has been managed according to the biochemical and imaging results obtained during his follow-up. The disease was not cured by the first surgery, but this is consistent with the evidence that when MTC is already extrathyroidal and associated to neck lymph node metastases, the possibility of a definitive cure is rare [6]. This is the rationale for making an early diagnosis of MTC, either by measuring serum Ct in patients with thyroid nodules [7] or performing *RET* screening in hereditary forms [8]. In 2006, the patient was enrolled in a clinical trial with motesanib because of the development of diarrhea, which is a common symptom in advanced MTC with very high levels of serum Ct. The clinical trial was of interest because motesanib was the first tyrosine kinase inhibitor (TKI) employed in thyroid cancer and in particular in MTC [9]. Tyrosine kinase inhibitors are multitargeted therapies, which mainly block the activation of vascular endothelial growth factor receptors (mainly type 2) but also interfere with the function of other tyrosine kinase receptors including, in some cases, the one coded by the *RET* oncogene. The patient had a clinical benefit from treatment, including full control of diarrhea, but unfortunately, a severe side effect such as the hydrops of the gallbladder required the discontinuation of the drug.

Thereafter, the patient was followed up for 7 years without any specific therapy, except for loperamide that was again necessary to control diarrhea. He went into an active surveillance with clinical and biochemical controls every 6–8 months. This is the strategy recommended by many experts since MTC is, in the majority of cases, a slowly progressive cancer, and systemic therapy with TKI should be initiated only when the disease is progressive according to RECIST, thus showing an increase of the metastatic target lesions of at least 20 % over 12–14 months [10]. Changes in serum markers alone, such as Ct and CEA, are not indications to start TKI. However, both serum Ct and CEA, and in particular their doubling times, are important to help define the schedule of follow-up visits and imaging [11].

According to the experts' opinions and RECIST, TKI therapy should be started when there are multiple metastases, larger than 2 cm and whose largest diameter has increased by more than 20 % over 12–14 months or less [12]. Therefore, in 2014, when the lung metastases and some lymph node metastases began to enlarge rapidly, we decided that it was time to begin therapy with another TKI. At that time, vandetanib had become available and had been demonstrated to significantly increase the time interval of progression-free survival and to reduce many of the symptoms related to the disease [13].

Unfortunately, vandetanib commonly causes severe cutaneous side effects mainly related to sun exposure, and although we informed the patient about this possible risk, he spent time in the sunlight. A few days later, he developed severe erythema (Fig. 41.2) that required the temporary suspension of the drug. The erythema was treated with steroids and antihistamines; few weeks later, when the erythema had almost completely resolved, the drug was restarted but at a lower daily dose (i.e., 100 mg/day). No side effects developed with this dose and the quality of life of our patient has been good. The control of side effects through the reduction of the daily dose or by using personalized protocols for drug administration is a validated method for managing patients on TKIs, since it has been demonstrated that they can continue to have a positive control on tumor growth [14] even at lower doses.

Several other side effects can be caused by vandetanib, including hypertension, QTc interval prolongation, fatigue, anorexia, and diarrhea. Whenever possible, the introduction of specific drugs such as calcium channel blockers to control blood pressure or loperamide to control diarrhea can be effective and allow continued use of the TKI. At the present time, vandetanib (commercial name Caprelsa) and cabozantinib (commercial name Cometriq), another multitarget TKI with the specificity to act against *MET*, in addition to *RET* and VEGFR, are the only drugs approved by the Food and Drug Administration (i.e., FDA) and European Medicines Agency (i.e., EMA) for the treatment of MTC. However, we know that after a median period of 14 months, almost all patients develop a kind of resistance to therapy, and the disease begins to progress. Fortunately, other TKIs that may stop MTC growth are currently under development and some are in clinical trials. Indeed, it has been shown that cabozantinib can be effective in patients who have been treated with other TKIs and developed progressive disease [15]. This is not yet the case with our patient who is still obtaining a clinical benefit with reduction of his lung and lymph node lesions (Fig. 41.3) by taking 100 mg/day of vandetanib.

Outcome

The quality of life of our patient is, at the present, rather good: he can work and perform his usual practice physical activities. Neither diarrhea nor erythema is present and vandetanib will be continued until there is no longer evidence of clinical benefit. If and when there is an increase in the size of the target lesions, the so-called escape phenomenon, we will likely substitute the vandetanib with cabozantinib or another drug that might be available at that time.

The escape phenomenon, due to the development of a resistance to the drug, commonly occurs with TKI treatment, regardless of tumor type. This is likely due to the method of action of TKIs, which are cytostatic and not cytotoxic drugs, and for this reason, surviving cells can develop resistance to the drug and then start to grow. Being cytostatic drugs, they should not be discontinued until there is evidence of disease progression. In some cases, if the progression is relatively limited, it could be clinically reasonable to continue the drug until the possibility of substitution with another drug.

Conclusions

MTCs that are already metastatic to the cervical nodes or extrathyroidal at the time of diagnosis have a low probability of cure with surgery alone. Patients can maintain a good quality of life, and the disease can grow rather slowly. However, when MTC metastases are multiple and rapidly growing, systemic therapy with a TKI should be considered. The management of patients with MTC who is receiving

TKI therapy should be done in tertiary care centers where there is experience in managing the frequent side effects of these drugs that often are the major limitation to this type of therapy. When side effects interfere with the quality of life of patients, the best initial strategy is to reduce the daily dose of the drug before the side effect becomes too severe or, in the latter situation, to stop the treatment until the recovery, possibly without any unnecessary prolonged interruption, to restart with a lower dose.

Clinical Pearls/Pitfalls

- *RET* genetic screening allows the identification of hereditary cases (approximately 7 %) that are initially diagnosed as apparently sporadic cases.
- The screening of first-degree relatives is strongly recommended if there is a *RET* mutation.
- The serum Ct and CEA doubling time can predict the growth rate of metastatic lesions but should not be used for the decision to start TKI therapy.
- Multimetastatic and progressive MTC should be treated with systemic therapy when progression is defined according to RECIST or if the patient develops symptoms.
- TKIs represent the first-line systemic therapy: adverse events should be managed by experts to avoid interruption of therapy.
- New TKIs are under evaluation which may provide improved efficacy and a better side effect profile than vandetanib or cabozantinib.

References

1. Romei C, et al. Genetic and clinical features of multiple endocrine neoplasia types 1 and 2. J Oncol. 2012;2012, 705036.
2. Eng C, et al. The relationship between specific RET proto-oncogene mutations and disease phenotype in multiple endocrine neoplasia type 2. International RET mutation consortium analysis. JAMA. 1996;276(19):1575–9.
3. Romei C, et al. Twenty years of lesson learning: how does the ret genetic screening test impact the clinical management of medullary thyroid cancer? Clin Endocrinol (Oxf). 2014;82(6): 892–9.
4. Elisei R, et al. The timing of total thyroidectomy in RET gene mutation carriers could be personalized and safely planned on the basis of serum calcitonin: 18 years experience at one single center. J Clin Endocrinol Metab. 2012;97(2):426–35.
5. Kloos RT, et al. Medullary thyroid cancer: management guidelines of the American Thyroid Association. Thyroid. 2009;19(6):565–612.
6. Machens A, et al. Prospects of remission in medullary thyroid carcinoma according to basal calcitonin level. J Clin Endocrinol Metab. 2005;90(4):2029–34.
7. Pacini F, et al. Routine measurement of serum calcitonin in nodular thyroid diseases allows the preoperative diagnosis of unsuspected sporadic medullary thyroid carcinoma. J Clin Endocrinol Metab. 1994;78(4):826–9.

8. Pacini F, et al. Early treatment of hereditary medullary thyroid carcinoma after attribution of multiple endocrine neoplasia type 2 gene carrier status by screening for ret gene mutations. Surgery. 1995;118(6):1031–5.
9. Schlumberger MJ, et al. Phase II study of safety and efficacy of motesanib in patients with progressive or symptomatic, advanced or metastatic medullary thyroid cancer. J Clin Oncol. 2009;27(23):3794–801.
10. Eisenhauer EA, et al. New response evaluation criteria in solid tumours: revised RECIST guideline (version 1.1). Eur J Cancer. 2009;45(2):228–47.
11. Meijer JA, et al. Calcitonin and carcinoembryonic antigen doubling times as prognostic factors in medullary thyroid carcinoma: a structured meta-analysis. Clin Endocrinol (Oxf). 2010; 72(4):534–42.
12. Schlumberger M, et al. Definition and management of radioactive iodine-refractory differentiated thyroid cancer. Lancet Diabetes Endocrinol. 2014;2(5):356–8.
13. Wells Jr SA, et al. Vandetanib in patients with locally advanced or metastatic medullary thyroid cancer: a randomized, double-blind phase III trial. J Clin Oncol. 2012;30(2):134–41.
14. Gori S, et al. Sunitinib therapy in metastatic papillary thyroid cancer. Tumori. 2013;99(6): 285e–7e.
15. Elisei R, et al. Cabozantinib in progressive medullary thyroid cancer. J Clin Oncol. 2013; 31(29):3639–46.

Chapter 42
Medical Treatment Decision-Making for Advanced, Progressive Medullary Thyroid Cancer

Ramona Dadu, Robert F. Gagel, and Mimi I. Hu

Introduction

There are currently two tyrosine kinase inhibitors (TKIs) (vandetanib and cabozantinib) approved by the US Food and Drug Administration (FDA) and the European Medicines Agency for the treatment of advanced, progressive, or symptomatic medullary thyroid cancer (MTC), with other therapies under investigation. The National Comprehensive Cancer Network Cancer Practice Guidelines for MTC recommends consideration of one of these two agents with unresectable disease that is symptomatic or structurally progressive (NCCN.org, accessed 10/2014). The approval of these agents has created new opportunities and challenges for clinicians treating patients with advanced MTC, necessitating a rethinking of how to integrate this new therapeutic modality into existing surgical and radiotherapeutic approaches to management. A great deal of clinical judgment needs to be applied toward identifying which patients to treat and with which agent; care providers should not treat patients with these agents simply because they are available.

An integration of these new agents into the management schema of MTC requires an understanding of the natural history of MTC. The availability of tumor markers, serum calcitonin and carcinoembryonic antigen, alerts the clinician to presence of disease long before it is clinically meaningful. As none of the current therapeutic approaches, other than surgical removal, is curative, it is important for the clinician to create a clear expectation that therapy will be introduced only when there is a clear expectation of benefit, usually years or even decades after the first appearance of an abnormal tumor marker. Active surveillance, or the "watch-and-wait"

R. Dadu, MD • R.F. Gagel, MD • M.I. Hu, MD (✉)
Department of Endocrine Neoplasia and Hormonal Disorders,
The University of Texas MD Anderson Cancer Center,
1515 Holcombe Boulevard, Houston, TX 77030-4009, USA
e-mail: mhu@mdanderson.org

D.S. Cooper, C. Durante (eds.), *Thyroid Cancer*,
DOI 10.1007/978-3-319-22401-5_42

approach, is an important component in the care of MTC patients as they can enjoy a good quality of life for many years without requiring systemic therapy. As available systemic therapies are not curative, have many side effects (some of which can be fatal), are administered chronically to control disease, and have not yet been shown to prolong overall survival, it is important to balance risk against benefit when considering initiating systemic therapy.

In contrast, in patients with rapidly progressive and/or symptomatic disease or disease in areas that are life threatening or have the potential to become life threatening, a more aggressive approach is warranted. Treatment options for these patients depend on the site of disease and tumor burden. Local therapy (such as surgical resection, radiotherapy, or embolization) should be employed when the disease burden is confined to one area and threatening quality of life or combined with systemic therapy when there is widespread, progressive disease.

The discussion in this chapter will use a case-based approach to understanding the elements involved in medical decision-making for patients with advanced MTC.

Case 1: Active Surveillance

A 57-year-old man presented at an outside institution with progressive back pain and was found to have a destructive bone lesion at the L3 spine. A laminectomy with excision identified metastatic MTC to the bone. Staging studies noted a 2.8 cm mass in the left thyroid with left lateral cervical adenopathy and metastatic lesions in the liver (up to 3.5 cm) but no pulmonary metastases; biopsies of the thyroid mass and a lymph node confirmed MTC. Baseline serum calcitonin (Ct) was 4723 pg/mL and serum carcinoembryonic antigen (CEA) was 15.3 ng/mL. The patient underwent external beam radiotherapy to the 3rd lumbar surgical bed followed by total thyroidectomy, bilateral central lymph node dissection, and left level III and IV lateral neck dissection. Thereafter, active surveillance was recommended. After 4 years, the patient remains asymptomatic with no demonstrable evidence of progression nor new lesions by periodic neck ultrasound and other imaging studies (Fig. 42.1). Serum Ct and CEA doubling times are 10.9 years and 3.9 years, respectively.

Active Surveillance for Progressive Disease

Evaluating serum tumor markers (Ct and CEA) over time in conjunction with obtaining serial cross-sectional imaging is an effective and objective strategy for monitoring for progression of MTC. Serum Ct is the primary biochemical marker used for postoperative surveillance and prediction of disease progression. CEA is a less specific biomarker for MTC but one whose magnitude can be useful in understanding extent of disease and prognosis. Ct and CEA doubling times correlate with

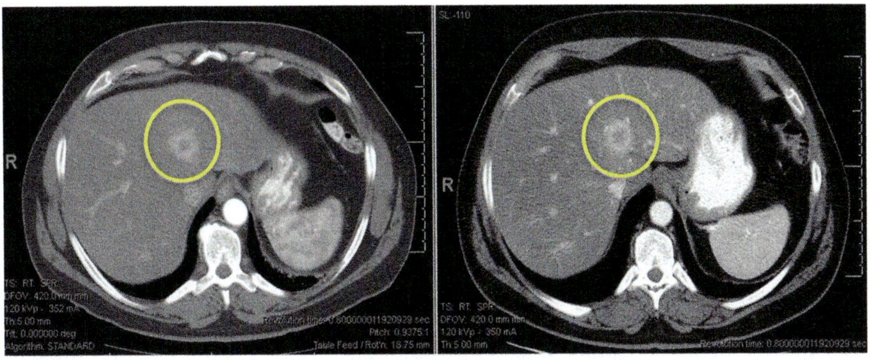

Fig. 42.1 Case no. 1: Stable liver metastases over 4 years demonstrated by high-resolution computerized tomography. *Left panel* August 2010. *Right panel* April 2014

rate of progression, recurrence, and survival [1]. Higher disease-specific survival and recurrence-free survival rates are associated with doubling times of over 1 year, with the CEA doubling time having a higher predictive value. Importantly, doubling times can be used to guide the frequency of imaging studies. In patients with prolonged doubling times of over 1 year, the time between imaging studies can be lengthened to every 6–12 months, thus lowering the cost of observation and reducing the radiation exposure risks associated with frequent imaging studies.

A broad spectrum of imaging modalities can be used to detect metastatic disease. Ultrasound of the neck is the most sensitive technique for detection of thyroid bed or nodal recurrence. Areas not easily imaged by ultrasound, such as the retropharyngeal region or superior mediastinum, can be best imaged by computed tomography (CT) or magnetic resonance imaging (MRI). Fine-section spiral CT or MRI of the chest or abdomen with liver protocol is useful for detection of pulmonary or hepatic metastasis. As case no. 1 clearly demonstrates, spinal metastases occur with some frequency in MTC. In patients with metastatic MTC, it is important to perform periodic bone scans or MRI examination of the spine; however, the presence of a spinal metastasis in the absence of concern about neurologic compressive symptoms is not an indication for therapeutic intervention and may be observed. Although ^{18}F-DOPA PET or a radiolabeled somatostatin analog has utility for detection of MTC, their usefulness for routine surveillance of MTC is unproven.

While RECIST (**R**esponse **E**valuation **C**riteria in **S**olid **T**umors) has its limitations, it is a standardized and broadly accepted set of published criteria for evaluating tumor size and determining response and progression in patients with solid tumors, including thyroid cancer (www.recist.org, accessed 10/2014). Progressive disease (PD) is defined as a 20 % increase in target lesion tumor measurements. A 30 % decrease in the size of target lesions defines a partial response (PR); stable disease (SD) is defined as any response in between (−29 to +19 %). A clinical dilemma in real-life practice is that radiologists often do not issue RECIST-based reports, making it incumbent upon the clinician to perform an accurate assessment to determine overall stability or progression.

Integration of Local Therapies into the Management of Progressive or Symptomatic Focal Metastases

Recurrent locoregional neck disease in the setting of distant metastases should be treated surgically if there is impending airway or other vital structural compromise. In selected cases, systemic therapy may be a consideration. For example, in a patient in whom the only surgical option for local airway involvement is total laryngectomy, it may be appropriate to delay surgery and initiate a TKI with the hope that surgery (and loss of voice) can be delayed or the procedure can be modified by reducing the size/extent of the metastatic lesion. Surgical wound healing is impaired by currently available antiangiogenic therapy; thus, such therapy must be stopped between 4 and 12 weeks before a surgical procedure.

It is unclear how targeted systemic therapy should be integrated with the use of external beam radiation therapy (EBRT). Prior to the availability of TKIs, EBRT was used postsurgically to control extensive nodal or soft tissue neck disease or bone metastases causing pain or neurologic deficit. Indeed, in a patient with localized but incurable disease, palliative EBRT may still be a useful adjuvant therapy, although there is no evidence for overall survival benefit. There is currently a bias (although there are no data supporting it) to defer EBRT to gross disease in the neck in the setting of other progressive, distant disease (and consequently, an indication for systemic therapy), given the risk of upper tracheoesophageal or tracheo-tumor fistula formation in the setting of EBRT to the neck and antiangiogenic therapy [2]. In patients with brain metastases, where there is an inherent risk for bleeding into the brain lesions during treatment with TKIs, which target vascular endothelial growth factor receptor (VEGFR), it is recommended that these lesions be irradiated (EBRT or stereotactic radiosurgery) prior to initiation of TKIs. For this reason, brain imaging should be performed prior to proceeding with systemic therapy. It is important to balance the risks and benefits of EBRT and TKI systemic therapy versus watchful waiting.

Distant metastases limited to the lung that are indolent and asymptomatic can usually be followed with serial imaging. Pulmonary metastases can occasionally cause symptoms such as dyspnea, obstructive pneumonia, and hemoptysis. In selected patients with isolated or localized pulmonary metastases, surgical resection or radiotherapy may offer palliation. For patients with liver metastases that are progressive or symptomatic, trans-arterial chemoembolization or radioembolization can be considered [3].

Skeletal metastases of MTC are often clinically silent. Skeletal related events (SREs) are defined as pain, spinal cord compression, or pathological fracture necessitating external beam irradiation or surgery. It is extremely important to identify bone metastases and initiate palliative treatment modalities before SREs occur. EBRT, stereotactic radiotherapy, vertebroplasty, radiofrequency ablation, cryosurgery, and arterial embolization can be considered to palliate painful metastases or to prevent further progression that could lead to fracture or neurological compromise. Metastasectomy is sometimes performed if there is only one site of bone involvement. Agents that inhibit osteoclast activity, such as bisphosphonates or denosumab, are used in patients with osteolytic bone metastases from several neoplasms (lung, breast, prostate, kidney, and multiple myeloma), and anecdotal experience supports their use in MTC. Zoledronic acid (4 mg) or denosumab (120 mg) given at the approved monthly dosing schedule, in our experience, has been effective in reducing pain and progression of disease associated with bone metastases, although there have been no controlled trials of their use in patients with MTC. Although less frequent dosing of these antiresorptive agents has not been evaluated formally for efficacy in thyroid cancer patients, it is reasonable to surmise that less frequent dosing while maintaining suppression of bone turnover may be as effective in reducing SREs with less risk for side effects, such as osteonecrosis of the jaw. Little is known about the efficacy of TKIs in treating metastatic bone lesions. RECIST excludes bone lesions as measureable targets; thus, bone metastases were not assessed in the phase III trials of vandetanib and cabozantinib although there are some reports of response with these agents [4]. Clinical trials in patients with MTC and bone metastases are needed to evaluate which agents are effective.

Case 2: Treating with a Systemic Agent and Management of Adverse Effects

A 60-year-old man with an indeterminate thyroid mass by fine needle aspiration underwent a total thyroidectomy 12 years ago, which identified sporadic medullary thyroid carcinoma. In that same year, he underwent central lymph node dissection for residual disease. Serum Ct remained detectable around 15 pg/mL (normal is undetectable) for many years. Coincident with rising Ct levels into the 1940s and the identification of recurrent central compartment disease, he underwent a second central lymph node dissection 9 years after original diagnosis. Over the course of the next year, the serum Ct continued to rise (doubling time of 1.5 years), with identification of cervical lateral lymph node metastases and subcentimeter pulmonary (biopsy proven as MTC) and mediastinal lymph node metastases. He was referred to MD Anderson for evaluation. A high-resolution hepatic CT identified suspicious hypervascular hepatic lesions (largest 1.1 cm). At the time, his Ct was 94.6 pg/mL and CEA was 9.4 ng/mL; thus, recommendation was for short-term surveillance for progressive rate. Over the next 7 months, his Ct rose to 250 pg/mL and CEA to 121.8 ng/mL, correlating with asymptomatic, progressive hepatic metastases (largest lesion measured 3 cm). Although systemic chemotherapy with vandetanib or cabozantinib was recommended, the patient elected to be treated with trans-arterial hepatic chemoembolization (TACE) of bilateral hepatic metastases with doxorubicin, as his pulmonary metastases were stable and he was asymptomatic. Reassessment 4 months after TACE identified progressive hepatic and intra-abdominal/cervical lymph node metastases by RECIST associated with rising tumor markers (serum Ct 1144 pg/mL, CEA 452.5 ng/mL). The patient agreed to initiate treatment with one of the approved TKI agents. Three months after TKI initiation, staging studies demonstrated tumoral and biomarker responses (Fig. 42.2).

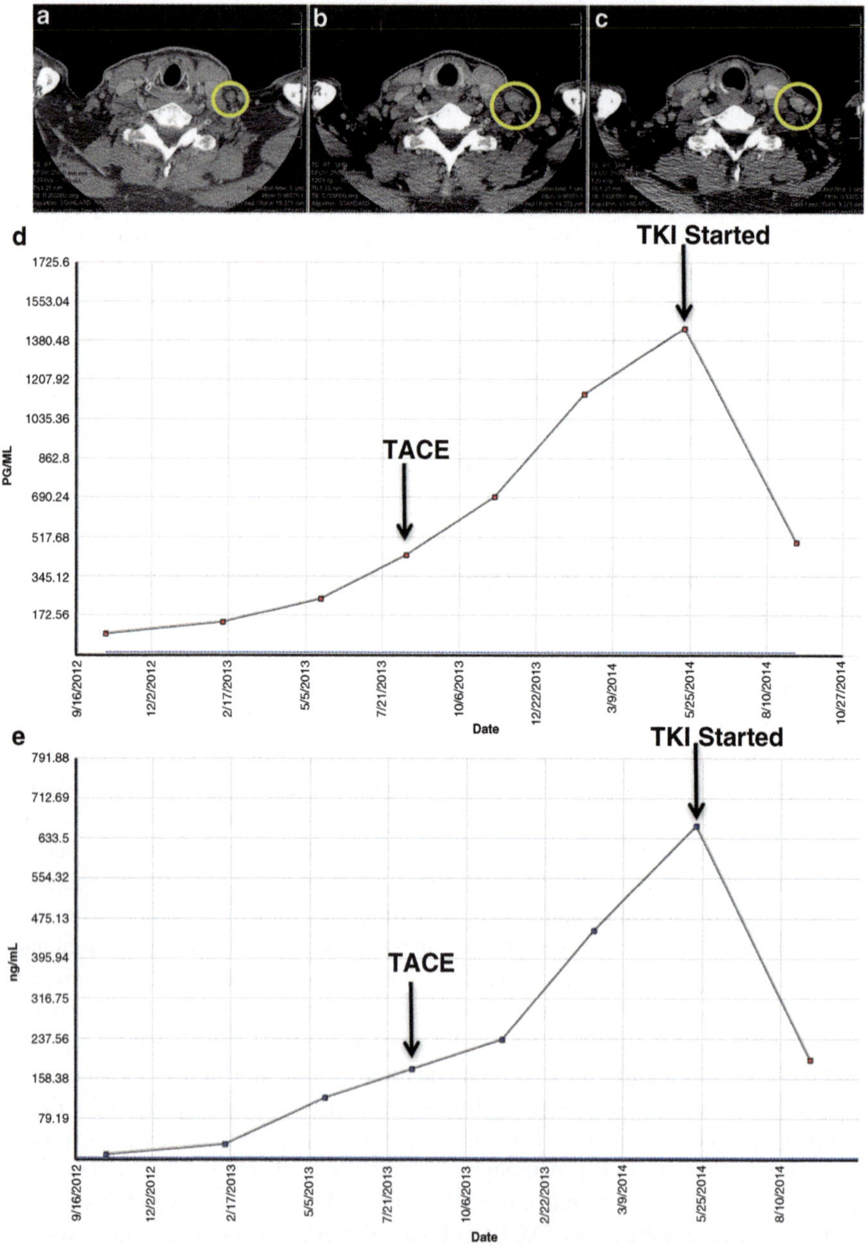

Fig. 42.2 Case no. 2: Cervical lymphadenopathy before and after initiating TKI. (Panel **a**). Left neck lymph node metastasis, 0.9 cm. (Panel **b**). Progressive left neck lymph node metastasis, 2.0 cm, 1 year later. TKI initiated. (Panel **c**) Regression of left neck lymph node metastasis, 1.5 cm, 3 months after initiating TKI. (**d**) Calcitonin change over time. (**e**) CEA change over time. *TACE* trans-arterial chemoembolization, *TKI* tyrosine kinase inhibitor, *CEA* carcinoembryonic antigen

Approved Agents for MTC: Cabozantinib and Vandetanib

On the basis of two randomized, placebo-controlled phase III trials that demonstrated efficacy (prolongation of progression-free survival), vandetanib and cabozantinib are now approved in the USA and Europe for the treatment of symptomatic or progressive MTC in patients with unresectable, locally advanced, or metastatic disease [5, 6]. The cabozantinib (EXAM) and vandetanib (ZETA) trials had some important differences (Table 42.1). The most notable differences are the requirement for progressive disease within 14 months in the cabozantinib trial and the presence of a crossover design in the vandetanib trial, making it impossible to compare outcomes in these two trials in any meaningful way.

The timing to initiate therapy varies greatly among physicians and practices. However, the recommended indications for initiation of systemic chemotherapy include [7]:

1. Progressive (based on RECIST criteria) and clinically significant disease. Most clinical trials in thyroid cancer require progression within 12–14 months in order to qualify for enrollment in a trial, and therefore this is the standard most centers use for initiating systemic therapy in asymptomatic patients.
2. Symptomatic metastatic disease that cannot be treated with local or symptom-specific therapies such as surgery, radiotherapy, embolization, cryoablation, or diarrhea management.
3. Bulky disease that compromises organ function and cannot be managed with localized therapies.

Table 42.1 Phase III trials for cabozantinib and vandetanib in patients with MTC

	Cabozantinib phase III (EXAM)		Vandetanib phase III (ZETA)	
Patients	Cabozantinib $N=219$	Placebo $N=111$	Vandetanib $N=231$	Placebo $N=100$
Inclusion criteria	Documented RECIST progression within 14 months of enrollment		Locally advanced or metastatic disease and serum Ct $\geq$ 500 pg/mL, with no requirement for progression	
Crossover design with progression during trial	Not allowed		Allowed	
Median PFS	11.2 months	4.0 months	Not reached (estimated 30.5 months)	19.3 months
OS	Immature analysis 44 % died at PFS cutoff		Immature analysis 15 % died at PFS cutoff	
Objective response rates	28 %	0 %	45 %	13 %[a]

[a]Twelve of the thirteen responses observed in patients randomized to the placebo group occurred while the patients were receiving open-label vandetanib

In selected cases, additional consideration for systemic therapy includes:

1. Calcitonin doubling time of less than 6 months and structural evidence of clinically significant disease that cannot be treated with local therapies. Rising tumor markers alone are not sufficient to demonstrate progression and warrant initiating systemic therapy [8].
2. Severe, intractable MTC-related diarrhea or Cushing's syndrome and lack of efficacy of other medical treatments and presence of structural and clinically significant disease.

Adverse Events Associated with Approved Agents

Compared with cytotoxic chemotherapeutic agents, the adverse events (AEs) associated with TKIs are generally manageable in the setting of a clinical trial or in the hands of physicians familiar with the toxicity profile of each TKI. Some AEs are serious or can cause a worsening of a patient's quality of life; therefore, it is extremely important to apply an individualized, patient-centered approach concerning when to initiate a systemic therapeutic agent and which drug to use [7]. While patients with progressive metastatic disease may benefit from the treatment, potential serious AEs of these drugs may outweigh the benefits in patients with indolent or stable disease. Here, we will describe the most common or rare but serious toxicities observed with vandetanib or cabozantinib.

Before starting treatment with vandetanib or cabozantinib, all patients should sign an informed consent after describing the common and serious AEs, symptoms of serious AEs, and the expected efficacy with medical therapy. Baseline AEs should be assessed prior to initiation of treatment with documentation of new and/or ongoing AEs throughout the treatment period [9]. The assessment and grading of each AE is performed at each visit using the Common Terminology Criteria for Adverse Events version 4.0 (CTCAE v4.0) [10]. Additionally, the Eastern Cooperative Oncology Group (ECOG) performance status (an assessment of general well-being) should be noted and be used as a basis for whether a patient can be safely treated with a proposed treatment or whether dose adjustment is necessary [11]. Of note, the EXAM and ZETA trials included patients with performance statuses between 0 and 2.

The most common AEs (>30 %) as reported in the phase III trial of vandetanib in MTC included diarrhea (56 %), rash (45 %), acne/dermatitis acneiform (35 %), nausea (33 %), and hypertension (32 %). Other less frequent AEs included constitutional symptoms (fatigue, headache, decreased appetite, weight changes, and asthenia), GI-related symptoms (vomiting, abdominal pain), upper respiratory complaints (cough, nasopharyngitis), QT prolongation (14 %), and photosensitivity (13 %). More serious AEs (grade 3+) were diarrhea (11 %), hypertension (9 %), QT prolongation (8 %), fatigue (6 %), decreased appetite (4 %), rash (4 %), and asthenia

(3 %) [5]. Vandetanib has a black box warning (reserved for serious side effects) for QT prolongation, torsade de pointes, and sudden death. Thus, vandetanib should not be given to patients with a history of congenital long QT syndrome, torsade de pointes, bradyarrhythmias, or uncompensated heart failure. Physicians who prescribe vandetanib must be certified by the Risk Evaluation and Mitigation Strategy (REMS) program, which educates prescribers about the risk of QT prolongation, appropriate monitoring and management of QT prolongation, and how to minimize serious cardiac arrhythmias or sudden death.

The most frequent (>30 %) **cabozantinib**-related AEs reported in the phase III MTC trial were diarrhea (63 %), stomatitis (51 %), palmar-plantar erythrodysesthesia (50 %), decreased weight (48 %), decreased appetite (46 %), nausea (43 %), fatigue (41 %), dysgeusia (34 %), hair color changes (34 %), and hypertension (33 %). Serious AEs reported as grade 3 or 4 were diarrhea (16 %), palmar-plantar erythrodysesthesia (13 %), fatigue (9 %), hypertension (8.4 %), venous thrombosis (3.7 %), hemorrhage (3.3 %), GI perforation (3.3 %), and GI/non-GI fistula (2.4 %) [6]. Cabozantinib has a black box warning for perforation, fistula, and hemorrhage; however, REMS certification is not required to prescribe this agent.

As neither agent is curative, chronic use is required for control of disease. Patient quality of life, compliance, and optimal response to drug therapy can all be limited without implementation of preventative strategies and aggressive management of AEs. The management of AEs associated with TKIs used for metastatic thyroid cancer is complex and beyond the scope of this article; it has been well described elsewhere [12].

Choosing a Therapeutic Agent Based on Adverse Event Risk Rather than Efficacy

Both cabozantinib and vandetanib have proven efficacy in patients with extensive MTC. At present, there are no efficacy data favoring one over another agent. A great deal of clinical judgment needs to be applied when deciding which drug to initiate. A systematic and patient-centered approach for deciding which drug to choose first was recently developed by our group [7]. This takes into account multiple factors including patient medical history, physical examination findings, baseline laboratory data, electrocardiogram, concomitant medications, and extension of tumor to surrounding tissues. From this evaluation, it is possible to assess the impact of a particular drug-related side effect for the individual patient. For example, a patient with a history of long QT syndrome or treatment with medications known to prolong the QT interval would be best treated with cabozantinib. On the other hand, a patient with a history of peptic ulcer disease, diverticulitis, or tumoral encroachment or invasion into the trachea/esophagus/major vascular structures might be better treated with vandetanib.

Clinical Pearls

- The majority of patients with residual MTC, after standard treatment with surgical resection, have indolent disease and can be actively monitored for objective progression on radiologic imaging performed at appropriate intervals.
- Systemic chemotherapy is not indicated in patients with indolent or structurally nonthreatening disease, even in the setting of distant metastases.
- In patients with progressive or symptomatic MTC without reasonable surgical or localized treatment options, cabozantinib or vandetanib should be considered to improve progression-free survival.
- A patient-centered approach must be used toward drug selection with diligent prevention and aggressive management strategies for adverse events.
- A patient with progressive MTC intolerant or unresponsive to the two approved agents should be referred for a clinical trial.
- Although these agents have had a significant impact on the management of MTC, more effective treatment options for this small but difficult to treat population are needed.

References

1. Meijer JA, le Cessie S, van den Hout WB, et al. Calcitonin and carcinoembryonic antigen doubling times as prognostic factors in medullary thyroid carcinoma: a structured meta-analysis. Clin Endocrinol (Oxf). 2009;72:534–42.
2. Blevins DP, Dadu R, Hu M, et al. Aerodigestive fistula formation as a rare side effect of anti-angiogenic tyrosine kinase inhibitor therapy for thyroid cancer. Thyroid. 2014;24:918–22.
3. Fromigue J, De Baere T, Baudin E, et al. Chemoembolization for liver metastases from medullary thyroid carcinoma. J Clin Endocrinol Metab. 2006;91:2496–9.
4. Cabanillas ME, Brose MS, Holland J, et al. A phase I study of cabozantinib (XL184) in patients with differentiated thyroid cancer. Thyroid. 2014;24:1508–14.
5. Wells Jr SA, Robinson BG, Gagel RF, et al. Vandetanib in patients with locally advanced or metastatic medullary thyroid cancer: a randomized, double-blind phase III trial. J Clin Oncol. 2012;30:134–41.
6. Elisei R, Schlumberger MJ, Muller SP, et al. Cabozantinib in progressive medullary thyroid cancer. J Clin Oncol. 2013;31(29):3639–46.
7. Cabanillas ME, Hu MI, Jimenez C. Medullary thyroid cancer in the era of tyrosine kinase inhibitors: to treat or not to treat-and with which drug-those are the questions. J Clin Endocrinol Metab. 2014;99(12):4390–6.
8. Tuttle RM, Haddad R, Ball DW, et al. NCCN Clinical practice guidelines in oncology: thyroid carcinoma. J Natl Compr Canc Netw. 2014;1.
9. Carhill AA, Cabanillas ME, Jimenez C, et al. The noninvestigational use of tyrosine kinase inhibitors in thyroid cancer: establishing a standard for patient safety and monitoring. J Clin Endocrinol Metab. 2013;98:31–42.
10. CTCAE v4.0. http://evs.nci.nih.gov/ftp1/CTCAE/CTCAE_4.03_2010-06-14_QuickReference_5x7.pdf. Accessed 10, 2014.
11. ECOG. http://www.ecog.org/general/perf_stat.html. Accessed 10, 2014.
12. Cabanillas ME, Hu MI, Durand JB, et al. Challenges associated with tyrosine kinase inhibitor therapy for metastatic thyroid cancer. J Thyroid Res. 2011;2011, 985780.

Part X
Medullary Thyroid Cancer: *Special Issues*

Chapter 43
Screening Leading to Diagnosis of C-Cell Hyperplasia

Giuseppe Costante

Case Presentation

A 58-year-old woman with history of hypertension was referred to the endocrinology outpatient clinic by her general practitioner in April 2010, following the discovery of a thyroid nodule on physical examination. At the endocrinology clinic, the patient was clinically euthyroid, the thyroid was slightly enlarged, and a nodule of approximately 2 cm was palpated in her left thyroid lobe.

Diagnosis/Assessment

Thyroid ultrasound (US) showed two hypoechoic nodules, one in the lower third of the left thyroid lobe (diameter 17.9 × 16.9 × 21.9 mm) and another (diameter 9.4 × 8.8 × 11.1 mm) adjacent to the isthmus in the right lobe.

The TSH was 1.7 mIU/l, anti-TPO antibodies were absent, and basal calcitonin (CT), which was routinely performed for the initial evaluation of nodular thyroid disease patients in our institution, was 39 pg/ml (n.v. <10 pg/ml). Due to the increased basal CT levels, the patient was also investigated by a pentagastrin (PG) stimulation test, which showed an increased response, with a 3-min CT peak at 284 pg/ml.

An US-guided fine-needle aspiration biopsy (FNAB) was performed on both nodules. Cytology of the para-isthmic right nodule was insufficient (class 1 of the Bethesda classification system), while the cytological findings of the lower left nodule were consistent with a benign lesion (class 2 of the Bethesda classification system).

G. Costante, MD (✉)
Endocrinology Clinic, Medicine Department, Institut Jules Bordet, Comprehensive Cancer Center, Boulevard de Waterloo, 121, 1000 Brussels, Belgium
e-mail: giuseppe.costante@bordet.be

D.S. Cooper, C. Durante (eds.), *Thyroid Cancer*,
DOI 10.1007/978-3-319-22401-5_43

Assessment and Literature Review

C-Cell Disease

The broad definition of *C-cell disease* indicates lesions deriving from the CT-secreting parafollicular cells (C cells) of the thyroid and includes medullary thyroid carcinoma (MTC) and C-cell hyperplasia (CCH) [1]. Both MTC and CCH are usually associated with increased circulating CT levels and may occur in sporadic or hereditary forms [1, 2].

MTC is a rare cancer, representing 4–10 % of all thyroid malignancies [2]. The great majority (approximately 75 %) of all MTCs are sporadic tumors [2], and their diagnosis occurs during the clinical workup of thyroid nodules. One out of four MTC cases is hereditary [2], associated with specific germline mutations of the *rearranged during transfection* (*RET*) proto-oncogene [2–4].

CCH was initially described in the 1970s as a lesion associated with familial MTC and multiple endocrine neoplasia (MEN) type 2 A and B [1–3]. In this context, CCH is prominently observed in the upper two thirds of the lateral thyroid lobes [3]. In some of these patients, the C cells may present cytologic and/or nuclear features of atypia. Importantly, C-cell hyperplasia in the familial setting must be considered a C-cell carcinoma in situ [3].

CCH histologically similar to that occurring in familial MTC has been described in individual cases of severe chronic lymphocytic thyroiditis [3]. Such an association is presently unexplained, and this sporadic CCH is considered idiopathic, even though it has been theorized that it could be secondary to C-cell stimulation by the elevated serum TSH [3]. Moreover, a morphometric study of C cells [4] has shown that 33 % of thyroids from normal subjects (15 % in women and 41 % in men) fulfilled the histologic criteria of CCH, but the exact significance of this sporadic CCH is unclear.

In terms of clinical relevance, it should be emphasized that while CCH represents a precancerous condition when observed within the MEN syndromes [3], the progression to MTC has never been demonstrated in sporadic CCH.

Diagnosis of C-Cell Disease

Early diagnosis in families known to harbor hereditary C-cell disease is now possible [5]. When it occurs in the context of MEN type 2 syndromes, the genetic screening for all members of families known to harbor germline *RET* proto-oncogene mutations allows early identification of carriers and radical prophylactic surgery may be offered as preventive care [5]. Depending on the specific genotype, which determines the age of onset and aggressiveness of MTC [5], appropriate timing and extent of surgery can be planned [1, 2, 5]. If thyroidectomy is performed in a timely manner, C-cell disease can be treated before clinical onset of cancer [5].

At surgical pathology, CCH is almost always observed in these patients, and micro-MTC may often occur [2, 5].

In the nonfamilial setting, MTC is the only form of C-cell disease that is clinically recognizable. A CCH diagnosis, in fact, can only take place at surgical pathology.

Sporadic MTC usually presents as a thyroid nodule. Although some clinical findings may suggest the possibility of MTC (its location in the upper third of a lobe, pain on palpation, the presence of enlarged lymph nodes), its diagnosis is often challenging. US typically reveals a hypoechogenic solid nodule with frequent microcalcifications, and there may be lymph node abnormalities. All these sonographic features are suspicious for malignancy but display low specificity and are unable to differentiate MTC from papillary thyroid carcinoma. FNAB is recommended in such cases. Cytology, however, displayed low sensitivity for preoperative MTC diagnosis, with consistent risk of misdiagnosis and inadequate initial treatment in most published studies [1]. Only two studies reported high FNAB sensitivity for MTC diagnosis [1]. A recent report from a study conducted in the USA and Europe among 12 centers and 7 countries demonstrated that an FNAB diagnosis of MTC could be made preoperatively in fewer than 50 % of cases, confirming its poor sensitivity for the diagnosis of sporadic MTC [6].

In MTC patients, serum CT levels rise early and increase with disease progression, thus representing a sensitive disease marker [1, 2]. They are also increased, to a limited extent, in CCH [1]. Nevertheless, in the original study by Guyetant et al. [4], sporadic CCH was not systematically associated with an elevation of serum CT levels.

It is recommended that two-site immunoassays using radioisotopic, enzymatic, or luminescent labeling should be employed, since they are the most sensitive tools for measuring serum CT levels [1]. They usually result <10 pg/ml in healthy subjects, but the normal cutoffs may widely vary among different laboratories [1]. CT values <5 pg/ml are seen in normal subjects with the most recent ultrasensitive methods [1]. It is also important that the cutoff values be defined taking into account sex and smoking habits. Basal CT levels are, in fact, higher in men than in women and are higher in smokers [1].

Increased CT Levels in Normal Subjects and in Other Pathological Conditions

Many CT elevations are unrelated to C-cell disease [1, 2] but are secondary to other conditions (Table 43.1). In particular, increased serum CT levels may be induced by pharmacological agents (e.g., proton pump inhibitors). Chronic renal failure, nonneoplastic hypergastrinemia, and a number of other pathological conditions can also cause hypercalcitoninemia (Table 43.1). Furthermore, falsely elevated CT levels can result from the interference by heterophilic antibodies (i.e., human antibodies that bind animal antibodies) used in the CT assay [1]. In such instances, performing a stimulation test may improve the specificity of CT determination [1].

Table 43.1 Causes of spurious elevations of serum calcitonin

Causes
Pharmacological
Proton pump inhibitors
Pathological conditions
Neoplastic
Small-cell lung carcinoma
Breast cancer
Neuroendocrine tumors of the lung or gastrointestinal tract
Zollinger's syndrome
Follicular thyroid tumors
Papillary thyroid microcarcinoma
Nonneoplastic
Chronic renal failure
Autoimmune thyroiditis
Pernicious anemia
Pancreatitis
Hyperparathyroidism
Nonneoplastic hypergastrinemia
Mastocytosis
Type 1A pseudohypoparathyroidism
Sepsis
Heterophilic antibodies

Increased CT levels have been reported in autoimmune thyroiditis, but this association is still controversial [1, 3]. Some studies have also reported decreased CT levels in smaller groups of Hashimoto's patients, possibly due to atrophy and/or fibrosis associated to destruction of both follicular and C cells [1, 3]. In a recent study [7] investigating the relationship between thyroid autoimmunity and CT levels, basal serum CT was not significantly higher in patients with positive anti-TPO than in control subjects (4.71 ± 6.46 vs. 4.84 ± 13.11 pg/ml; $P > 0.05$). Importantly, the rate of "suspicious" CT values (above the 10 pg/ml cutoff) did not significantly differ between patients with or without thyroid autoimmunity (3.9 vs. 3.0 %) [7].

Increased CT Levels and Preoperative MTC Diagnosis

The preoperative CT determination displays a much higher diagnostic performance than FNAB for preoperative diagnosis of MTC [1]. In most published studies, basal CT levels >100 pg/ml have a positive predictive value (PPV) for MTC approximating 100 % [1]. For basal CT increases <100 pg/ml, the PPV for MTC diagnosis drops to approximately 10 % [8]. In such instances, performing a stimulation test may improve the specificity of an elevated basal CT level [1].

CT Stimulation Testing for Diagnosis of C-Cell Disease

The most widely used CT stimulation testis performed by a slow intravenous injection of PG (0.5 μg/kg body weight) [1, 9]. Serum CT levels are measured in basal condition and 3 and 5 min after initiation of PG infusion [1, 9]. The test may cause potentially dangerous or unpleasant side effects (i.e., tachycardia, bradycardia, substernal tightness, nausea, vomiting, dizziness, flushing). It is not recommended in subjects over 60 years of age, and it is contraindicated in patients with hypertension and/or those with coronary artery disease [1, 9].

Similar to basal CT, stimulated CT levels are also higher in men than women [1]. A great proportion (80 %) of normal subjects have peak CT levels <10 pg/ml, and the maximal response is <30 pg/ml in 95 % of normals [1]. Stimulated CT levels >100 pg/ml suggest C-cell disease, even though milder elevations may occur in adults with other thyroid abnormalities [1, 9]. In MTC patients, the CT peak after PG stimulation is usually 5–10 times higher than basal levels [1]. Importantly, PG stimulation produces no or more limited increases (zero to twofold rise in CT levels) in other neuroendocrine tumors displaying elevated CT values [10].

A short intravenous calcium infusion may also provoke CT secretion [9]. This approach represents an alternative to PG in areas of the world where PG is not available and may also be combined with PG testing to enhance sensitivity [9]. Serum CT levels measured after a 30 s infusion of calcium gluconate are very similar to those observed after PG administration [9, 11]. In a recent report, the procedure, cutoffs, and the safety of CT testing by calcium gluconate have accurately been defined [11]. The dose of calcium gluconate of 25 mg (i.e., 2.3 mg or 0.12 mEq of elemental calcium)/kg body weight has been shown to be well tolerated and safe. The calculation of the adjusted body weight (www.manuelsweb.com/IBW.htm for ideal body weight and adjusted body weight calculator) has been recommended, to avoid an overdose in obese patients. After a basal CT determination, calcium gluconate should be administered i.v. (5 ml/min) and a 3-min minimum infusion time should be utilized. CT determination should be performed 2, 5, and 10 min after stopping the infusion [11]. In one report, the optimal CT threshold peaks for MTC diagnosis were >79 pg/ml in females and >544 pg/ml in males [11].

CT Determination for MTC Screening

Early diagnosis and radical surgical treatment are considered critical for reducing MTC-related morbidity and mortality [2]. Since virtually all MTC patients have elevated circulating CT levels at the time of diagnosis, several studies performed during the last decade of the past century have suggested that universal screening of patients with thyroid nodular disease by routine measurement of serum CT might improve early diagnosis and improve the long-term prognosis of MTCs [1]. Indeed, a major caveat to the suitability of this approach relates to the discrepancy between the low prevalence of MTC among patients with thyroid nodules (0.26–1.30 %) and the much higher (0.6–6.8 %) frequencies of increased CT levels reported in the majority of published studies [1]. Thus, the PPV of increased basal CT levels resulted rather low (10–40 %), even in those studies in which appropriate selection criteria excluded patients presenting known causes of spurious CT elevations [1]. For this reason, confirmatory testing by CT stimulation was necessary in most studies [1]. Only two reports, by the same group, presented higher (>90 %) PPVs of basal CT measurement [12, 13]. Overall, the stimulated CT levels displayed a greater sensitivity and specificity for MTC diagnosis than basal CT [1]. Nonetheless, the basal cutoff levels used to perform CT stimulation testing varied greatly (5–20 pg/ml) [1]. Similarly, there has been a wide variation among studies concerning the stimulated (either by PG or calcium gluconate) CT values regarded as an indication for surgery (30–1000 pg/ml) [1].

In 2009, the American Thyroid Association (ATA) published specific guidelines for MTC [14] and revised their recommendations for thyroid nodules and differentiated thyroid cancer management [15]. Focusing on CT screening in thyroid nodular disease patients, the ATA declined to recommend for or against the universal CT screening approach, while specifying that (if measured) a CT value >100 pg/ml would be suspicious and necessitate further evaluation and appropriate treatment [14, 15]. Shortly after, the European Thyroid Association (ETA) released new guidelines [16], in collaboration with the American Association of Clinical Endocrinologists (AACE) and with the Italian *Associazione Medici Endocrinologi* (AME) which called for mandatory CT measurement only in patients suspected to have MTC or with a family history of MTC. In short, the designed task forces from ATA and ETA did not consider the level of available evidence strong enough to support the systematic CT screening of patients with thyroid nodular disease. Possibly, large, long-term, prospective, randomized multicenter studies, with standard enrollment criteria, CT assay techniques, and homogeneous cut points for interpreting the results, could answer the question of whether routine CT screening of nodular thyroid disease patients should be adopted, based on its impact on MTC-related morbidity and mortality. It would not be surprising, however, that even the most accurate CT assay would still yield a low PPV. As a general rule in clinical epidemiology, in fact, the disease prevalence in the population under study constitutes the major determinant of the PPV. For uncommon diseases (like MTC), positive results would mostly be false positives, no matter how sensitive and specific the employed assay method.

Back to the Patient

Management of the Case

Due to the PG stimulation test indicating C-cell disease and an inconclusive cytology in a sonographically suspicious thyroid nodule, the patient refused a repeated FNAB and preferred to directly undergo surgery. A total thyroidectomy with prophylactic central neck dissection was performed.

Surgical pathology showed nodular thyroid hyperplasia in both thyroid nodules, and immunohistochemistry revealed low-power microscopic fields containing at least 50 C cells, consistent with histological findings of CCH.

All 13 dissected lymph nodes were normal.

CT Screening and Diagnosis of Sporadic CCH

In the present case, both basal and PG-stimulated CT levels were consistent with C-cell disease, and FNAB could not exclude the presence of an MTC. Histological verification was, therefore, recommended and indicated benign thyroid nodules and sporadic CCH.

Should this situation be included among the causes of false-positive results in the CT screening of thyroid nodules? If we assume that the screening would be aimed at identifying true malignant disease, CCH could be considered a false positive. Unless future studies will provide evidence that sporadic CCH represents a precancerous lesion evolving to MTC, surgical treatment is actually unnecessary in such patients.

How often does this situation take place during the screening for MTC in thyroid nodular disease patients? The frequency of CCH in prospective screening studies varied from 0.12 to 1.56 % [1]. Importantly, when analyzing the proportion of CCH versus MTC patients in these series, CCH accounted for 30–75 % of the cases with basal CT levels between 20 and 100 pg/ml and positive PG stimulation testing [1, 17]. It would, therefore, be extremely helpful if CCH could be distinguished from MTC preoperatively, to avoid unnecessary surgery. In this respect, some reports have suggested that the magnitude of the stimulated CT peak may help to distinguish between CCH and MTC, even though the proposed threshold for discriminating the benign from the malignant lesion varies among different reports [1]. In particular, one study observed that a PG-stimulated CT peak >100 < 1000 pg/ml exhibited an 80 % PPV for CCH, while values >1000 pg/ml exhibited a 100 % PPV for MTC [8]. Another study found that a peak of CT of 275 pg/ml after PG had a 100 % PPV value for diagnosis of MTC, while PG-stimulated CT levels <275 pg/ml had an 89 % PPV for the diagnosis of CCH [17]. Although encouraging, these PPV values cannot be considered definitive, and further studies are needed to more precisely define the threshold windows of stimulated CT levels allowing the differentiation of MTC from CCH.

Patient Outcome

L-thyroxine replacement therapy was started immediately after surgery.

Three months after thyroidectomy, the patient was euthyroid, her serum TSH was 1.9 mIU/l, and the basal CT levels fell to <0.5 pg/ml.

The patient is presently in good health.

Clinical Pearls

- Serum calcitonin is a highly sensitive marker for C-cell disease.
- Increased basal calcitonin levels are frequently associated to C-cell hyperplasia rather than to MTC.
- CCH does not represent a malignant condition in the nonfamilial setting.
- Differentiation between MTC and CCH is often difficult, even after provocative testing (e.g., PG or calcium stimulation).
- There is insufficient evidence supporting systematic calcitonin screening in the initial management of thyroid nodular disease patients.

References

1. Costante G, Durante C, Francis Z, Schlumberger M, Filetti S. Determination of calcitonin levels in C-cell disease: clinical interest and potential pitfalls. Nat Clin Pract Endocrinol Metab. 2009;5(1):35–44.
2. Leboulleux S, Baudin E, Travagli JP, Schlumberger M. Medullary thyroid carcinoma. Clin Endocrinol (Oxf). 2004;61:229–31.
3. LiVolsi VA. C cell hyperplasia/neoplasia. J Clin Endocrinol Metab. 1997;82:39–41.
4. Guyétant S, Rousselet MC, Durigon M, Chappard D, Franc B, Guerin O, Saint-André JP. Sex-related C cell hyperplasia in the normal human thyroid: a quantitative autopsy study. J Clin Endocrinol Metab. 1997;82:42–7.
5. Waguespack SG, Rich TA, Perrier ND, Jimenez C, Cote GJ. Management of medullary thyroid carcinoma and MEN2 syndromes in childhood. Nat Rev Endocrinol. 2011;7:596–607.
6. Essig Jr GF, Porter K, Schneider D, Debora A, Lindsey SC, Busonero G, et al. Fine needle aspiration and medullary thyroid carcinoma: the risk of inadequate preoperative evaluation and initial surgery when relying upon FNAB cytology alone. Endocr Pract. 2013;19:920–7.
7. Grani G, Nesca A, Del Sordo M, Calvanese A, Carbotta G, Bianchini M, et al. Interpretation of serum calcitonin in patients with chronic autoimmune thyroiditis. Endocr Relat Cancer. 2012;19(3):345–9.
8. Costante G, Meringolo D, Durante C, Bianchi D, Nocera M, Tumino S, et al. Predictive value of serum calcitonin levels for preoperative diagnosis of medullary thyroid carcinoma in a cohort of 5817 consecutive patients with thyroid nodules. J Clin Endocrinol Metab. 2007;92:450–5.
9. Colombo C, Verga U, Mian C, Ferrero S, Perrino M, Vicentini L, et al. Comparison of calcium and pentagastrin tests for the diagnosis and follow-up of medullary thyroid cancer. J Clin Endocrinol Metab. 2012;97:905–13.
10. Leboulleux S, Baudin E, Young J, Caillou B, Lazar V, Pellegriti G, et al. Gastroenteropancreatic neuroendocrine tumor metastases to the thyroid gland: differential diagnosis with medullary thyroid carcinoma. Eur J Endocrinol. 1999;140:187–91.
11. Mian C, Perrino M, Colombo C, Cavedon E, Pennelli G, Ferrero S, et al. Refining calcium test for the diagnosis of medullary thyroid cancer: cutoffs, procedures, and safety. J Clin Endocrinol Metab. 2014;99:1656–64.
12. Pacini FF, Fontanelli M, Fugazzola L, Elisei R, Romei C, Di Coscio G, et al. Routine measurement of serum calcitonin in nodular thyroid diseases allows the preoperative diagnosis of unsuspected sporadic medullary thyroid carcinoma. J Clin Endocrinol Metab. 1994;78:826–9.
13. Elisei R, Bottici V, Luchetti F, Luchetti F, Di Coscio G, Romei C, Grasso L, et al. Impact of routine measurement of serum calcitonin on the diagnosis and outcome of medullary thyroid

cancer: experience in 10,864 patients with nodular thyroid disorders. J Clin Endocrinol Metab. 2004;89(1):163–8.

14. American Thyroid Association Guidelines Task Force, Kloos RT, Eng C, Evans DB, Francis GL, Gagel RF, et al. Medullary thyroid cancer: management guidelines of the American Thyroid Association. Thyroid. 2009;19:565–612.
15. American Thyroid Association (ATA) Guidelines Taskforce on Thyroid Nodules and Differentiated Thyroid Cancer, Cooper DS, Doherty GM, Haugen BR, Kloos RT, Lee SL, et al. Revised American Thyroid Association management guidelines for patients with thyroid nodules and differentiated thyroid cancer. Thyroid. 2009;19:1167–214.
16. Gharib H, Papini E, Paschke R, Duick DS, Valcavi R, Hegedüs L, et al. American Association of Clinical Endocrinologists, Associazione Medici Endocrinologi, and European Thyroid Association medical guidelines for clinical practice for the diagnosis and management of thyroid nodules: executive summary of recommendations. J Endocrinol Invest. 2010;33:1–50.
17. Milone F, Ramundo V, Chiofalo MG, Severino R, Paciolla I, Pezzullo L, et al. Predictive value of pentagastrin test for preoperative differential diagnosis between C-cell hyperplasia and medullary thyroid carcinoma in patients with moderately elevated basal calcitonin levels. Clin Endocrinol (Oxf). 2010;73:85–8.

Chapter 44
Increased Basal Calcitonin in Nodular Goiter: Is It Micromedullary Thyroid Cancer?

Andreas Machens and Henning Dralle

Case Presentation

A 64-year-old woman with a 17-year history of thyroid nodules was referred in 2013 with elevated basal calcitonin serum levels for a second opinion regarding the need for thyroidectomy.

Evaluation for Surgery

In July 2004, outside thyroid ultrasonography had identified a 22 × 13 mm hypoechoic nodule in the left lobe, for which the patient had been placed on a daily levothyroxine dose of 75 μg to suppress serum TSH.

In October 2012, the left lobe hypoechoic nodule, measuring 28 × 12 mm, appeared hypofunctional on thyroid scintigraphy carried out elsewhere. Thyroid ultrasonography at that hospital identified two additional 3 and 5 mm nodules in an otherwise normal-appearing thyroid gland. The patient's basal calcitonin serum level was slightly elevated: 15.2 pg/mL (unspecified calcitonin assay; upper normal assay limit 11.8 pg/mL).

A. Machens, MD (✉) • H. Dralle, MD FRCS, FACS, FEBS
Department of General, Visceral, and Vascular Surgery, University Hospital, Halle (Saale), Germany

Medical Faculty, University of Halle-Wittenberg, Ernst-Grube-Str. 40, 06097 Halle (Saale), Germany
e-mail: AndreasMachens@aol.com

D.S. Cooper, C. Durante (eds.), *Thyroid Cancer*,
DOI 10.1007/978-3-319-22401-5_44

In February 2013, high-resolution thyroid ultrasonography at the same facility uncovered, apart from the large left nodule (now measuring 26×16 mm), two hypoechoic nodules in the left lobe, measuring 10×6 mm and 7×4 mm, respectively, and a 3×1 mm hypoechoic, calcified nodule in the right lobe. Ultrasound-guided fine-needle aspiration of the large left nodule yielded a cytological diagnosis of follicular neoplasia (Bethesda class IV). Using a more sensitive calcitonin assay (IMMULITE 2000, Diagnostic Products Corporation, USA; normal upper assay limit <5 pg/mL), serum calcitonin was 25 pg/mL basally and peaking at 256 pg/mL 2 min after intravenous stimulation with 0.5 μg of pentagastrin per kilogram body weight. Carcinoembryonic antigen serum levels were normal (1.6 and 1.5 μg/L; upper normal limit <5.0 μg/L).

In March 2013, upon first presentation to our institution, calcitonin serum level was 16.5 pg/mL basally and peaked at 194 pg/mL 5 min (IMMULITE 2000, Diagnostic Products Corporation, USA; normal upper assay limit <5 pg/mL) after intravenous stimulation at 10 mL/min with 2.5 mg of calcium gluconate per kg body weight. Repeat ultrasonography confirmed the cytologically indeterminate left hypoechoic nodule at 25×16 mm (Fig. 44.1) and the small right calcified nodule measuring 4.8 mm (Fig. 44.2).

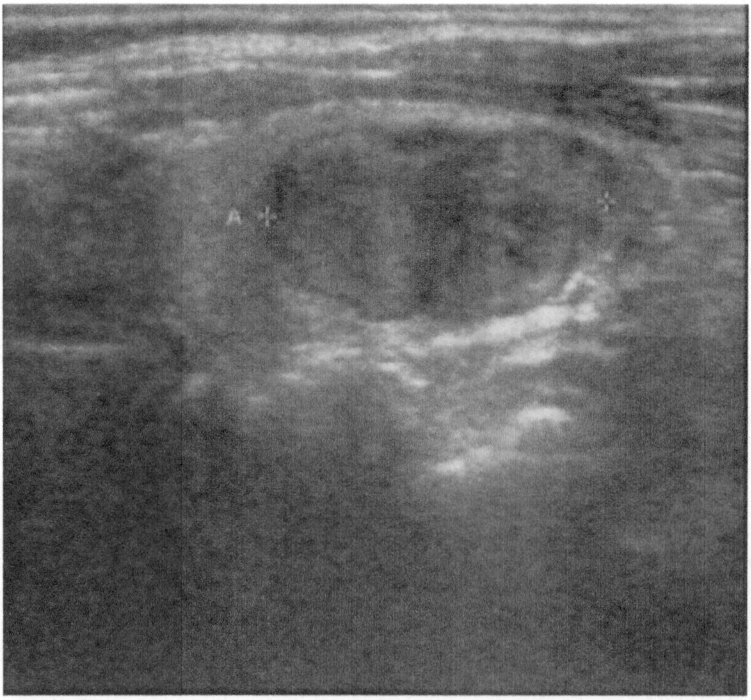

Fig. 44.1 Ultrasound of the left thyroid lobe showing a hypoechoic nodule 25×16 mm in size

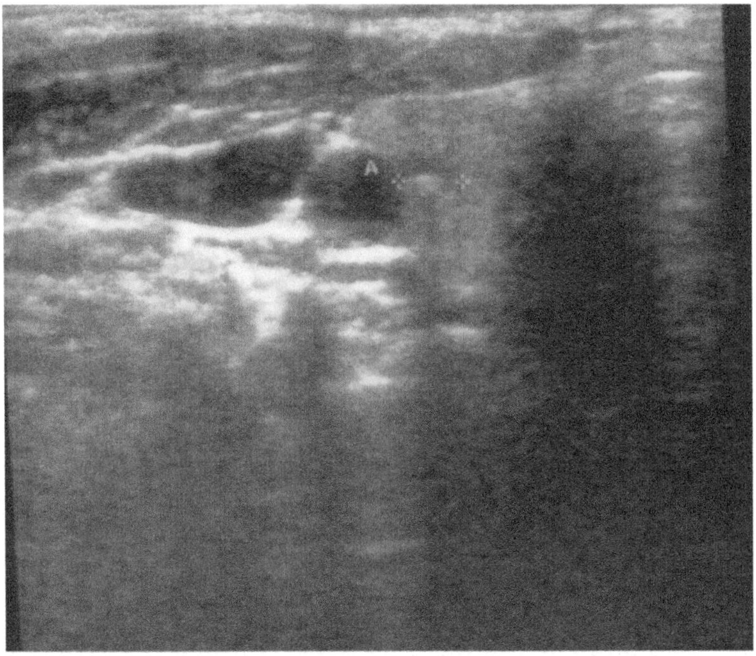

Fig. 44.2 Ultrasound of the right thyroid lobe showing a small calcified nodule 4.8 mm in size

Assessment and Literature Review

Is It Medullary Thyroid Cancer?

Medullary thyroid cancer affects 0.3–1.4 % of patients with thyroid nodules [1–4]. They synthesize and secrete calcitonin proportional to overall tumor mass into the bloodstream. In the setting of nodular thyroid disease, an elevated basal calcitonin ≤ 100 pg/mL can pose a diagnostic dilemma that becomes more problematic as the serum calcitonin levels move lower and lower. Because male thyroid glands contain larger numbers of parafollicular C cells than female thyroids, males have higher serum calcitonin levels. Thus, there are gender-specific basal calcitonin thresholds for thyroidectomy: 20 pg/mL for women (positive predictive value, PPV 88 %) and 80–100 pg/mL for men (PPV 100 %) [5]. Corresponding absolute calcitonin thresholds after stimulation with pentagastrin are 250 pg/mL for women and 500 pg/mL for men (PPV 100 % each) [5]. Interestingly, our patient's calcitonin serum levels, ranging from 15.2 pg/mL to 25 pg/mL basally depending on the assay and reaching 256 pg/mL after stimulation with pentagastrin, crossed the absolute calcitonin thresholds for women of 20 pg/mL basally and 250 pg/mL after stimulation with pentagastrin by a narrow margin. Although it may be a more suitable provocative agent than calcium, pentagastrin has been unavailable since 2005 in many countries, including the USA. In the era of more sensitive immunochemiluminometric calcitonin assays, the need for provocative testing is dwindling. It is important to note that our patient required thyroid surgery for the cytological diagnosis of follicular neoplasia from the indeterminate left nodule, which is what prompted calcitonin screening in the first place.

If It Is Medullary Thyroid Cancer, Will It Be Confined to the Thyroid Gland?

The diagnosis of sporadic medullary thyroid cancer raises the question of whether the tumor is limited to the thyroid gland or has already spread beyond the thyroid capsule. On preoperative neck ultrasonography, more than one-third of patients with MTC have false-negative findings [6]. This is why basal calcitonin serum levels provide important clues as to the presence of occult lymph node metastases [7].

The overall risk of lymph node metastases is estimated at:

- 0 %—when basal calcitonin is ≤20 pg/mL
- 11 %—when basal calcitonin is 20.1–50 pg/mL
- 17 %—when basal calcitonin is 50.1–100 pg/mL
- 35 %—when basal calcitonin is 100.1–200 pg/mL

Lymph node metastases begin to appear in the:

- Ipsilateral central and lateral neck—when basal calcitonin exceeds 20 pg/mL
- Contralateral central neck—when basal calcitonin exceeds 50 pg/mL
- Contralateral lateral neck—when basal calcitonin exceeds 200 pg/mL

Absent clinical and ultrasonographic evidence of suspicious lymph nodes, the patient's most recent basal calcitonin of 16.5 pg/mL argued against the presence of lymph node metastases.

If Basal Calcitonin Fails to Normalize, Will Reoperation Be Worthwhile for Minimal Disease?

The prospect of biochemical cure after a second neck operation is contingent on the residual basal calcitonin level, as long as no more than five lymph node metastases were removed at the initial operation [8]:

- 75–77 % for a residual basal calcitonin <10 pg/mL
- 35–36 % for a residual basal calcitonin of 10.1–100 pg/mL

The pros and cons of reoperation in a scarred neck (high chance of definitive cure versus expectant observation of minimal residual disease) need to be detailed to the patient. Reoperations in a scarred neck, as a matter of principle, should not be embarked on outside specialist centers to keep surgical morbidity to a minimum. The one-time cost of reaching a definitive cure and the cost of daily levothyroxine supplementation may be smaller from a societal perspective than the need for continual biochemical follow-up and imaging studies, some of which may prompt additional operations at incremental costs [5].

Management of the Case

After informed consent, the patient opted for thyroidectomy under intraoperative nerve monitoring as a minimum procedure, with possible lymph node dissection depending on intraoperative evidence of nodal disease. Inside the dorsal portion of the right lobe, a small firm nodule was identified. The central neck was explored for suspicious nodes but none were found, as to be expected with a basal calcitonin level ≤20 pg/mL, so that no neck dissection was performed.

Histopathological examination revealed a 15 mm follicular adenoma in the left lobe and a 5 mm medullary thyroid cancer surrounded by normal thyroid parenchyma in the absence of C-cell hyperplasia.

The patient made an uneventful recovery. Video laryngoscopy confirmed normal vocal cord function after the operation. On the second postoperative day, basal and calcium gluconate-stimulated calcitonin levels were below the assay's detection limit (<2 pg/mL; IMMULITE 2000, Diagnostic Products Corporation, USA) reflecting biochemical cure. Follow-up examinations 4 weeks later showed normal parathyroid hormone serum levels, whereas serum calcitonin remained below the assay's detection limit.

RET (rearranged during transfection) screening (exons 5, 8, 10, 11, 13, 14, 15, and 16) was negative, excluding hereditary medullary thyroid cancer with a probability of 99 %.

Importance of Identifying Occult Medullary Thyroid Cancer

For any medical intervention, there is a continuum of benefit vs. harm. The net benefit of surgical intervention for medullary thyroid microcarcinoma is a continuous function of the:

- Risk of morbidity if left untreated (the risk of which is unknown)
- The relative risk reduction of treatment (surgical cure, likely to be high)
- The risk of harm from the treatment (surgical morbidity, likely to be low in expert hands)

Sporadic micromedullary thyroid cancer is found pathologically in 0.3–0.4 % of patients with nodular thyroid disease [2]. In the absence of good natural history data, it is important to note the close relationships between primary tumor diameter [9] and:

- Preoperative basal calcitonin serum levels: means of 136.5 pg/mL (≤2 mm) to 926.0 pg/mL (9–10 mm)
- The rates of lymph node metastases: from 13 % (≤2 mm) to 43 % (9–10 mm)
- The biochemical cure rate: from 85 % (≤2 mm) to 77 % (9–10 mm)

Although cancer-specific death is extremely uncommon, as many as 24 % of patients harboring micromedullary thyroid cancer are not biochemically cured, perhaps reflecting locally metastatic or systemic disease [9].

Owing to the lack of long-term follow-up data, the same body of scientific evidence has led to different conclusions. In Europe, the Thyroid Section of the German Society for Endocrinology in 2004 [10] and the European Thyroid Association in 2006 [11] started supporting calcitonin screening in patients with nodular thyroid disease. In a decision model developed for a hypothetical group of adult patients presenting for evaluation of thyroid nodules in the USA, serum calcitonin screening, which is sensitive to age and gender, appeared to be cost effective in patients undergoing evaluation for thyroid nodules [12]. The American Thyroid Association, raising concerns of cost-effectiveness and unproven benefit, advises neither for nor against calcitonin screening [4, 13].

Despite these professional disagreements, a strong consensus exists to actively detect and, in most cases, to resect involved nodes [2].

Clinical Pearls/Pitfalls

- Gender-specific basal calcitonin thresholds for sporadic medullary thyroid cancer are 20 pg/mL for women and 80–100 pg/mL for men.
- Lymph node metastases begin to appear in the ipsilateral central and lateral neck when basal calcitonin exceeds 20 pg/mL, in the contralateral central neck when basal calcitonin exceeds 50 pg/mL, and in the contralateral lateral neck when basal calcitonin exceeds 200 pg/mL.
- In sporadic micromedullary thyroid cancer, there are significant relationships between primary tumor diameter and (1) preoperative basal calcitonin serum levels (means of 136.5–926.0 pg/mL), (2) the rates of lymph node metastases (from 13 to 43 %), and (3) biochemical cure rates (85–77 %).

References

1. Costante G, Meringolo D, Durante C, Bianchi D, Nocera M, Tumino S, Crocetti U, Attard M, Maranghi M, Torlontano M, Filetti S. Predictive value of serum calcitonin levels for preoperative diagnosis of medullary thyroid carcinoma in a cohort of 5817 consecutive patients with thyroid nodules. J Clin Endocrinol Metab. 2007;92:450–5.

2. Ahmed SR, Ball DW. Clinical review: incidentally discovered medullary thyroid cancer: diagnostic strategies and treatment. J Clin Endocrinol Metab. 2011;96:1237–45.
3. Chambon G, Alovisetti C, Idoux-Louche C, Reynaud C, Rodier M, Guedj AM, Chapuis H, Lallemant JG, Lallemant B. The use of preoperative routine measurement of basal serum thyrocalcitonin in candidates for thyroidectomy due to nodular thyroid disorders: results from 2733 consecutive patients. J Clin Endocrinol Metab. 2011;96:75–81.
4. Wells SA Jr, Asa SL, Dralle H, Elisei R, Evans DB, Gagel RF, Lee NY, Machens A, Moley JF, Pacini F. Raue F, Frank-Raue K, Robinson B, Rosenthal MS, Santoro M, Schlumberger M, Shah MH, Waguespack SG, The American Thyroid Association Guidelines Task Force on Medullary Thyroid Carcinoma. Revised American Thyroid Association guidelines for the management of medullary thyroid cancer. Thyroid. 2015;25:567-610.
5. Machens A, Hoffmann F, Sekulla C, Dralle H. Importance of gender-specific calcitonin thresholds in screening for occult medullary thyroid cancer. Endocr Relat Cancer. 2009;16:1291–8.
6. Kouvaraki MA, Shapiro SE, Fornage BD, Edeiken-Monro BS, Sherman SI, Vassilopoulou-Sellin R, Lee JE, Evans DB. Role of preoperative ultrasonography in the surgical management of patients with thyroid cancer. Surgery. 2003;134:946–55.
7. Machens A, Dralle H. Biomarker-based risk stratification for previously untreated medullary thyroid cancer. J Clin Endocrinol Metab. 2010;95:2655–63.
8. Machens A, Dralle H. Benefit-risk balance of reoperation for persistent medullary thyroid cancer. Ann Surg. 2013;257:751–7.
9. Machens A, Dralle H. Biological relevance of medullary thyroid microcarcinoma. J Clin Endocrinol Metab. 2012;97:1547–53.
10. Karges W, Dralle H, Raue F, Mann K, Reiners C, Grussendorf M, Hüfner M, Niederle B, Brabant G, German Society for Endocrinology (DGE). Thyroid section. Calcitonin measurement to detect medullary thyroid carcinoma in nodular goiter: German evidence-based consensus recommendations. Exp Clin Endocrinol Diabetes. 2004;112:52–8.
11. Pacini F, Schlumberger M, Dralle H, Elisei R, Smit JW, Wiersinga W, European Thyroid Cancer Taskforce. European consensus for the management of patients with differentiated thyroid carcinoma of the follicular epithelium. Eur J Endocrinol. 2006;154:787–803.
12. Cheung K, Roman SA, Wang TS, Walker HD, Sosa JA. Calcitonin measurements in the evaluation of thyroid nodules in the United States: a cost-effectiveness and decision analysis. J Clin Endocrinol Metab. 2008;93:2173–80.
13. American Thyroid Association (ATA) Guidelines Taskforce on Thyroid Nodules and Differentiated Thyroid Cancer, Cooper DS, Doherty GM, Haugen BR, Kloos RT, Lee SL, Mandel SJ, Mazzaferri EL, McIver B, Pacini F, Schlumberger M, Sherman SI, Steward DL, Tuttle RM. Revised American Thyroid Association management guidelines for patients with thyroid nodules and differentiated thyroid cancer. Thyroid. 2009;19:1167–214.

Chapter 45
Timing and Extent of Surgery for a Pediatric Patient with Hereditary MTC and Positive Screening for the S891A *RET* Mutation

Henning Dralle and Andreas Machens

Case Presentation

A 17-year-old male non-index patient (patient 3.1.2; Table 45.1, Fig. 45.1) was referred for surgical intervention with positive screening for the S891A *RET* mutation, which had been prompted by a positive *RET* gene test in his father (index patient 2.1; Fig. 45.1) after outside surgery for medullary thyroid cancer (MTC). Familial screening uncovered eight additional gene carriers.

Evaluation for Surgery

On stimulation with pentagastrin, the adolescent carrier's calcitonin serum levels rose from 24 pg/mL basally (upper normal limit <8.4 pg/mL; Immulite 2000 assay, Diagnostic Products Corp., Los Angeles, CA) to a peak level of 510 pg/mL after 5 min (patient 3.1.2; Table 45.1, Fig. 45.1). Physical examination of the thyroid gland and high-resolution neck ultrasonography were negative. Thyroid examination of the other eight non-index patients, including ultrasonography, identified multinodular goiter disease without evidence of lymph node metastases in the 78-year-old grandmother (patient 1.1) and a suspicious small hypoechoic lesion in her 46-year-old son (patient 2.3) (Fig. 45.2). With the exception of two 5- and 8-year-old children (patients 3.2.1 and 3.1.3), all non-index patients exhibited

H. Dralle, MD, FRCS, FACS, FEBS (✉) • A. Machens, MD
Department of General, Visceral, and Vascular Surgery, University Hospital, Halle (Saale), Germany

Medical Faculty, University of Halle-Wittenberg, Ernst-Grube-Str. 40, 06097 Halle (Saale), Germany
e-mail: henning.dralle@uk-halle.de

D.S. Cooper, C. Durante (eds.), *Thyroid Cancer*,
DOI 10.1007/978-3-319-22401-5_45

Table 45.1 Clinical histopathological characteristics of all eight non-index patients carrying the S891A *RET* mutation

Patient no., gender, age (years)	Preoperative calcitonin (pg/mL)		Extent of surgery	Histopathology; pTNM	Postoperative calcitonin (pg/mL)	
	Basal	Peak			Basal	Peak
1.1; f; 78	312	2634	TT, LND central and lateral	Bilateral MTC (10 mm, 11 mm); 1/45 LNM; pT1bpN1aM0	7	48
2.3; m; 46	60	nd	TT, LND central and lateral	Bilateral MTC (3 mm, 5 mm), unilateral PTC (1 mm); 0/31 LNM; pT1apN0M0	<2	<2
3.1.2; m; 17	24	510	TT, LND central	Bilateral MTC (3 mm, 3 mm), 0/7 LNM; pT1apN0M0	<2	<2
3.2.4; f; 10	9	27	TT	Bilateral CCH, no MTC, 0/1 LNM	<2	<2
3.1.3; m; 8	4	79	TT	No CCH, no MTC; 0/1 LNM	<2	<2
3.2.3; m; 8	9	nd	TT	Bilateral CCH, no MTC	<2	<2
3.2.2; m; 6	9	57	TT	Bilateral CCH, no MTC, 0/1 LNM	<2	<2
3.2.1; f; 5	3	nd	TT	Bilateral CCH, no MTC, 0/1 LNM	<2	<2

Patient numbers are the same as in Fig. 45.1. The calcitonin assay's upper normal limit was <5.0 pg/mL for women and <8.4 for men (Immulite 2000 assay, Diagnostic Products Corp., Los Angeles, CA)

pTNM according to Sobin LH, Gospodarowicz MK, Wittekind Ch (eds.): TNM Classification of Malignant Tumors, 7th Edition, 2009

TT total thyroidectomy, *LND* lymph node dissection, *CCH* C-cell-hyperplasia, *f* female, *m* male, *MTC* medullary thyroid cancer, *LNM* lymph node metastasis, *nd* not determined

elevated basal calcitonin levels. All family members who had a pentagastrin stimulation test performed showed peak calcitonin levels markedly increased over baseline (Table 45.1). None of the eight non-index patients had biochemical or imaging evidence for adrenal medullary or parathyroid disease.

Assessment and Literature Review

The p.S891A missense mutation affects 2–9 % of all *RET* gene carriers across geographic boundaries [1–3], depending on the intensity of national screening programs (every patient diagnosed with MTC as opposed to no more than family screening for confirmation of clinically manifest disease). Within the spectrum of hereditary C-cell disease, the S891A mutation is part of a group of intracellular *RET*

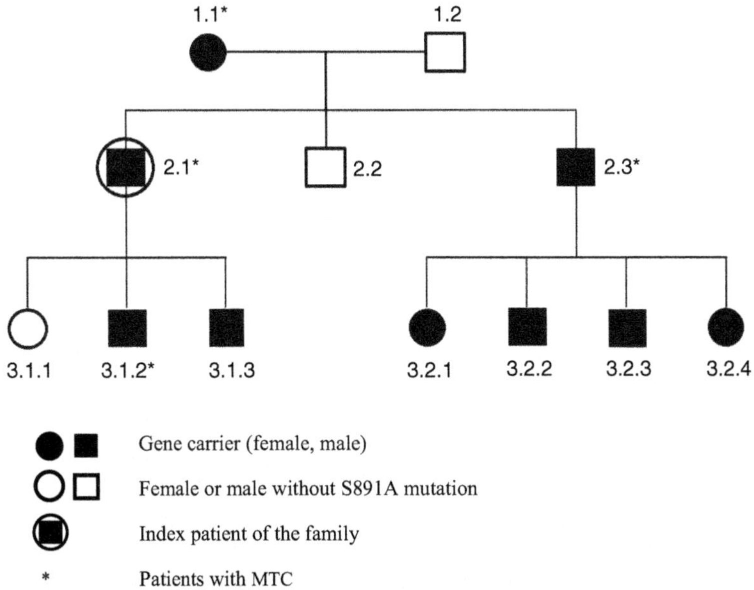

Fig. 45.1 Pedigree of the 3-generational family carrying the heterozygous S891A *RET* mutation. *Filled circle, filled square* Gene carrier (female, male). *Open circle, open square* Kindred (female, male) without S891A mutation. *Open circle with filled square* Male index patient of the family. *Asterisk* Patients with MTC

mutations (tyrosine kinase sub-domain 2) and carries a low risk for aggressive MTC [American Thyroid Association (ATA) risk level A] [1, 4]. Carriers of the S891A mutation have a <10 % risk of pheochromocytoma or hyperparathyroidism [5].

Because of the weaker genotype-phenotype relationship and the C cells' need to acquire additional mutations (dubbed "second hits") for malignant transformation, there is more variability in the onset of MTC (range 13–48 years) among carriers of the S891A mutation [1, 2, 5], reflecting the play of chance. This variability hampers predictions regarding the age by which tumors will have developed. This is why a carrier's age is less useful than his or her calcitonin levels to determine the optimum time for prophylactic thyroidectomy [3, 6]. Basal calcitonin levels within the upper normal range of the assay can reliably distinguish between C-cell diseases limited to, or spreading beyond, the confines of the thyroid capsule so that these patients can safely forego central lymph node dissection, sparing them incremental surgical morbidity [3]. For an individual patient with S891A ATA A low-risk mutation as in the presented family, prophylactic parathyroid preserving thyroidectomy without node dissection should be performed before basal calcitonin levels are exceeding the upper normal limit. Lymph node metastases have only been observed in patients with calcitonin levels beyond the upper normal limit (3). It is important to note that basal calcitonin levels as high as 40 pg/mL in children younger than 6 months and as high as 15 pg/mL in children younger than 3 years can be normal [7]. Because it

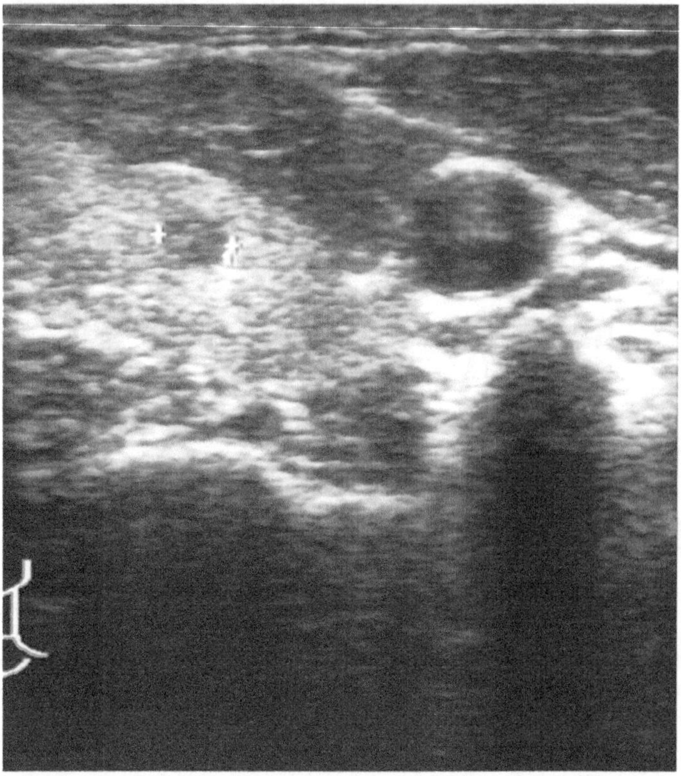

Fig. 45.2 Ultrasound of the left thyroid lobe visualizing a medullary thyroid microcarcinoma of 5 mm in size (patient 2.3)

is less sensitive than calcitonin to spot MTC in hereditary C-cell disease, ultrasonography is only of limited use for the clinical work-up of pediatric *RET* mutation carriers [8].

Management of the Cases

After informed consent, balancing the pros and cons, all eight non-index patients (including those children who had normal or slightly elevated basal calcitonin levels only) opted for surgical treatment. As detailed in Table 45.1 and Fig. 45.1, MTC or CCH was present in seven of eight patients and in all three generations, including in our 17-year-old adolescent gene carrier (patient 3.1.2; Table 45.1 and Fig. 45.1). No lymph node metastases were seen up to a basal calcitonin serum level of 60 pg/mL. One carrier (patient 2.3) also harbored a 1 mm papillary thyroid microcarcinoma in addition to bilateral MTC, in all likelihood a chance occurrence [9].

Intriguingly, it was the 78-year-old grandmother, displaying high basal calcitonin serum levels, who had node-positive MTC (patient 1.1), and not the index patient who was operated on elsewhere.

Outcome

All non-index patients with node-negative C-cell disease were biochemically cured, as shown in Table 45.1, and made an uneventful recovery without recurrent laryngeal nerve palsy or postoperative hypoparathyroidism. As long as basal calcitonin serum levels did not exceed the upper limit of the assay reference range, total thyroidectomy alone was adequate to reach biochemical cure.

Clinical Pearls/Pitfalls

- The S891A *RET* mutation carries a low risk for aggressive MTC. Manifestation of MTC has not been described before age 17.
- Owing to the considerable variation in the time of malignant transformation from C-cell hyperplasia to MTC and tumor spread to the lymph nodes, preoperative calcitonin levels, being more sensitive than ultrasonography in detecting pediatric MTC, should be considered for the timing of prophylactic thyroidectomy.
- As long as calcitonin serum levels are still within the normal range, prophylactic parathyroid preserving thyroidectomy alone is adequate, sparing gene carriers the incremental surgical morbidity attendant to lymph node dissection.
- Elevated basal calcitonin levels in excess of 60 pg/mL are associated with an increased risk of lymph node metastases, warranting compartmental lymph node dissection.

References

1. Machens A, Niccoli-Sire P, Hoegel J, Frank-Raue K, van Vroonhoven TJ, Roeher HD, Wahl RA, Lamesch P, Raue F, Conte-Devolx B, Dralle H, European Multiple Endocrine Neoplasia (EUROMEN) Study Group. Early malignant progression of hereditary medullary thyroid cancer. N Engl J Med. 2003;349:1517–25.
2. Machens A, Lorenz K, Dralle H. Constitutive RET tyrosine kinase activation in hereditary medullary thyroid cancer: clinical opportunities. J Int Med. 2009;266:114–25.
3. Machens A, Lorenz K, Dralle H. Individualization of lymph node dissection in RET (rearranged during transfection) carriers at risk for medullary thyroid cancer. Ann Surg. 2009;250:305–10.
4. Kloos RT, Eng C, Evans DB, Francis GL, Gagel RF, Gharib H, Moley JF, Pacini F, Ringel MD, Schlumberger M, Well Jr SA. Medullary thyroid cancer: management guideline of the American Thyroid Association. Thyroid. 2009;19:565–612.

5. Schulte KM, Machens A, Fugazzola L, McGregor A, Diaz-Cano S, Izatt L, Aylwin S, Talat N, Beck-Peccoz P, Dralle H. The clinical spectrum of multiple endocrine neoplasia type 2a caused by the rare intracellular RET mutation S891A. J Clin Endocrinol Metab. 2010;95:E92–7.
6. Elisei R, Romei C, Renzini G, Bottici V, Cosci B, Molinaro E, Agate L, Cappagli V, Miccoli P, Berti P, Faviana P, Ugolini C, Basolo F, Vitti P, Pinchera A. The timing of total thyroidectomy in RET gene mutation carriers could be personalized and safely planned on the basis of serum calcitonin: 18 years experience at one single center. J Clin Endocrinol Metab. 2012;97:426–35.
7. Basuyau JP, Mallet E, Leroy M, Brunelle P. Reference intervals for serum calcitonin in men, women, and children. Clin Chem. 2004;50:1828–30.
8. Morris LF, Waguespack SG, Edeiken-Monroe BS, Lee JE, Rich TA, Ying AK, Warneke CL, Evans DB, Perrier ND, Grubbs EG. Ultrasonography should not guide the timing of thyroidectomy in pediatric patients diagnosed with multiple endocrine neoplasia syndrome 2A through genetic screening. Ann Surg Oncol. 2013;20:53–9.
9. Machens A, Dralle H. Simultaneous medullary and papillary thyroid cancer: a novel entity? Ann Surg Oncol. 2012;19:37–44.

Part XI
Thyroid Lymphoma

Chapter 46
Thyroid Lymphoma: Differential Diagnosis and Management

Salem I. Noureldine, Emad Kandil, and Ralph P. Tufano

Case Presentation

A 60-year-old woman presented with a rapidly increasing right-sided neck swelling over a 3-week period. The enlargement was associated with significant dysphagia, specifically for solid foods. No hoarseness or neck tenderness was reported. The patient denied having fever, chills, weight loss, or other constitutional symptoms. Her past medical history was significant for chronic autoimmune thyroiditis and hypothyroidism treated with levothyroxine. She denied any past history of radiation exposure or family history of thyroid cancer. Physical examination was remarkable for a significant enlargement of the right thyroid lobe with tracheal deviation to the left side.

A computed tomography (CT) scan of the neck revealed an irregular shaped mass in the right thyroid lobe measuring 8.7 × 7.1 × 7.0 cm in size extending around the esophagus and narrowing the airway (Fig. 46.1). The patient underwent a fine needle aspiration (FNA) biopsy of the thyroid mass and the cytology was highly suspicious for lymphoma. Flow cytometry studies were done and confirmed the diagnosis.

In order to classify the subtype of the lymphoma, an open biopsy of the thyroid was performed under local anesthesia. Immunohistochemistry revealed the tumor to be consistent with B-cell lymphoma, with features intermediate between diffuse

S.I. Noureldine, MD • R.P. Tufano, MD, MBA, FACS (✉)
Division of Head and Neck Endocrine Surgery, Department of Otolaryngology–Head and Neck Surgery, The Johns Hopkins University School of Medicine, 601 N. Caroline Street, 6th floor, Baltimore, MD 21287, USA
e-mail: snourel1@jhmi.edu; rtufano@jhmi.edu

E. Kandil, MD, FACS, FACE
Division of Endocrine Surgery, Department of Surgery, Tulane University School of Medicine, New Orleans, LA 70118, USA
e-mail: ekandil@tulane.edu

D.S. Cooper, C. Durante (eds.), *Thyroid Cancer*,
DOI 10.1007/978-3-319-22401-5_46

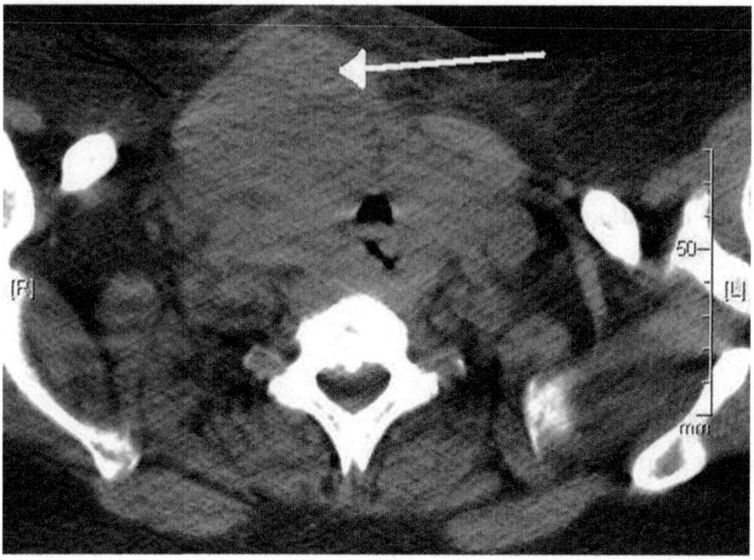

Fig. 46.1 Pretreatment computed tomography scan of the soft tissues of the neck. An irregular shaped mass in the right thyroid lobe measuring 8.7 cm in largest dimension extending around the esophagus and narrowing the airway can be appreciated. Multiple enlarged lymph nodes can also be noted

large B-cell lymphoma (DLBCL) and a variant of Burkitt's lymphoma (Fig. 46.2). As part of the work-up, the patient also underwent a bone marrow biopsy which showed no morphologic evidence of lymphoma.

Background of the Disease

Primary thyroid lymphoma (PTL) is rare and accounts for 1–5 % of thyroid malignancies and approximately 2 % of extranodal lymphomas [1, 2]. The mean age of onset is from 60 to 70 years with 50 % of patients presenting later in life in their seventh or eighth decade. There is a distinct female predominance with a female-to-male ratio of 3–4:1 [2, 3]. This is similar to the female predominance in autoimmune Hashimoto's thyroiditis, and there appears to be a distinct etiologic relationship with PTL. More than 90 % of patients with PTL have elevated circulating thyroidal autoantibodies, noted either before or after the onset of PTL [4–6]. Although the risk of developing PTL is 67- to 80-fold increased in people with Hashimoto's thyroiditis, it is exceedingly rare for any person with Hashimoto's thyroiditis to develop PTL [5, 7].

The vast majority of PTLs are non-Hodgkin's lymphomas of B-cell origin. Nonetheless, there have been rare reports of Hodgkin's and T-cell thyroid lymphomas in the literature [1]. There are several histologic subtypes of PTL including

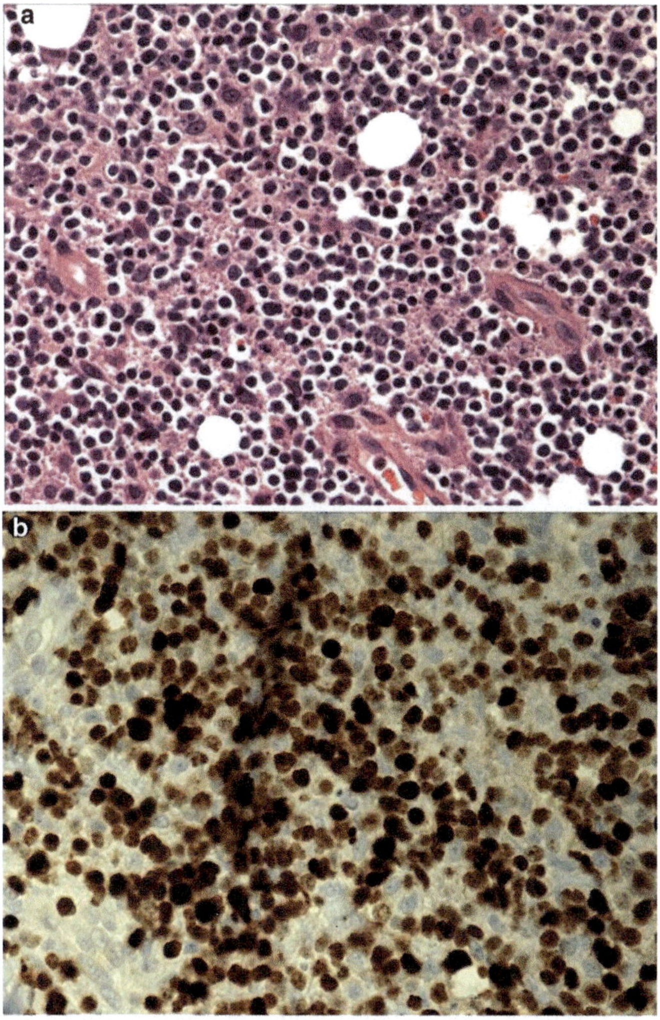

Fig. 46.2 (**a**) Incisional thyroid biopsy revealed evidence of small-to medium-sized lymphoid infiltrate. (**b**) Immunohistochemical studies with staining with 100 % labeling with Ki 67 (pattern seen in Burkitt's lymphoma)

DLBCL constituting 50–70 % of cases, marginal zone B-cell lymphoma of the mucosa-associated lymphoid tissue (MALT) (10 %), follicular lymphoma (12 %), small lymphocytic lymphoma (4 %), Hodgkin's disease (2 %), and Burkitt's lymphoma (4 %) [3, 8, 9]. The most common and most aggressive subtype, DLBCL, is associated with a fivefold higher mortality compared to MALT lymphomas that tend to have an indolent clinical course with an excellent prognosis [4, 9, 10]. Therefore, histologic distinction is of paramount importance for determining the best treatment option.

Clinical Presentation, Differential Diagnosis, and Assessment

Most, if not all, PTLs are diagnosed due to a painless)thyroid mass, and greater than 70 % of cases are diagnosed due to a rapidly enlarging mass in the neck [4]. The most common symptoms are consequent to the mass, including hoarseness, dysphagia, and dyspnea. Occasionally, stridor or superior vena cava syndrome may occur [4, 9]. As expected, with its intrinsic association with autoimmune thyroid disease, it is common for patients to be hypothyroid and require thyroid hormone replacement therapy [11]. Some patients also have constitutional symptoms (classified as “B”) of fevers, night sweats, and unexplained weight loss of more than 10 % body weight in the preceding 6 months.

This abrupt clinical presentation with the associated symptoms not only raises the possibility of PTL but also a soft tissue abscess or infection of the neck, hemorrhage into a thyroid nodule, subacute thyroiditis, anaplastic thyroid carcinoma, and metastatic cancer. Therefore, immediate diagnostic discrimination, via history and physical examination, in addition to laboratory, radiology, and cyto-histopathology assessment, is needed due to the significant differences in therapy.

Ultrasonography is often the first imaging modality employed to evaluate a patient with a thyroid nodule or goiter since it is readily accessible, inexpensive, and noninvasive. Ultrasound is effective at delineating intrathyroidal architecture, distinguishing cystic from solid lesions, determining if a nodule is solitary or part of a multinodular gland, and accurately locating and measuring it [12]. Thyroid lymphoma should be suspected in patients with Hashimoto’s thyroiditis when the thyroid begins to rapidly grow. The initial assessment of such patients must be cytologic or histologic. Ultrasound-guided FNA biopsy can suggest or diagnose PTL in a majority of cases [13]. FNA biopsy alone can easily diagnose high-grade lymphomas based on morphologic features, such as noncohesive large-sized cells with basophilic cytoplasm and coarse chromatin pattern within the nuclei. MALT lymphomas and mixed large-cell lymphomas are difficult to diagnose on morphology alone; thus, immunophenotypic analyses must be frequently applied [14]. Nonetheless, the rates of achieving a positive diagnosis via FNA biopsy range from 25 to 80 % [1, 15, 16]. Therefore, in the context of concomitant Hashimoto’s thyroiditis and the potential risk of nondiagnostic FNA, it is sometimes useful to utilize ultrasound-guided core-needle biopsy or even open surgical biopsy under local anesthesia [17].

Thyroid lymphomas may be confused with poorly differentiated thyroid carcinomas on clinical as well as histologic and cytologic grounds. Immunophenotypic analyses, including flow cytometry and immunohistochemistry staining, are usually key to distinguishing between a poorly differentiated epithelial malignancy of the thyroid and a thyroid lymphoma [18]. With the addition of immunophenotypic analyses to FNA biopsy, pathologic studies have reported an improved accuracy rate of 80–100 % [4, 13, 19, 20]. The diagnosis and subtyping of PTLs is made with a combination of morphologic features, immunophenotyping indicating B-cell linage of lymphocytes with tumor clonality, immunohistochemical staining for CD20, restrictive expression of lambda or kappa light chains, and immunoglobulin gene rearrangements [4, 5, 13, 19, 21].

Once a cytologic or histologic diagnosis of PTL is made, full clinical staging is needed. Neck ultrasound is easily performed and can often provide useful information, but magnetic resonance imaging (MRI) is far more useful in denoting involvement of other vital structures in the neck [22, 23]. The imaging characteristics of extranodal involvement can be subtle or absent at conventional computed tomography (CT) [24]. Imaging of tumor metabolism with 2-[fluorine-18]fluoro-2-deoxy-d-glucose (FDG) positron emission tomography (PET) has facilitated the identification of affected extranodal sites, even when CT has demonstrated no lesions. More recently, hybrid PET/CT has become the standard imaging modality for initial staging, follow-up (restaging, detection of recurrence), and treatment response assessment in patients with Hodgkin's lymphoma and non-Hodgkin's lymphoma and has proved superior to CT in these settings [25]. FDG-PET is even recommended for identifying areas suspicious for tumor transformation (increasing FDG avidity), repeating biopsy, and changing chemotherapy regimens [26]. Bone marrow biopsy should also be performed to rule out marrow involvement [27]. Laboratory assessments should include standard blood work including a complete blood count with differential and a metabolic panel to include albumin, electrolytes, blood urea nitrogen, and creatinine, in addition to measurements of serum lactate dehydrogenase (LDH) levels [26]. Prior history of immunosuppressive therapy should also be assessed.

The staging system used for PTL is based on the Ann Arbor modification of the Rye classification system for Hodgkin's lymphoma. This system is not as predictive of outcomes in non-Hodgkin's lymphomas or in MALT lymphomas; however, it remains the convention for PTL staging [28]. In this system, the subscript "E" applies to a lymphoma arising in an extralymphoid site, as in all PTL cases. Approximately 50 % of patients with PTL have disease confined to the thyroid gland (stage IE), and 45 % have disease in locoregional nodes (stage IIE) [3]. Stage IIIE cases involve nodal disease on both sides of the diaphragm, and stage IVE cases reflect diffuse or disseminated disease.

Management and Outcome

Because PTL is typically responsive to radiation and chemotherapy, the role of surgery is limited [16]. However, surgery continues to play an important role, especially in confirming the diagnosis through open biopsy in those patients in whom core-needle biopsy provided insufficient confirmation of an initial FNA biopsy. Surgery can also provide local control in more indolent subtypes and aid in the palliation of symptoms for large obstructive lymphomas [27, 29].

In general, the best clinical outcomes are seen with multimodal therapy, using sequential systemic chemotherapy and local external beam radiation [30]. The combination chemotherapy regimen usually consists of cyclophosphamide, doxorubicin, vincristine, and prednisolone (CHOP). Nearly 30 % of patients with clinically localized PTL treated solely with radiation therapy relapse at distant sites, demonstrating the need for systemic therapy [31].

Rituximab is a monoclonal B-cell antibody that selectively binds to the CD20 antigen found on the surface of pre-B and mature B lymphocytes [32]. It is used as first-line therapy both in MALT and in DLBCL patients in combination with CHOP (the so-called R-CHOP regimen) and other anthracycline-based or anthracycline-free chemotherapy regimens [26]. Meta-analysis of published reports on primary nodal lymphoma patients verifies the superiority of adding rituximab to combination chemotherapy [33], and it has been shown to be cost effective when used for that purpose [34]. A number of other monoclonal antibody drugs are entering clinical practice (obinutuzumab, ofatumumab, ibritumomab) [35]. The survival rates range from 13 to 92 % at 5 years [27]. Patients over 65 years of age with large, rapidly growing tumors with high-grade histology have the worst prognosis.

Management of the Case

Due to the aggressive histologic subtype, the patient was started on rituximab, cyclophosphamide, vincristine, and doxorubicin. This resulted in a rapid shrinkage of the mass over 1 week. The patient reported resolution of compressive symptoms. A CT scan was performed at the end of the treatment period and revealed no evidence of residual disease (Fig. 46.3).

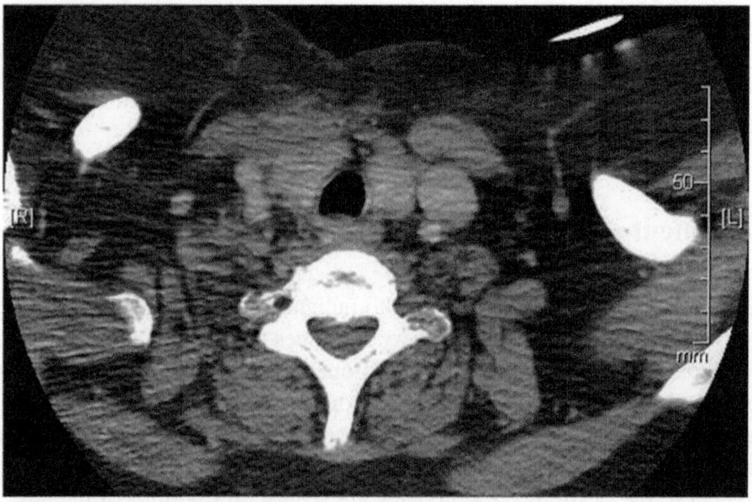

Fig. 46.3 Posttreatment computed tomography scan of the soft tissues of the neck reveals no evidence of obvious residual disease

Clinical Pearls

Thyroid lymphoma should be suspected in patients with Hashimotos thyroiditis when the thyroid begins to rapidly grow.

- The initial assessment of such patients must be cytologic or histologic.
- Ultrasound-guided FNA biopsy can suggest or diagnose PTL in a majority of cases.
- FNA alone can easily diagnose high-grade lymphomas based on morphologic features, such as noncohesive large-sized cells with basophilic cytoplasm and coarse chromatin pattern within the nuclei.
- MALT lymphomas and mixed large-cell lymphomas are difficult to diagnose on morphology alone; thus, immunophenotypic analyses must be frequently applied.
- Open biopsy may be necessary to subtype the PTL.
- The most effective treatment is radiation in combination with systemic chemotherapy.

Conflicts of Interest Disclosures All authors report no conflicts of interest.

References

1. Ansell SM, Grant CS, Habermann TM. Primary thyroid lymphoma. Semin Oncol. 1999;26(3):316–23.
2. Pedersen RK, Pedersen NT. Primary non-Hodgkin's lymphoma of the thyroid gland: a population based study. Histopathology. 1996;28(1):25–32.
3. Graff-Baker A, Roman SA, Thomas DC, Udelsman R, Sosa JA. Prognosis of primary thyroid lymphoma: demographic, clinical, and pathologic predictors of survival in 1,408 cases. Surgery. 2009;146(6):1105–15.
4. Derringer GA, Thompson LD, Frommelt RA, Bijwaard KE, Heffess CS, Abbondanzo SL. Malignant lymphoma of the thyroid gland: a clinicopathologic study of 108 cases. Am J Surg Pathol. 2000;24(5):623–39.
5. Kossev P, Livolsi V. Lymphoid lesions of the thyroid: review in light of the revised European-American lymphoma classification and upcoming World Health Organization classification. Thyroid. 1999;9(12):1273–80.
6. Rossi D. Thyroid lymphoma: beyond antigen stimulation. Leuk Res. 2009;33:607–9.
7. Holm LE, Blomgren H, Lowhagen T. Cancer risks in patients with chronic lymphocytic thyroiditis. N Engl J Med. 1985;312(10):601–4.
8. Kandil E, Safah H, Noureldine S, Abdel Khalek M, Waddadar J, Goswami M, et al. Burkitt-like lymphoma arising in the thyroid gland. Am J Med Sci. 2012;343(1):103–5.
9. Thieblemont C, Mayer A, Dumontet C, Barbier Y, Callet-Bauchu E, Felman P, et al. Primary thyroid lymphoma is a heterogeneous disease. J Clin Endocrinol Metab. 2002;87(1):105–11.
10. Tsang RW, Gospodarowicz MK, Pintilie M, Wells W, Hodgson DC, Sun A, et al. Localized mucosa-associated lymphoid tissue lymphoma treated with radiation therapy has excellent clinical outcome. J Clin Oncol. 2003;21(22):4157–64.
11. Pasieka JL. Hashimoto's disease and thyroid lymphoma: role of the surgeon. World J Surg. 2000;24(8):966–70.
12. Harvey HK. Diagnosis and management of the thyroid nodule. An overview. Otolaryngol Clin North Am. 1990;23(2):303–37.

13. Cha C, Chen H, Westra WH, Udelsman R. Primary thyroid lymphoma: can the diagnosis be made solely by fine-needle aspiration? Ann Surg Oncol. 2002;9(3):298–302.
14. Stein SA, Wartofsky L. Primary thyroid lymphoma: a clinical review. J Clin Endocrinol Metab. 2013;98(8):3131–8.
15. Skarsgard ED, Connors JM, Robins RE. A current analysis of primary lymphoma of the thyroid. Arch Surg. 1991;126(10):1199–203. discussion 203–4.
16. Pyke CM, Grant CS, Habermann TM, Kurtin PJ, van Heerden JA, Bergstralh EJ, et al. Non-Hodgkin's lymphoma of the thyroid: is more than biopsy necessary? World J Surg. 1992;16(4):604–9. discussion 9–10.
17. Kwak JY, Kim EK, Ko KH, Yang WI, Kim MJ, Son EJ, et al. Primary thyroid lymphoma: role of ultrasound-guided needle biopsy. J Ultrasound Med. 2007;26(12):1761–5.
18. Ruggiero FP, Frauenhoffer E, Stack Jr BC. Thyroid lymphoma: a single institution's experience. Otolaryngol Head Neck Surg. 2005;133(6):888–96.
19. Young NA, Al-Saleem T. Diagnosis of lymphoma by fine-needle aspiration cytology using the revised European-American classification of lymphoid neoplasms. Cancer. 1999;87(6):325–45.
20. Jeffers MD, Milton J, Herriot R, McKean M. Fine needle aspiration cytology in the investigation on non-Hodgkin's lymphoma. J Clin Pathol. 1998;51(3):189–96.
21. Yamauchi A, Tomita Y, Takakuwa T, Hoshida Y, Nakatsuka S, Sakamoto H, et al. Polymerase chain reaction-based clonality analysis in thyroid lymphoma. Int J Mol Med. 2002;10(1):113–7.
22. Ota H, Ito Y, Matsuzuka F, Kuma S, Fukata S, Morita S, et al. Usefulness of ultrasonography for diagnosis of malignant lymphoma of the thyroid. Thyroid. 2006;16(10):983–7.
23. Takashima S, Nomura N, Noguchi Y, Matsuzuka F, Inoue T. Primary thyroid lymphoma: evaluation with US, CT, and MRI. J Comput Assist Tomogr. 1995;19(2):282–8.
24. Kostakoglu L, Goldsmith SJ. Fluorine-18 fluorodeoxyglucose positron emission tomography in the staging and follow-up of lymphoma: is it time to shift gears? Eur J Nucl Med. 2000;27(10):1564–78.
25. Paes FM, Kalkanis DG, Sideras PA, Serafini AN. FDG PET/CT of extranodal involvement in non-Hodgkin lymphoma and Hodgkin disease. Radiographics. 2010;30(1):269–91.
26. National Comprehensive Cancer Network, Inc. Practice guidelines in oncology—Non-Hodgkin's lymphomas version 4. 2014. http://www.nccn.org/about/nhl.pdf. Accessed Dec 2014.
27. Widder S, Pasieka JL. Primary thyroid lymphomas. Curr Treat Options Oncol. 2004;5(4):307–13.
28. Sobin LH, Gospodarowicz MK, Wittekind C, International Union against Cancer. TNM classification of malignant tumours. 7th ed. Chichester, West Sussex/Hoboken, NJ: Wiley-Blackwell; 2010.
29. Earnest LM, Cooper DS, Sciubba JJ, Tufano RP. Thyroid MALT lymphoma in patients with a compressive goiter. Head Neck. 2006;28(8):765–70.
30. Logue JP, Hale RJ, Stewart AL, Duthie MB, Banerjee SS. Primary malignant lymphoma of the thyroid: a clinicopathological analysis. Int J Radiat Oncol Biol Phys. 1992;22(5):929–33.
31. Doria R, Jekel JF, Cooper DL. Thyroid lymphoma. The case for combined modality therapy. Cancer. 1994;73(1):200–6.
32. Keating GM. Rituximab: a review of its use in chronic lymphocytic leukaemia, low-grade or follicular lymphoma and diffuse large B-cell lymphoma. Drugs. 2010;70(11):1445–76.
33. Gao G, Liang X, Jiang J, Zhou X, Huang R, Chu Z, et al. A systematic review and meta-analysis of immunochemotherapy with rituximab for B-cell non-Hodgkin's lymphoma. Acta Oncol. 2010;49(1):3–12.
34. Johnston KM, Marra CA, Connors JM, Najafzadeh M, Sehn L, Peacock SJ. Cost-effectiveness of the addition of rituximab to CHOP chemotherapy in first-line treatment for diffuse large B-cell lymphoma in a population-based observational cohort in British Columbia, Canada. Value Health. 2010;13(6):703–11.
35. Stathis A, Ghielmini M. New agents for the treatment of lymphoma. Ann Oncol. 2012;23 Suppl 10:x92–8.

Part XII
Anaplastic Thyroid Cancer

Chapter 47
Anaplastic Thyroid Cancer: Surgery or Not in Locally Advanced Disease

Robert C. Smallridge and Keith C. Bible

Introduction

Anaplastic thyroid carcinoma (ATC) is one of the most aggressive and lethal of all malignancies, accounting for approximately 1.7 % of all thyroid cancers in the United States and a median of 3.6 % (range, 1.3–9.8 %) worldwide [1]. By the American Joint Committee on Cancer (AJCC) TNM classification, ATC is always stage IV at presentation; stage IVA tumors are intrathyroidal, IVB tumors have extrathyroidal extension and may involve locoregional lymph nodes, and IVC tumors are distantly metastatic.

Survival correlates inversely with TNM stage and, in most (but not all) reports, correlates directly/positively with extent of surgery, administration of high-dose radiotherapy, and absence of distant metastases [2]. The American Thyroid Association management guidelines for ATC recommends initial surgery in potentially grossly resectable (R0, negative surgical margins; R1, microscopically involved margins) stage IVA or IVB disease in patients who are in reasonably good health and who elect aggressive treatment [1]. The role of R2 (gross residual disease)/debulking/resection is less certain.

R.C. Smallridge, MD (✉)
Mayo Clinic, 4500 San Pablo Rd, Jacksonville, FL 32224, USA
e-mail: smallridge.robert@mayo.edu

K.C. Bible, MD, PhD
Mayo Clinic, 200 First St SW, Rochester, MN 55905, USA

D.S. Cooper, C. Durante (eds.), *Thyroid Cancer*,
DOI 10.1007/978-3-319-22401-5_47

Case Report

A 57-year-old man presented with a rapidly growing left neck mass, first noticed while shaving. He noted fatigue, neck pain, and change in his voice and swallowing ability without shortness of breath. Quality of life (QOL) was rated 10 (as good as can be). He had no history of radiation exposure. His mother and one sister had a history of hyperthyroidism, another sister had breast cancer and follicular thyroid cancer, and his daughter had a multinodular goiter. On physical exam, an 8 cm left neck mass was noted, with tracheal deviation to the right. Vocal cords were mobile and there were no mucosal pharyngeal lesions visualized.

Neck ultrasound showed a large, 5.8 cm, left thyroid mass with two right lobe nodules (up to 1.1 cm) and a 2.4 cm isthmus nodule; fine needle aspirate was non-diagnostic. An 18-gauge needle core biopsy showed a sarcomatoid anaplastic thyroid carcinoma. Immunohistochemistry was positive for KRT-OSCAR and KRTAE1/AE3 and negative for S100, Melan-A, HMB-45, KRT-7, KRT-20, TTF-1, and thyroglobulin. These stains were felt to support epithelial derivation consistent with ATC.

An 18 F-fluorodeoxyglucose (FDG) positron emission tomography–computed tomography (PET–CT) scan demonstrated a 5 cm hypermetabolic left thyroid mass [max. standardized uptake value (SUV) = 30.8] which eroded the left side of the thyroid cartilage and extended medially to the prevertebral area posterior to the larynx (Fig. 47.1). A mass of lymph nodes extended superiorly along the parapharyngeal area at the level of the oropharynx, with hypermetabolic uptake in the left internal jugular vein consistent with tumor thrombus. There were no macroscopic distant metastases.

The patient underwent total thyroidectomy and left modified radical neck dissection, partial upper sternal split, and removal of thrombus from the internal jugular to innominate veins. The tumor invaded the vasculature adjacent to the pharynx, necessitating resection of pharyngeal musculature but with preservation of mucosal integrity; gross residual disease was left after surgery (R2 resection).

Pathology revealed an 8.5 × 4.8 × 4.0 cm, 184.5 g left thyroid mass extending into perithyroidal soft tissue with perineural involvement; deep soft tissue margins positive. Seven of twenty-one lymph nodes were involved with ATC, with extranodal extension present. TNM classification was pT4bN1bM0, AJCC stage IVB.

Early postoperative locoregional complications included a chyle leak, an abscess requiring drainage, an infected sternal wound requiring debridement, and an esophageal stricture. QOL decreased to 5 postoperatively.

Intensity-modulated radiotherapy (IMRT) to the neck and upper mediastinum was administered over 6 weeks (200 cGy 5 days a week, 33 fractions, total dose = 6600 cGy). He received doxorubicin and docetaxel (each at 20 mg/m^2/week for 7 weeks, pre-and concurrently administered with IMRT) followed by two cycles of 60 mg/m^2 each every 3 weeks.

At 3 months post-op, his QOL = 3. PET/CT scan showed no apparent recurrence or metastases. Three months later, a PET/CT scan demonstrated a new 11 mm right

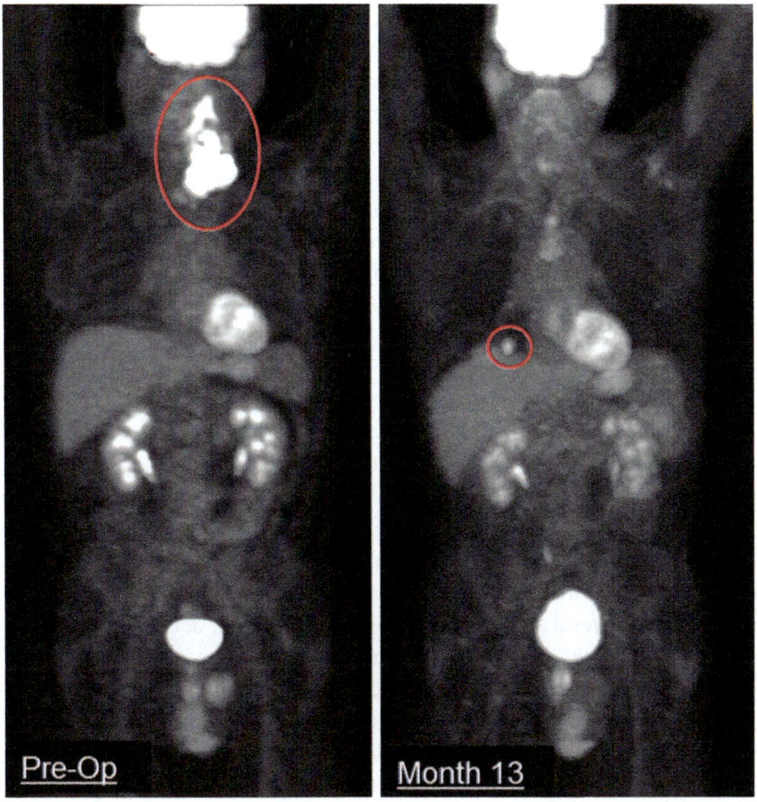

Fig. 47.1 Preoperative and month 18 FDG-PET whole-body imaging of the presented patient. *Areas highlighted in red* indicate observed macroscopic disease at each time point

lower lung lesion (max. SUV = 4.2) and an indeterminate hypermetabolic focus in the right hilum (SUV = 2.8). The right lower lung lesion was treated with stereotactic body radiotherapy (SBRT), 54 Gy in 3 fractions.

Ten months after surgery, quality of life had increased to seven. PET/CT showed increased size and intensity of a C6 spinous process lesion (max. SUV = 8.1, formerly 4.9 on imaging 5 weeks earlier); he received 3000 cGy SBRT. Thirteen months following surgery, quality of life had increased to nine, and the patient was active in carpentry work related to the construction of a new home. PET/CT, however, indicated a new right lower lung nodule proximal to the previously treated lung lesion (1.4 cm, max. SUV 5.2); this was treated with CT-directed cryoablation with good tolerance of the procedure.

Three months later, a left lower lung lesion had increased from 0.5 to 1.7 cm and SUV from 1.8 to 8.7. A new lesion in the right back (levator scapulae) musculature (SUV = 8.3) was also identified. Cryoablations of the musculoskeletal lesions were uneventful. Subsequent cryoablation of the lung lesion, however, resulted in a pneumothorax (requiring chest tube decompression), air embolization (including coronary arteries and requiring hyperbaric therapy), ventricular tachycardia (requiring cardioversion), and transient neurologic deficits (expressive aphasia and right upper extremity weakness). Nineteen months after surgery, a scalp lesion was biopsied (IHC stain was negative for ALK expression) and the following month systemic therapy (weekly docetaxel and doxorubicin) was resumed. Quality of life score decreased to 2. At most recent follow-up, 22 months after initial surgery, the QOL score had increased to 6, and the patient had resumed carpentry work on his home under construction. PET/CT showed asymptomatic and globally stable lung and levator scapulae lesions, but new suspicious levels 3 and 5 neck lymph nodes.

Literature Review

A review of 34 series from 1987 to 2009 showed that in 27, R2 or debulking resections were performed [3]. In another review of prognosis, 17 of 21 series reported that extent of surgery correlated significantly with outcomes, as patients with R0 or R0/R1 resections survived longer [2], presumably due to tumors being less aggressive and more resectable.

More recently, several authors have provided additional detailed results on extent of surgery and outcomes. Ito et al. [4] reported on 40 patients with stage IVB ($n=25$) or IVC ($n=15$) disease further dividing the former group into IVB-a (extension into the soft tissue, trachea, larynx, recurrent laryngeal nerve, or esophagus) or IVB-b (encasement of the carotid artery or mediastinal vessels or invasion of the prevertebral fascia). Table 47.1 depicts their results by stage and extent of surgery. Only one of the six IVB 1-year survivors had an R1 resection (still alive after 4.5 years); the other five long-term survivors had R2 resections, with median survival of 546 days (range, 386–716). All six had received external radiation, and five were given chemotherapy. The lone stage IVC long-term survivor (684 days) received only radiation therapy.

Akaishi et al. [5] retrospectively reviewed 100 cases of ATC from 1993 to 2009, including stages IVA ($n=11$), IVB ($n=31$), and IVC ($n=58$). One-year survivals for each stage were 73, 23, and 7 %, respectively; the authors noted that "survival after complete resection was significantly better than after incomplete resection or no resection." Nine patients survived more than 1 year (Table 47.2). As expected, those with IVA disease had the longest median and overall survival; however, 8 of the 19 patients had less than complete surgical resection. All 19 had received adjuvant radio- and chemotherapy.

Sugitani et al. [6] reviewed the results of the ATC Research Consortium of Japan. Their registry of 38 institutions contained 677 patients, of which 547 cases were not incidental findings of ATC nor ATC transformation found only in metastatic lesions. In evaluating the extent of surgery in 534 patients, the 1-year survival rate was 10 % on 389 patients who received no or palliative surgery and 39 % in 145 patients receiving radical surgery; in a multivariate analysis, the hazard ratio was 0.35 (0.28–0.43, $p<0.0001$) for radical surgery. Table 47.3 summarizes the effect of surgery on

Table 47.1 Extent of surgical resection and survival in 40 patients with stages IVB and IVC anaplastic thyroid carcinoma

	Surgery extent			Survival	
Stage (no.)	*R1*	*R2*	None	1 year (%)	Median (days)
IVB-a (12)	2	10	0	5 (42 %)	287
IVB-b (13)	0	3	10	1 (8 %)	119
IVC (15)	0	5	10	1 (7 %)	125

Modified from Ito et al. [4]

R1 microscopic residual tumor, *R2* macroscopic residual tumor

Table 47.2 Extent of surgery in 19 patients with anaplastic thyroid carcinoma surviving more than 1 year

Stage (no.)	Resection complete	Debulk	Survival (months)	Still alive
IVA (8)	8	–	38.6 (12.8–84.9)	5
IVB (7)	3	4	20.5 (13.0–151.3)	2
IVC (4)	–	4	16.1 (15.3–19.2)	2

Modified from Akaishi et al. [5]

Table 47.3 Effect of extent of surgery on 1-year survival in 534 patients with anaplastic thyroid carcinoma

	1-year survival (%) Surgery extent		
Stage (no.)	None/palliative	Radical	HR (95 % CI)
IVA (69)	26	43*	0.25 (0.12–0.50)
IVB (242)	12	41*	0.39 (0.28–0.53)
IVC (233)	7	31*	0.43 (0.27–0.68)

Modified from Sugitani et al. [6]

HR hazard ratio, *CI* confidence interval

*$p<0.005$

1-year survival for each stage of disease, indicating a benefit of more surgery for all stages. Further analysis of the additional benefits of adjuvant therapies in those undergoing radical surgery revealed the following: (a) for patients with stage IVA disease, neither external radiation nor radiation plus chemotherapy statistically improved 1-year survival versus surgery alone, although the numbers were small and there was a trend toward better outcomes with adjuvant therapies; (b) for stage IVB patients, the combination of radiation and chemotherapy was associated with greater 1-year survival (from 21 to 57 %, $p=0.0062$) and reduced death hazard ratio (0.45; 0.25–0.81).

In a recent report, Sugitani et al. [7] provided more details on the extent of surgery in 224 of their stage IVB patients. Twenty-three patients underwent super-radical surgery, including total pharyngolaryngectomy, laryngectomy, tracheal or esophageal resection, or mediastinal surgery, while 49 patients underwent restricted radical surgery (thyroidectomy, lymph node removal, and occasionally resection of recurrent laryngeal nerve, muscle, vein, or superficial shaving of trachea or esophagus). Palliative surgery was performed in 72 cases and no surgery in 80. One-year survival rates were 30, 39, 13, and 8 %, respectively. The authors proposed that although super-radical surgery may help in selected cases, these patients had a high likelihood of requiring a tracheostomy and were less likely to receive external radiation or chemotherapy.

In another recent study of 83 patients, 1-year disease-specific survival was 54 % for patients with an R0/R1 resection and 28 % with an R2/X resection, but only 8 % with no surgery/treatment [8]. In contrast, Segerhammar et al. [9] found no effect of extent of resection on survival in 59 patients, but they had only 5 who had R2 resections. Age has often been a predictive factor for survival, with older patients faring less well [2]. Polistena et al. [10] reported their experience in 79 patients, 42<75 years old and 37≥75 years. Although fewer patients in the older age group underwent surgery (32 % vs. 78 %), older patients whose tumor was >5 cm and who had surgery (mostly total thyroidectomy) lived significantly longer than those without surgery. Thus, older age should not exclude patients from surgery if otherwise they are deemed healthy.

A general exclusion criterion for offering surgery has been presenting with stage IVC disease, as reflected in the ATA guidelines which recommends radiotherapy and chemotherapy for those desiring aggressive treatment [1]. However, Brignardello et al. [11] observed that surgery may have a role in patients presenting with distant metastases. They had 55 patients (31 with stage IVC disease) who underwent either "maximal debulking" (R0, R1, or R2 resection with only minimal residual macroscopic tumor) or "partial debulking." Patients were excluded if they had overt involvement of pharynx, larynx, trachea, or esophagus, if mediastinal vessels were involved, or if prevertebral fascia and paraspinous muscles were involved. Almost all received radiochemotherapy. Of note, maximal debulking was associated with improved median survival in both stage IVB (10.9 vs. 3.0 months) and IVC (6.5 vs. 3.2 months) patients [11]. One-year survival was 36.4 % and 27.8 %, respectively, in stages IVB and IVC who underwent "maximal debulking" surgery, whereas no patients lived >1 year in either stage in response to only partial debulking. The authors attributed the improvement due to fewer deaths from locoregional tumor progression [11].

Summary

The preponderance of the literature supports the notion that patients with anaplastic thyroid carcinoma have longer survival if they undertake complete or near complete surgical resection. However, no studies to date have been prospective and randomized, with elderly and/or more debilitated patients and/or those who have extensive unresectable locoregional disease or widespread distant metastases less likely to be offered surgery. Given the severe molecular dysregulation in ATC [3], the recognition that almost all patients eventually die from their disease (suggesting micrometastases on presentation), and the observation that some patients have prolonged responses with only radiation and chemotherapy, it is apparent that the landscape of molecular abnormalities and how they may correlate with outcomes must be much better defined. For instance, two gain-of-function mutations of the anaplastic lymphoma kinase (ALK) gene have been reported [12], and one patient with stage IVC ATC and an ALK rearrangement had a prolonged response to crizotinib, an ALK inhibitor [13]. Once better molecular characterization is accomplished, then multicenter prospective studies can be designed to better characterize and optimize the individual contributions of surgery, external radiation, and systemic therapies (both cytotoxic and targeted).

Back to the Patient

Returning to our patient, he remains alive and active with a reasonable quality of life, but with persistent disease. We propose that aggressive multimodal therapy directed at both locoregional control and the almost inevitable systemic disease currently offers the best opportunity for prolonging survival, but with considerable complication risks. We have, however, much to learn about this horrific tumor.

Pearls

In most series, maximal surgical resection appears to improve 1-year survival, but resectability depends on the extent of the primary tumor at presentation.

- Aggressive multimodal therapy presently offers the most successful approach to attempt to prolong survival in patients with anaplastic thyroid cancer but imposes risks of complications.
- Older age, extensive locoregional disease, and stage IVC disease should not exclude the possibility of surgery.

References

1. Smallridge RC, Ain KB, Asa SL, Bible KC, Brierley JD, Burman KD, et al. American Thyroid Association guidelines for management of patients with anaplastic thyroid cancer. Thyroid. 2012;22(11):1104–39.
2. Smallridge RC, Abate EG. Anaplastic thyroid carcinoma: prognosis. In: Wartofsky L, Van Nostrand D, editors. Thyroid cancer: a comprehensive guide to clinical management. 3rd ed. New York, NY: Springer; 2015 (in press).

3. Smallridge RC, Copland JA. Anaplastic thyroid carcinoma: pathogenesis and emerging therapies. Clin Oncol. 2010;22(6):486–97.
4. Ito KI, Hanamura T, Murayama K, Okada T, Watanabe T, Harada M, et al. Multimodality therapeutic outcomes in anaplastic thyroid carcinoma: improved survival in subgroups of patients with localized primary tumors. Head Neck. 2012;34:230–7.
5. Akaishi J, Sugino K, Kitagawa W, Nagahama M, Kameyama K, Shimizu K, et al. Prognostic factors and treatment outcomes of 100 cases of anaplastic thyroid carcinoma. Thyroid. 2011;21:1183–9.
6. Sugitani I, Miyauchi A, Sugino K, Okamoto T, Yoshida A, Suzuki S. Prognostic factors and treatment outcomes for anaplastic thyroid carcinoma: ATC Research Consortium of Japan cohort study of 677 patients. World J Surg. 2012;36(6):1247–54.
7. Sugitani I, Hasegawa Y, Sugasawa M, Tori M, Higashiyama T, Miyazaki M, et al. Super-radical surgery for anaplastic thyroid carcinoma: a large cohort study using the anaplastic thyroid carcinoma research consortium of Japan database. Head Neck. 2014;36(3):328–33.
8. Mohebati A, Dilorenzo M, Palmer F, Patel SG, Pfister D, Lee N, et al. Anaplastic thyroid carcinoma: a 25-year single-institution experience. Ann Surg Oncol. 2014;21(5):1665–70.
9. Segerhammar I, Larsson C, Nilsson IL, Backdahl M, Hoog A, Wallin G, et al. Anaplastic carcinoma of the thyroid gland: treatment and outcome over 13 years at one institution. J Surg Oncol. 2012;106(8):981–6.
10. Polistena A, Monacelli M, Lucchini R, Triola R, Conti C, Avenia S, et al. The role of surgery in the treatment of thyroid anaplastic carcinoma in the elderly. Int J Surg. 2014;12 Suppl 2:S170–6.
11. Brignardello E, Palestini N, Felicetti F, Castiglione A, Piovesan A, Gallo M, et al. Early surgery and survival of patients with anaplastic thyroid carcinoma: analysis of a case series referred to a single institution between 1999 and 2012. Thyroid. 2014;24(11):1600–6.
12. Murugan AK, Xing M. Anaplastic thyroid cancers harbor novel oncogenic mutations of the ALK gene. Cancer Res. 2011;71(13):4403–11.
13. Godbert Y, Henriques de Figueiredo B, Bonichon F, Chibon F, Hostein I, Perot G, et al. Remarkable response to crizotinib in woman with anaplastic lymphoma kinase-rearranged anaplastic thyroid carcinoma. J Clin Oncol. 2014;33(20):e84–7.

Index

D.S. Cooper, C. Durante (eds.), *Thyroid Cancer*,
DOI 10.1007/978-3-319-22401-5

Printed by Printforce, the Netherlands